Pulmonary Adenocarcinoma: Approaches to Treatment

Pulmonary Adenocarcinoma: Approaches to Treatment

LEORA HORN, MD, MSC
Associate Professor of Medicine
Medicine - Hematology Oncology
Vanderbilt Univeristy
Nashville, TN, United States

ELSEVIER

ELSEVIER

3251 Riverport Lane
St. Louis, Missouri 63043

Pulmonary Adenocarcinoma: Approaches to Treatment   ISBN: 978-0-323-66209-3

Publisher: Dolores Meloni
Acquisition Editor: Robin R Carter
Editorial Project Manager: Jennifer Horigan
Production Project Manager: Poulouse Joseph
Designer: Alan Studholme

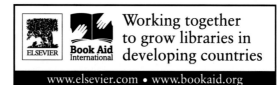

Working together
to grow libraries in
developing countries

www.elsevier.com • www.bookaid.org

List of Contributors

Leora Horn, MD, MSc
Associate Professor of Medicine
Medicine — Hematology Oncology
Vanderbilt Univeristy
Nashville, TN, United States

Erin A. Gillaspie, MD, MPH
Assistant Professor of Thoracic Surgery
Thoracic Surgery
Vanderbilt University Medical Center
Nashville, TN, United States

Ming-Sound Tsao, MD, FRCPC
Professor
Laboratory Medicine and Pathobiology
University of Toronto
Consultant Pathologist and Senior Scientist
    Princess Margaret Cancer Centre
Toronto, ON, Canada

Heather A. Wakelee, MD
Professor of Medicine, Oncology
Stanford University/Stanford Cancer Institute
Stanford, CA, United States

Jeffrey R. Zweig, MD
Fellow in Hematology/Oncology
Department of Medicine
Divisions of Hematology and Oncology
Stanford Cancer Institute
Stanford University
Stanford, CA, United States

Hak Choy, MD
Chair
Radiation Oncology
UT Southwestern
Dallas, TX, United States

Michael J. Jelinek, MD
Hematology/Oncology Fellow
Department of Medicine
University of Chicago
Chicago, IL, United States

Stephen V. Liu, MD
Associate Professor of Medicine
Division of Oncology
Georgetown University
Lombardi Comprehensive Cancer Center
Washington, DC, United States

Bhavisha A. Patel, MD
Hematology/Oncology Fellow
Department of Hematology/Oncology
Medstar Washington Hospital Center
Washington, MD, United States

Lecia V. Sequist, MD, MPH
The Landry Family Associate Professor of Medicine
Harvard Medical School
Boston, MA, United States

Director
Center for Innovation in Early Cancer Detection
Massachusetts General Hospital Cancer Center
Boston, MA, United States

Rina Hui, MBBS, PhD
Associate Professor
Department of Medical Oncology
Westmead Hospital and the University of Sydney
Sydney, NSW, Australia

J. Travis Mendel, MD
Resident
Radiation Oncology
UT Southwestern
Dallas, TX, United States

Shirish Gadgeel, MD
Professor
Department of Internal Medicine, Division
    of Hematology & Oncology
University of Michigan
Ann Arbor, MI, United States

Jyoti D. Patel, MD, FASCO
Professor of Medicine
University of Chicago
Chicago, IL, United States

Michael Millward, MBBS, MA
Professor
Cancer Council Professor of Clinical Cancer Research
Consultant Medical Oncologist
Sir Charles Gairdner Hospital and the University of
    Western Australia
Perth, WA, Australia

Emily Dickinson
Student
Cognitive Sciences
Rice University
Houston, TX, United States

Karen L. Reckamp, MD, MS
Professor
Department of Medical Oncology
City of Hope Comprehensive Cancer Center
Duarte, CA, United States

Dan Zhao, MD, PhD
Fellow
Hematology/Oncology
City of Hope Comprehensive Cancer Center
Duarte, CA, United States

Prodipto Pal, MD, PhD
Assistant Professor
Thoracic Pathology Service
Department of Laboratory Medicine and Pathobiology
University Health Network - University of Toronto
Toronto, ON, Canada

Michael Cabanero, MD
Assistant Professor
Thoracic Pathology Service
Department of Laboratory Medicine and Pathobiology
University Health Network - University of Toronto
Toronto, ON, Canada

Nicolas Marcoux, MD, FRCPC
Research Fellow
Massachusetts General Hospital Cancer Center
Boston, MA, United States

Medical Oncologist, Hematologist
CHU de Québec
Quebec City, Canada

Preface

Lung cancer is the leading cause of cancer-related mortality worldwide. The past three decades have seen the therapeutic approach to lung cancer evolve from a tactic of one size fits all to classifying the tumor into small cell lung cancer or non–small cell lung cancer (NSCLC) based on immunohistochemical stains. Approximately 85% of patients with lung cancer will have NSCLC, which can be further subclassified into adenocarcinoma, squamous cell carcinoma, or large cell neuroendocrine histology.

All histologic types of lung cancer can develop in current and former smokers. However, with the decline in cigarette consumption, adenocarcinoma has become the most frequent histologic subtype of lung cancer diagnosed in the United States. It also tends to be the most common form of lung cancer diagnosed in lifetime never smokers or former light smokers (<15 pack-year history), women, and younger adults (<60 years).

A diagnosis of adenocarcinoma alone has become insufficient to make therapeutic recommendations. The identification of actionable driver mutations and knowledge of to programmed death ligand 1 (PD-L1) status has changed the landscape of treatment options and trajectory of outcomes for a cohort of patients, and testing patients at diagnosis has become the standard of care.

In this book, we describe the optimal treatment approach to patients with adenocarcinoma of the lung from diagnosis to end-of-life care. We describe the appropriate testing required to make a pathologic diagnosis of NSCLC adenocarcinoma histology, including molecular and PD-L1 testing. We also review the optimal surgical approaches and adjuvant therapy recommendations for patients diagnosed with early-stage disease and radiation approaches for patients with locally advanced disease.

The majority of patients, however, will present with advanced stage disease that may be treatable but not curable with current systemic therapies. We have seen rapid advances made in the treatment landscape for patients with tumors that harbor the EGFR or BRAF mutation and the ALK or ROS1 fusion. For this cohort of patients, which account for less than 20% of North American patients with advanced stage disease, tyrosine kinase inhibitors (TKIs) are approved as first-line therapy based on studies that have demonstrated an improved response rate, progression-free survival (PFS), and overall survival (OS) compared with chemotherapy or historical controls. Moreover, for patients with tumors that are HER2, MET, RET, and NTRK positive, each accounting for less than 2% of NSCLC adenocarcinoma, there are exciting agents in clinical development that will further expand on oral treatment options for patients with NSCLC adenocarcinoma histology. For the majority of patients with no oncogenic driver, or for a driver for which there is no targeted therapy at this time, such as the 25% of patients with KRAS mutation positive NSCLC, chemotherapy for many years was the standard of care with important patient considerations required in selecting the optimal first- and second-line treatment option. With the introduction of immune checkpoint inhibitors into the treatment armamentarium, we have seen rapid improvements in outcomes for patients with advanced stage disease.

Adenocarcinoma of the lung provides a comprehensive overview of the rapidly evolving treatment paradigm for patients with NSCLC, providing a valuable resource to all interested in this disease.

Leora Horn
July 2018

Contents

1 **The Surgical Management of Pulmonary Adenocarcinoma**, *1*
Erin A. Gillaspie, MD, MPH

2 **Pulmonary Adenocarcinoma— Pathology and Molecular Testing**, *13*
Prodipto Pal, MD, PhD, Michael Cabanero, MD, and Ming-Sound Tsao, MD, FRCPC

3 **Adjuvant and Neoadjuvant Therapy in Non—Small-Cell Lung Cancer**, *35*
Jeffrey R. Zweig, MD, Heather A. Wakelee, MD

4 **Management of Locally Advanced Lung Cancer**, *57*
Hak Choy, MD, Jameson Travis Mendel, MD

5 **First-Line Therapy for Wild-Type Patients**, *87*
Michael J. Jelinek, MD, Jyoti D. Patel, MD

6 **Lung Adenocarcinoma: Second-Line Treatment**, *103*
Bhavisha A. Patel, MD, Stephen V. Liu, MD

7 **Epidermal Growth Factor Receptor— Mutant Non—Small-Cell Lung Cancer**, *115*
Nicolas Marcoux, MD, FRCPC, Lecia V. Sequist, MD, MPH

8 **Approach to Anaplastic Lymphoma Kinase (ALK) Gene Rearranged Non—Small Cell Lung Cancer (NSCLC)**, *133*
Shirish Gadgeel, MD

9 **Targeted Therapy in Non—Small-Cell Lung Cancer (Beyond Epidermal Growth Factor Receptor and Anaplastic Lymphoma Kinase)**, *143*
Emily Dickinson, Dan Zhao, MD, PhD, and Karen L. Reckamp, MD, MS

10 **Treatment of Pulmonary Adenocarcinoma With Immune Checkpoint Inhibitors**, *151*
Rina Hui, MBBS, PhD, Michael Millward, MBBS, MA

INDEX, *173*

The Surgical Management of Pulmonary Adenocarcinoma

ERIN A. GILLASPIE, MD, MPH

INTRODUCTION

The management of lung cancer has evolved dramatically over the last two decades. Importantly, research has established that a multidisciplinary approach is essential to help achieve optimal long-term outcomes.

Surgery plays an important role in early, locally advanced, and select advanced stages of lung cancer. While surgical approach continues to transition to more and more minimally invasive options, the principles remain the same.

This chapter will focus on establishing patient candidacy and surgical considerations for the treatment of pulmonary adenocarcinoma.

STAGING

The accurate staging of lung cancer is crucial in helping to guide treatment recommendations. This often includes a combination of imaging modalities and biopsies to determine size, location, nodal involvement, and histology. Even with a thorough preoperative workup there will be a subset of patients who will have unanticipated findings at the time of surgery.

Initial Staging: Imaging

Computed tomography (CT) scanning is a standard part of the workup for lung cancer and in determining the candidacy for resection. While excellent in delineating the extent of primary disease and some sites of metastatic disease, it is the least sensitive and specific modality for the identification of lymph node involvement.[1]

The utility of positron emission tomography (PET) scan has evolved over time and now holds an important role in extrathoracic staging to rule out distant metastasis which would in many cases render a patient unresectable. PET is also helpful in assessing the mediastinum for lymph node involvement. Confirmation of PET scan abnormalities with tissue diagnosis remains important as the imaging also carries a significant rate of false-positive upstaging in particular regions where histoplasmosis is prevalent.[1,2]

Imaging and staging should ideally be completed as quickly as possible and should not be any older than 60 days prior to the initiation of therapy or there is a risk of progression in the interim.

Pathologic Staging: Tissue Diagnosis for Suspected Lung Cancer

Tissue diagnosis may be accomplished through a range of procedures including conventional bronchoscopy, CT-guided transthoracic needle biopsy, navigational bronchoscopy, and resectional biopsy (surgery). Resectional biopsy has largely been supplanted by navigational bronchoscopy, which is less invasive than endobronchial methods.[3]

Endobronchial and Transbronchial Biopsy

Endobronchial and transbronchial approaches to biopsy are minimally invasive with low morbidity and low cost.

Biopsies are obtained through a flexible, fiber-optic bronchoscope. Generally, four to five pieces of tissue are collected, each measuring approximately 1−2 mm in diameter. Samples may be submitted as a frozen section or in formalin fixative for permanent section analysis. Although the procedure is low risk, a careful physical history should be obtained ahead of time to ensure no anesthetic or bleeding risks exist for a patient.

Endobronchial lesions are visible within the bronchial tree and may be sampled directly using a biopsy forceps though a flexible or rigid bronchoscope.

Transbronchial biopsy is also performed with the assistance of a flexible bronchoscopy. At minimum, a chest X-ray is required, and preferably, a CT scan is

Pulmonary Adenocarcinoma: Approaches to Treatment. https://doi.org/10.1016/B978-0-323-55433-6.00001-8

performed prior to the procedure to help guide tissue sampling. Fluoroscopy is commonly used intraprocedurally to help localize a target lesion to improve accuracy of the diagnostic yield. The most common complication associated with the biopsy of peripheral nodules is pneumothorax.[4]

Electromagnetic navigational bronchoscopy (ENB) is a newer technology that allows a practitioner to use CT scan to plot a course through the bronchial tree to a lung nodule or desired biopsy location.[5] This technology is particularly effective in more difficult-to-reach nodules and smaller nodules. Zhang et al. performed a metaanalysis to evaluate the overall diagnostic yield and accuracy of ENB and a pooled sensitivity of 82% and specificity of 100%.[6] In a metaanalysis, Gex et al. identified the variables favorably influencing the performance of ENB include greater size of the nodule, nodule visualization using a radial-probe EBUS, presence of a bronchus sign, lower registration error, and catheter suction technique. Overall, the technique has been demonstrated to be safe and effective.[7]

Fine needle aspiration (FNA) and needle biopsy are alternative methods for sampling nodules.[8] CT scan is the imaging modality of choice to visualize the needle advancing within the nodule or area of abnormality.[9] The accuracy for CT-guided biopsies range from 64% to 97%. A trend toward lower diagnostic accuracy was noted for smaller lesions less than 1.5 cm in diameter and in a subpleural location.[8] The most common complications are pneumothorax and hemorrhage. Risk factors for complications include smaller size of lesions, length of intrapulmonary needle path, and trans-fissure course.[10,11]

In 2014, Capalbo et al. compared FNA and core needle biopsy in 121 of their patients. FNA resulted in fewer complications—pneumothorax in 18% versus 31% and parenchymal hemorrhage in 9% versus 34%—and diagnostic accuracy of FNA was 94.8% when performed in the presence of a pathologist who could confirm adequacy of tissue sampling.[12]

Surgical Lung Biopsy

Open lung biopsy has taken on new meaning in the minimally invasive surgical era. Standard video-assisted thoracoscopic surgery (VATS) and uniportal VATS have replaced open thoracotomy as the approach of choice.

Early in the experience, outcomes were compared between diagnostic efficacies of thoracotomy and VATS approach. No matter the surgical approach,

diagnostic yielded has been demonstrated to be equivalent.[4,13,14]

An open lung biopsy allows surgeons to palpate and visualize the whole lung and directly select the lesions to biopsy. Palpating lesions is more challenging in a VATS approach. For small lesions or ground-glass opacities where identification can be difficult, localization may be performed preoperatively to assist using ENB to inject blue dye or place a fiducial prior to thoracoscopy. An alternative and equally effective method as described in a paper by Grogan et al. is preoperative CT-guided radionucleotide labeling of a lesion with technetium 99. Intraoperatively, a collimated probe connected to a γ detector can be used to isolate the lesion. The lesion may be wedged out, and then background counts can then be assessed to confirm specimen removal. Localization has been described to be successful in 95% of cases.[15]

An open lung biopsy specimen may be reviewed intraoperatively, and if malignancy is confirmed, a definitive resection can be performed in the same setting if appropriate. Surgical considerations will be discussed in more detail later in the chapter.

Pathologic Mediastinal Assessment

Imaging can be informative and is an important first step in the assessment of mediastinal nodes. CT has a sensitivity of 55% and specificity of 81%, while PET-CT has a sensitivity of 62% and specificity of 90%.[16]

Mediastinoscopy has long been considered the gold standard diagnostic technique for the assessment of mediastinal lymph nodes. Mediastinoscopy can evaluate level 2, 4, and 7 nodes and can send large tissue samples for analysis. This has been replaced in many centers by endobronchial ultrasound (EBUS) as the first line. Despite this, mediastinoscopy does maintain an important role in diagnosis of suspicious lymphadenopathy or mediastinal restaging and carries a sensitivity of 89% and specificity of 100%.[1]

EBUS with transbronchial needle aspiration has increasingly been used as a favored method for diagnosis of suspicious mediastinal nodes. EBUS is unique in that it offers the ability to sample both N1 and N2 nodes. Caution should be exercised when considering resectability for left upper lobe tumors as they have the most unpredictable pattern of lymph node metastasis and frequently involve level 5 and 6 nodes which are inaccessible to mediastinoscopy and EBUS. Review of available publications reveals a median sensitivity of 89% and has a very low risk of complications.[1,17,18]

Rapid onsite cytologic evaluation confirms adequacy of samplings at the time of procedure to enhance overall yield.[19]

The number of lymph node stations to assess is debated among experts with some favoring the routine sampling of all lymph node stations while others favoring only the sampling of those nodes that are suspicious on imaging.[18,20]

Even with negative imaging, negative surgical biopsy, and a small (T1) cancer, there will still be a subset of patients found to have occult N2 disease either on frozen section at the time of lung resection or discovered later on final pathology. The rate of occult N2 disease with T1 primary tumors and negative imaging is in the range of 6.1%−6.5% and 8.7% for T2 tumors.[21,22] Although prediction models to try to determine the risk of N2 disease have been developed and tested, they are not widely accepted and adopted.[23,24]

ASSESSING SURGICAL CANDIDACY

After establishing the stage of cancer, a meticulous preoperative evaluation should be performed prior to recommending resection. Workup should include history and physical examination, pulmonary function tests, a nutritional assessment, and cardiac clearance.

Smoking Cessation

Smokers should be counseled to stop immediately. In a study by Mason et al. in 2009 from the General Thoracic Surgery Database, the risk of in-hospital death and pulmonary complications was higher in patients who were actively smoking at the time of surgery and could be mitigated by preoperative smoking cessation.[25]

Assessment of Cardiovascular Risk

Major cardiac-related adverse events occur in approximately 2%−3% of patients after pulmonary resection. The thoracic revised cardiac risk index is a validated tool that can be used to help guide which patients should be sent for additional, preoperative consultation. Patients who score more than 1.5 in the cardiac index or those describing limited exercise capacity or a recent diagnosis of active heart disease all warrant evaluation.[26,27]

Assessment of Pulmonary Function

Patients undergoing pulmonary resection commonly have a number of coexisting conditions and exposures which can perturb pulmonary function. It is therefore essential to ensure adequate pulmonary reserve prior to proceeding with resection.

Spirometry and measurement of diffusion capacity for carbon monoxide (DLCO) are recommended for all patients undergoing pulmonary resection and are calculated as a percentage of normal.[28]

The forced expiratory volume in 1 s (FEV1), measured during spirometry, determines the mechanical function of the lung, i.e., the airflow limitations of medium to large airways. DLCO value provides a gross estimate of the function of the alveolar-capillary membrane.

A preoperative predicted value of 60% or less for FEV1 has been shown to be an important cut-off value for predicting respiratory complications.[29] DLCO is a second, independent functional parameter that can separately predict surgical risk and is currently ordered as a standard part of workup along with pulmonary function testing. If this is also less than 60%−70% on preoperative predictive value, additional testing is warranted to help determine the safety of resection.[30−32]

A postoperative predicted value of DLCO and FEV1 may be calculated directly by subtracting the number of segments that would be resected at the time of surgery, assuming that each contributes equally. A more accurate method would be to obtain a quantitative lung scan to directly determine the contribution from each portion of the lung.[27,32]

DLCO postoperative predicted value of less than 60% in some studies and 40% in others denotes a significant risk for perioperative morbidity and mortality. For FEV1 values of less than 40% and DLCO of less than 40%, exercise stress testing should be performed.[32−34]

Options for secondary testing include a shuttle walk test, stair climbing, exercise stress test or a perfusion scan. The former are more subjective, while later are more quantitative and have established thresholds associated with surgical risk.

A quantitative radionucleotide scan uses inhaled radioactive xenon and the intravenous administration of technetium-labeled macroaggregates to determine the fraction of total perfusion for the upper, middle, and lower zones of the lung.[35]

Cardiopulmonary exercise testing is a physiologic testing technique that provides an evaluation of functional capacity of both the heart and lungs.

The risk for perioperative complications has been reported to be higher with the lower measured value of VO2 max. Values over 20 mL/kg min can safely undergo a planned resection. A value between 10 and 15 mL/kg min indicates an increased risk of perioperative death.[27,36] Brunelli et al. observed a mortality rate of 13% with a VO2 max of <12%, while no mortality was observed with >20.[36]

Licker et al. found in their study that VO2 max of <10 mL/kg min is at very high risk and considered a contraindication to anatomic resection—total morbidity 5%, cardiac morbidity 39%.[29]

SURGICAL MANAGEMENT OF LUNG CANCER

Stage, histology, and patient candidacy determine the treatment modalities that will confer the best overall survival. Surgery plays an important role in the management of lung cancer, and this approach has evolved significantly over the last two decades.

Early-Stage Lung Cancer

Surgery is considered to be a standard part of the treatment for stage I and II non—small cell lung cancers (NSCLCs) (Table 1.1). The eighth edition staging system comprehends tumors that are node negative and up to 7 cm in size and tumors that involve the chest wall, pericardium, or satellite nodules in the same lobe. Surgery is also performed for patients who have smaller tumors up to 5 cm or involving the main bronchus, ipsilateral, hilar nodes.[37,38]

Locally Advanced Lung Cancer

The treatment of locally advanced lung cancer is complex and requires a multidisciplinary approach. The presentations in which surgery can play a role in therapy are described below.[39]

TABLE 1.1 Early-Stage Lung Cancer				
	N0	**N1**	**N2**	**N3**
T1	IA	IIB	IIIA	IIIB
T2a	IB	IIB	IIIA	IIIB
T2b	IIA	IIB	IIIA	IIIB
T3	IIB	IIIA	IIIB	IIIC
T4	IIIA	IIIA	IIIB	IIIC

Adapted from Detterbeck et al. Eighth edition lung cancer staging.

T3N1 Tumors

T3N1 is a relatively infrequent stage of lung cancer but surgery has a well-defined role as the primary treatment for these tumors. T3 lung cancers range in size from 5 to 7 cm or invade structures that can be routinely taken en bloc with the lung—the chest wall, pericardium, or a single phrenic nerve. Often, hilar nodal involvement is discovered at the time of resection. The surgical goal is an en bloc resection with microscopically negative margins.[39,40]

The most common presentation is with chest wall involvement. Chest wall resection can be performed en bloc with a pulmonary resection. At least 2—3 cm margins or one rib above and below the involved area should be included in the resection to achieve a complete microscopic resection. As thoracoscopic equipment has evolved and thoracic surgeon experience has increased, more complex cases are able to be completed minimally invasively. Small chest wall defects and those hidden by the scapula do not require reconstruction. A defect greater than 5 cm should be reconstructed along with resection of the fifth to sixth ribs near the tip of the scapula to prevent entrapment and to maintain chest wall integrity.

There is currently no clear evidence for neoadjuvant chemotherapy in these patients; however, adjuvant chemotherapy is recommended for tumors that are determined on final pathology to be greater than 5 cm or have positive ipsilateral hilar lymph nodes. Postoperative radiation is usually reserved for patients in whom there is a concern for residual disease.[39,40]

N2 Disease

Approximately, 15% of patients with pulmonary adenocarcinoma will present with stage IIIA (N2) disease. The optimal management of N2 disease is perhaps the most controversial in thoracic oncology. Ipsilateral mediastinal lymph node involvement ranges from occult disease to single station, microscopic disease to multistation bulky disease, and everything in between.

Even with negative imaging and negative pathologic mediastinal staging, there is a subset of patients who are discovered to have N2 disease at the time of lung resection. The rate ranges from 6.1% to 8.7%.[21,22] When confronted with unseen N2 disease at the time of surgery, many surgeons will complete resection of the tumor and refer the patient for consideration of adjuvant therapy as the patient has already been subjected to the risk of anesthesia and thoracic surgery.

For preoperatively identified N2 disease, there is no consensus among surgeons as to what defines resectable N2 disease and who should be considered for surgery as part of a multimodal treatment regimen. However, the INT0139 trial firmly established that surgery alone was insufficient for the management of N2 disease.

As a part of a multimodal treatment regimen, studies suggest that surgery can enhance disease-free and overall survival in patients who do not present with bulky mediastinal disease, those who are able to complete neoadjuvant therapy and pathologic partial or complete response at the time of resection.[21,22]

Additional research is required to help establish a more structured treatment plan for patients presenting with N2 disease.

T4 Tumors

T4 tumors are locally aggressive with invasion of critical mediastinal structures such as the PA, heart, aorta, superior vena cava (SVC), trachea, esophagus, spine, or the diaphragm. In many institutions, these advanced-stage tumors are considered unresectable and relegated to chemotherapy and radiation.

Several nonrandomized series have shown that highly selected patients may have 5-year survival rates as high as 48%. Most reported experience involves tumors invading the SVC, left atrium, carina, intrapericardial pulmonary vessels, and vertebral bodies. Prognosis is associated with achieving en bloc survival and limited or no nodal involvement (N0–N1).[41–43]

Surgery should be performed in high, volume thoracic centers. Meticulous preoperative planning and in some cases multidisciplinary surgical approach is necessary to ensure complete resection.[42]

Due to the heterogeneity of this population, it is difficult to accumulate sufficient evidence to clearly define the role of surgery in this group of patients.

Superior Sulcus Tumors

Superior sulcus tumors, also known as Pancoast tumors, arise from the apex of the right upper or left upper lobe. These tumors may invade any of the structures in the thoracic inlet (Fig. 1.1).

As with other locally advanced tumors, multidisciplinary approach is the mainstay of management of superior sulcus tumors with chemoradiotherapy administration followed by restaging to determine resectability.

The factors associated with poor prognosis include incomplete resection, lack or response to neoadjuvant treatment, invasion into the brachial plexus, >50% of the vertebral body and great vessels as well as lymph node involvement.[43]

Oligometastatic Disease

The concept of oligometastatic disease was first proposed in 1995 and then further defined in 2006 by Niibe et al., who classified oligometastatic disease by prognosis. They described oligorecurrence or oligometastatic disease in the adrenal or brain as actually having

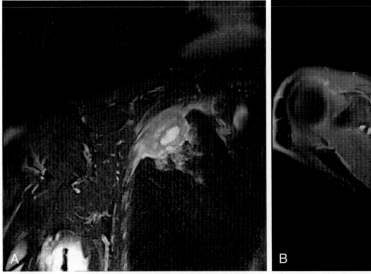

FIG. 1.1 Right-sided superior sulcus tumor seen in coronal **(A)** and axial **(B)** views. The tumor is invading the posterior chest wall.

a relatively favorable prognosis. For these lesions, the standard of care includes surgical resection of both the primary and metastasis or recurrence.[44,45] Generally for synchronous disease, the metastatic site is treated first. If this is not able to be successfully addressed, there is no benefit to resecting the primary.

SURGICAL APPROACH TO LUNG CANCER

The conduct of the operation begins with the administration of anesthesia and placement of an endotracheal tube that allows for pulmonary isolation. This may be accomplished with a double-lumen endotracheal tube or a bronchial blocker.

The approach to surgery and extent of pulmonary resection is determined by the size and location of the tumor and experience of the surgeon.

Open Lobectomy

The majority of pulmonary resections continue to be performed in open fashion. An open lobectomy is performed through a thoracotomy: axillary, anterolateral, or posterolateral.

A posterolateral thoracotomy is the most standard approach and is performed using a semi-muscle-sparing approach by dividing the latissimus and sparing the serratus anterior muscle. If the latissimus can be retracted, rather than divided, then this is preferred.

The chest is entered and a rib can be shingled to assist with exposure. The lung is rendered atelectatic, and the chest and lung are inspected for unexpected findings and to confirm resectability.

Surgery begins with the removal of N1 and N2 lymph nodes which are sent to pathology. A lobectomy is performed by isolating the arteries, vein, and bronchus associated with the lobe and dividing each, along with the fissure that connects the upper, middle (right), and lower lobes. Once the lobectomy is completed, the remaining lung is reinflated to fill the pleural space, and chest tubes are positioned to help drain fluid and air while the patient recovers.

Lung resections carry a significant risk of perioperative morbidity with 37% of patients experiencing some form of postoperative complications—atrial arrhythmia and prolonged air leak being the most common. Other complications can include infection, bleeding, hypoxia, and death.[46]

Video-Assisted Thoracoscopic Surgery Lobectomy

The first reports of VATS lobectomy were in 1992 and 1993.[47,48] Adoption across the United States has been slow, but now approximately 44% of cases are

being performed minimally invasively with this approach being available in 80% of hospitals across the nation.[49,50]

A VATS lobectomy is conducted in similar fashion to an open lobectomy but utilizes 2–3 small ports in the chest, each measuring approximately 1 cm, and a slightly larger utility incision measuring 3 cm that is used to remove the specimens (Fig. 1.2). VATS differs from open surgery in both the length of incisions and that there is minimal muscular division and no rib spreading (Fig. 1.3).

A camera allows visualization of the whole hemithorax and special instruments have been designed to allow for uses a camera to provide visualization of the whole chest and special instruments to facilitate.

Comparison of the outcomes of VATS versus open lobectomies have shown VATS to be a safe surgery with oncologically equivalent outcomes.[46,51,52] Both VATS and open surgery have similar patterns of

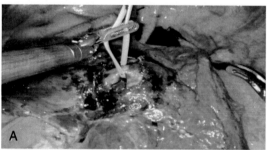

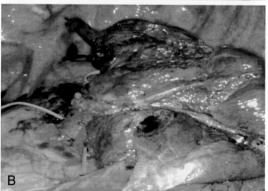

FIG. 1.2 Isolation of a branch of the left upper lobe pulmonary artery **(A)** and left upper lobe pulmonary vein **(B)** during a left upper lobectomy. **(A)** The anatomy of the left upper lobe pulmonary artery is highly variable. The branches are dissected out and divided with serial applications of a vascular load stapling device. **(B)** The superior pulmonary vein drains the upper lobe of the lung. The vein is isolated, but not divided until a separate inferior pulmonary vein is confirmed.

postoperative complications, although VATS occurs at a lesser rate.[53–55] Additional benefits include earlier recovery, less pain, less impact on pulmonary function, better quality of life, and increased delivery of adjuvant therapy.[56–60]

Despite the evidence to support benefits to patients, VATS lobectomy has had variable uptake across the United States with some institutions performing only open procedures while others are performing in excess of 90% of cases thoracoscopically. The ideal proportion of VATS lobectomy is not yet well defined. There equally is no great explanation for the significant variability in practice patterns. Initial safety concerns have been put to rest and excellent training pathways have been developed to help with the adoption of new technology.[46]

Alternative methods to perform minimally invasive surgery have emerged since the advent of VATS lobectomy, and this may help to increase the overall volume of minimally invasive surgery.

Robotic Lobectomy

Robotic lobectomies were first performed by Morgon et al. and Ashton et al. in 2003, and the use of this technology has continued to increase with time.[61,62]

Much like VATS, robotic lobectomy is performed through small (8 mm) incisions with a slightly different configuration (Fig. 1.4).

This newer technology allows several advantages over traditional thoracoscopic surgery in that it provides a three-dimensional high-definition field and the instruments have 9 degrees of freedom and include the ability to stable and seal vessels.

Studies have demonstrated equal safety and operative times with comparable morbidity, mortality, and benefits to VATS including survival. Cost studies have demonstrated that while upfront cost is more, ultimately minimally invasive surgery including robotic surgery ultimately provide cost savings both intra-operatively and post-operatively.[60,63–66]

As with any new technology, there is a learning curve but the da Vinci robots (Intuitive Surgical, Sunnyvale,

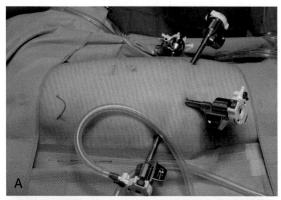
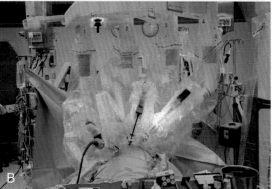

FIG. 1.4 Robotic lobectomy port sites **(A)** and docking of the robotic arms **(B)**. **(A)** Four incisions were created to perform the robotic lobectomy, each measuring 8 mm. At the end of the case, the anteriormost incision is lengthened slightly to allow the removal of the lobe. A separate incision is used for the chest tube. **(B)** Once the ports are placed, the robotic arms are docked, and instruments are inserted into the chest. The surgeon can then sit at the console and perform the surgery using the robotic instruments.

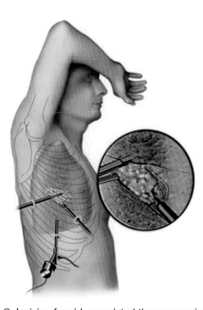

FIG. 1.3 Incision for video-assisted thoracoscopic surgery lobectomy. The incisions are generally placed in the fifth intercostal space, anterior axillary line, and the eighth intercostal space anterior and posterior axillary line. There are, however, variations depending on the lobe that is being resected and surgeon preference. (Photo credit Dominic M Doyle, Ms for Vanderbilt.)

CA, USA) company has developed comprehensive training programs and certification processes including on-site proctoring for cases.

Uniportal and Subxiphoid Lobectomy

Uniportal lobectomy is single-incision VATS lobectomy, which became another natural extension of VATS lobectomy. Developed by Dr. Rocco and Dr. Gondolas-Rivas, this procedure required improvement in articulating staplers and the development of other reticulating instruments to improve angles of dissection. Uniportal VATS is cited to have better visualization and operative conditions similar to an open approach.[67]

Subxiphoid is another iteration of uniportal lobectomy with an incision just below the xiphoid rather than in the chest wall. This is to help eliminate postoperative pain and chest wall numbness that are associated with instrumentation of the intercostal spaces. A 4-cm incision is created in the subxiphoid space, and the pleural cavity is accessed. The lobectomy is performed in an identical fashion to a VATS lobectomy. The procedure is more challenging due to the longer tunnel and more limited view but can be accomplished safely and with significant reduction in postoperative pain.[68]

IMPORTANT SURGICAL CONSIDERATIONS
Extent of Resection

Lobectomy has long been considered the standard of care and the most optimal oncologic procedure in the management of early-stage NSCLC. More limited resections (including segmentectomy or wedge resection) were thought to be associated with higher risk of recurrence and historically were reserved for patients with limited cardiopulmonary reserve.

The advent of CT screening for lung cancer and improvements in imaging technology have led to the identification of a large number of patients with small (<2 cm) peripheral nodules. This prompted a renewed interest in the possibility of more limited resection.

The advantages of sublobar resection include preservation of pulmonary function, which can preserve a patient's ability to undergo subsequent resections and diminished morbidity and mortality.

Current evidence supporting sublobar resection is mostly single institution; retrospective studies and many are in patients who have insufficient cardiopulmonary reserve to tolerate a lobectomy. Studies are summarized in Table 1.2.

The factors identified as potentiating higher recurrence were larger tumors (stage IB), inadequate margins (less than 1 cm) highlighting the importance of tumor size influencing local recurrence.[78]

A large American study by the Cancer and Leukemia Group B (CALGB) is currently underway to try to help definitively answer the question as to whether a sublobar resection for tumors <2 cm without any lymph node involvement is oncologically sufficient.

Extent of Lymph Node Resection
The accuracy of lymph node staging is important to help determine stage and thereby guide adjuvant treatment decisions.

TABLE 1.2
Outcomes of Single-Center Studies Lobectomy Versus Sublobar Resection

Study	Size of Study	Stage	SURVIVAL (5 YEARS)	
			Lobectomy	Sublobar
Campione et al.[69]	121 patients	IA	65	62
Ucar et al.[70]	34	IA and B	64	70
El-Sherif[71]	784	IA	HR 1.39 (favoring sublobar resection)	
Kilik[72]	184	IA and B	447	46
Koike[73]	223	IA	90	89
Iwasaki[74]	86	I, II, IIIA	73	70
Cao[75]	2745	IA and B	HR 0.91 (favoring lobectomy)	
Okada[76]	567	IA and B	89.6	89.1
Altorki[77]	347	IA	86	85

Does removing more nodes in a mediastinal lymph node dissection detect more disease than systematic sampling of each lymph node station? The answer may depend on the T stage of the tumor.

The ACOSOC Z0030 trial demonstrated that in T1 and T2 tumors, a complete lymph node dissection identified occult N2 disease missed on sampling in 4% of cases. It should be noted that this study had low utilization of preoperative mediastinal pathologic staging and even PET-CT was not used until the later part of the study, potentially reducing the accuracy of preoperative staging.[46] In addition, despite identifying the occult N2 disease, this did not confer a survival benefit to patients.

Sentinel lymph node biopsy (SNLB) has been occasionally gained traction in thoracic surgery to help guide lymphadenectomy. The hypothesis was based on the same rationale that led to the use of SNLB for both melanoma and breast cancer. Unfortunately, studies have not justified the use of SLNB for NSCLC.[79]

Hopefully this question will soon be answered by the Japanese Clinical Oncology Group Trial (JCOG 1413) which is a randomized phase III clinical trial looking at lobe-specific versus systemic nodal dissection for clinical stage I and II NSCLCs. They plan to enroll 1700 patients from 44 institutions with primary endpoint of overall survival.[80]

CONCLUSION

Surgery continues to play an important role in the management of lung cancer. Surgery alone, for many stages, is insufficient and the multidisciplinary approach to therapy requires a coordinated approach by medical oncology and radiation oncology.

REFERENCES

1. Silvestri GA, Gonzalez AV, Jantz MA, et al. Methods for staging non-small cell lung cancer: Diagnosis and management of lung cancer, 3rd ed: American College of Chest Physicians evidence-based clinical practice guidelines. *Chest.* 2013;143(5):50S–211S.
2. Deppen S, Putman JB, Andrade G, et al. Accuracy of FDG-PET to diagnose lung cancer in a region of endemic granulomatous disease. *Ann Thorac Surg.* 2011;92(2):428–433.
3. Khan KA, Nardelli P, Jaeger A, O'Shea C, Cantillon-Murphy P, Kennedy MP. Navigational bronchoscopy for early lung cancer: a road to therapy. *Adv Ther.* 2016;33(4):580–596.
4. Bensard DD, McIntyre RC, Waring BJ, Simon JS. Comparison of video thoracoscopic lung biopsy to open lung biopsy in the diagnosis of interstitial lung disease. *Chest.* 1993;103:7651.
5. Wells AU, Hirani N. Interstitial lung disease guideline. *Thorax.* 2008;63(1):v1–v58.
6. Zhang W, Chen S, Dong X, Lei P. Meta-analysis of the diagnostic yield and safety of electromagnetic navigation bronchoscopy for lung nodules. *J Thorac Dis.* 2015;7(5):799–809.
7. Gex G, Pralong JA, Combescure C, Seijo L, Rochat T, Soccal PM. Diagnostic yield and safety of electromagnetic navigation bronchoscopy for lung nodules: a systematic review and meta-analysis. *Respiration.* 2014;87(2):165–176.
8. Birchard KR. Transthoracic needle biopsy. *Semin Intervent Radiol.* 2011;28(1):L87–97.
9. Yao X, Gomes MM, Tsao MS, Allen CJ, Geddie W, Sehkon H. Fine-needle aspiration biopsy versus core-needle biopsy in diagnosing lung cancer: a systematic review. *Curr Oncol.* 2012;19(1):e16–e27.
10. Rizzo S, Preda L, Raimondi S, et al. Risk factors for complications of CT-guided lung biopsies. *Radiol Med.* 2011;116(4):548–563.
11. Saji J, Nakamura H, Tsuchida T, et al. The incidence and risk of pneumothorax and chest tube placement after percutaneous CT-guided lung biopsy: the angle of the needle trajectory is a novel predictor. *Chest.* 2002;121(5):1521–1526.
12. Capalbo E, Peli M, Lovisatti M, et al. Trans-thoracic biopsy of lung lesions: FNAB or CNB? Our experience and review of the literature. *Radiol Med.* 2014;199(8):572–594.
13. Allen MS, Deschamps C, Jones DM, Trastek VF, Pairolero PC. Video-assisted thoracic procedures: the mayo experience. *Mayo Clin Proc.* 1996;71:351.
14. Kadokura M, Colby TV, Myers JL, et al. Pathologic comparison of video-assisted thoracic surgical lung biopsy with traditional open lung biopsy. *J Thorac Cardiovasc Surg.* 1995;109:494.
15. Grogan EL, Jones DR, Kozower BD, Simmons WD, Daniel TM. Identification of small lung nodules: technique of radiotracer-guided thoracoscopic biopsy. *Ann Thorac Surg.* 2008;85(2):S772–S777.
16. Gelberg J, Grondin S, Trembley A. Mediastinal staging for lung cancer. *Can Respir J.* 2014;21(3):159–161.
17. Yasafuku K, Pierre A, Darling G, et al. *A Prospective Controlled trial of Endobronchial Ultrasound-Guided Transbronchial Needle Aspiration Compared with Mediastinoscopy for Mediastinal Lymph Node Staging of Lung Cancer.* Philadelphia, Pennsylvania: 91st Annual Meeting of The American Association for Thoracic Surgery; 2011.
18. Darling GE, Dickie AJ, Malthaner RA, Kennedy EB, Tey R. Invasive mediastinal staging of non-small-cell lung cancer: a clinical practice guideline. *Curr Oncol.* 2011;18(6):e304–e310.

19. Wong RWM, Thai A, Khor YH, Ireland-Jenkin K, Lanteri CJ, Jennings BR. the utility of rapid on-Site evaluation on endobronchial ultrasound guided transbronchial needle aspiration: does it make a difference? *J Resp Med*. 2014.

20. Kinsey CM, Arenberg DA. Endobronchial ultrasound-guided transbronchial needle aspiration for non-small cell lung cancer staging. *Am J Respir*. 2015;189(6).

21. Lee PC, Port JL, Korst RJ, Liss Y, Meherally DN, Altorki NK. Risk factors for occult mediastinal metastases in clinical stage I non-small cell lung cancer. *Ann Thorac Surg*. 2007; 84(1):177–181.

22. Al-Sarraf N, Aziz R, Gately K, et al. Pattern and predictors of occult mediastinal lymph node involvement in non-small cell lung cancer patients with negative mediastinal update on positron emission tomography. *Eur J Cardio-thorac Surg*. 2008;33(1):104–109.

23. Jiang L, Jiang S, Lin Y, et al. Nomogram to predict occult N2 lymph nodes metastases in patients with squamous non-small cell lung cancer. *Medicine*. 2015;94(46):e2054.

24. Defranchi SA, Cassivi SD, Nichols FC, et al. N2 Disease in T1 non-small cell lung cancer. *Ann Thor Surg*. 2009;88(3): 924–928.

25. Mason DP, Subramanian S, Nowicki ER, et al. Impact of smoking cessation before resection of lung cancer: a society of thoracic surgeons general thoracic surgery database study. *Ann Thorac Surg*. 2009;88(2):362–370.

26. Thomas DC, Blasberg JD, Arnold BN, et al. Validating the thoracic revised cardiac risk index following lung resection. *Ann Thorac Surg*. 2017;104(2):389–394.

27. Spyratos D, Zarogoulidis P, Porpodis K, Angelis N, et al. Preoperative evaluation for lung cancer resection. *J Thorac Dis*. 2014;6(supp1):S162–166.

28. Mazzone PJ. Preoperative evaluation of the lung cancer resection candidate. *Expert Rev Respir Med*. 2010;4(1): 97–113.

29. Licker MJ, Widikker I, Robert J, et al. Operative mortality and respiratory complications after lung resection for cancer: impact of chronic obstructive pulmonary disease and time trends. *Ann Thorac Surg*. 2006;81:1830–1837.

30. Berry MF, Hanna J, Tong BC, et al. Risk factors for morbidity after lobectomy for lung cancer in elderly patients. *Ann Thorac Surg*. 2009;88:1093–1099.

31. Brunelli A, Sabbatini A, Xiume F, et al. A model to predict the decline of the forced expiratory vlume in one second and the carbon monoxide lung diffusion capacidty after major lung resection. *Interact Cardiovasc Thorac Surg*. 2005;4:61–65.

32. Salati M, Brunelli A. Risk stratification in lung resection. *Curr Surg Rep*. 2016;4(37):1–9.

33. Ferguson MK, Reeder LB, Mick R. Optimizing selection of patients for major lung resection. *J Thorac Cardiovasc Surg*. 1995;109:275–281.

34. Brunelli A, Refai MA, Salati M, Sabbatini A, Morgan-Hughes NJ, Rocco G. Carbon monoxide lung diffusion capacity improves risk stratification in patients without airflow limitation: evidence for systematic measurement before lung resection. *Eur J Cardiothorac Surg*. 2006;29: 567–570.

35. Gould G, Pearce A. Assessment of suitability for lung resection. *Crit Care Pain*. 2006;6(3):98–100.

36. Brunelli A, Belardinelli R, Refai M, et al. Peak oxygen consumption during cardiopulmonary exercise test improves risk stratification in candidates to Major lung resection. *Chest*. 2009;135:1260–1267.

37. Lackey A, Donington JS. Surgical management of lung cancer. *Semin Intervent Radiol*. 2013;30(2):133–140.

38. Detterbeck FC, Boffa DJ, Kim AW, Tanoue LT. The eighth edition lung cancer stage classification. *Chest*. 2017; 151(1):193–203.

39. Donington JS, Pass HI. Surgical approach to locally advanced non-small cell lung cancer. *Cancer J*. 2013; 19(3):217–221.

40. Lanuti M. Surgical management of lung cancer involving the chest wall. *Clinics*. 2017;27(2):195–199.

41. Reardon ES, Schrump DS. Extended resections of non-small cel lung cancers invading the aorta, pulmonary artery, left atrium, or esophagus: can they be justified? *Thorac Surg Clin*. 2014;24(4):457–464.

42. Van Schil PE, Berzenji L, Yogeswaran SK, Hendriks JM, Lauwers P. Surgical management of stage IIIA non-small cell lung cancer. *Front Oncol*. 2017;7:249.

43. Farjah F, Wood DE, Varghese TK, Symons RG, Flum DR. Trends in the operative management and outcomes of T4 lung cancer. *Ann Thorac Surg*. 2008;86(2):368–374.

44. David EA, Clark JM, Cooke DT, Melnikow J, Kelly K, Canter RJ. The role of thoracic surgery in the therapeutic management of metastatic non-small cell lung cancer. *J Thorac Oncol*. 2017;12(11):1636–1645.

45. Varela G, Thomas PA. Surgical management of advanced non-small cell lung cancer. *J Thorac Dis*. 2014;6(2): S217–223.

46. Allen MS, Darling GE, Pechet TT, et al. Morbidity and mortality of major pulmonary resections in patients with early-stage lung cancer: initial results of the randomized, prospective ACOSOC Z0030 trial. *Ann Thorac Surg*. 2006; 81(3):1013–1019.

47. Hazelrigg SR, Nunchuck SK, LoCicero J. Video assisted thoracic surgery study group data. *Ann Thorac Surg*. 1993; 56:1039–1043.

48. Roviaro G, Rebuffat C, Varoli F, Vergani C, Mariani C, Maciocco M. Videoendoscopic assisted pulmonary lobectomy for cancer. *Surg Laparosc Endosc*. 1992;2: 244–247.

49. Abdelsattar ZM, Allen MS, Shen KR, et al. Variation in hospital adoption Rates of video-assisted thoracoscopic lobectomy for lung cancer and the effects on outcomes. *Ann Thorac Surg*. 2017;103(2):454–460.

50. Blasberg JD, Seder CW, Leverson G, Shan Y, Maloney JD, Mackle RA. Video-assisted thoracoscopic lobectomy for lung cancer: current practice patterns and predictors of adoption. *Ann Thorac Surg*. 2016;102(6):1854–1862.

51. Boffa DJ, Allen MS, Grab JD, Gaissert HA, Harpole DH, Wright CD. Data from the society of thoracic surgeons general thoracic surgery database: the surgical management of primary lung tumors. *J Thorac Cardiovasc Surg*. 2008;135: 247–254.

52. Flores RM, Ihekweazu U, Dycoco J. Video-assisted thoraco-scopic surgery (VATS) lobectomy: catastrophic intraoperative complications. *Thorac Cardiovasc Surg.* 2011;142:1412–1417.

53. McKenna Jr RJ, Houck W, Fuller CB. Video-assisted thoracic surgery lobectomy: experience with 1,100 cases. *Ann Thorac Surg.* 2006;81(2):421–425.

54. Onaitis MW, Petersen RP, Balderson S, et al. Thoracoscopic lobectomy is a safe and versatile procedure: experience with 500 consecutive patients. *Ann Surg.* 2006;244(3):420–425.

55. Ali MK, Mountain CF, Ewer MS, Johnston D, Haynie TP. Predicting loss of pulmonary function after pulmonary resection for bronchogenic carcinoma. *Chest.* 1980;77(3):337–342.

56. Rocco G, Internullo E, Cassivi SD, Van Raemdonck D, Ferguson MK. The variability of practice in minimally invasive thoracic surgery for pulmonary resections. *Thorac Surg Clin.* 2008;18(3):235–247.

57. Demmy TL, Curtis J. Minimally invasive lobectomy directed toward frail and high-risk patients: a case-control study. *Ann Thorac Surg.* 1999;68(1):194–200.

58. Sugiura H, Morikawa T, Kaji M, Sasamura Y, Kondo S, Katoh H. Long-term benefits for the quality of life after video-assisted thoracoscopic lobectomy in patients with lung cancer. *Surg Laparosc Endosc Percutan Tech.* 1999;9(6):403–408.

59. Petersen RP, Pham D, Burfeind WR, et al. Thoracoscopic lobectomy facilitates the delivery of chemotherapy after resection for lung cancer. *Ann Thorac Surg.* 2007;83(4):1245–1249.

60. Dylewski MR, Ohaeto AC, Pereira JF. Pulmonary resection using a total endoscopic robotic video-assisted approach. *Semin Thorac Cardiovasc Surg.* 2011;23(1):36–42.

61. Morgan JA, Ginsburg ME, Sonett JR, et al. Advanced thoracoscopic procedures are facilitated by computer-aided robotic technology. *Eur J Cardiothorac Surg.* 2003;23:883–887.

62. Ashton Jr RC, Connery CP, Swistel DG, DeRose JJ. Robot-assisted lobectomy. *J Thorac Cardiovasc Surg.* 2003;126:292–293. https://doi.org/10.1016/S0022-5223(03)00201-0.

63. Gharagozloo F, Margolis M, Tempesta B. Robot-assisted thoracoscopic lobectomy for early-stage lung cancer. *Ann Thorac Surg.* 2008;85(6):1880–1885.

64. Cerfolio RJ, Bryant AS, Skylizard L, Minnich DJ. Initial consecutive experience of completely portal robotic pulmonary resection with 4 arms. *J Thorac Cardiovasc Surg.* 2011;142(4):740–746.

65. Giulianotti PC, Buchs NC, Caravaglios G, Bianco FM. Robot-assisted lung resection: outcomes and technical details. *Interact Cardiovasc Thorac Surg.* 2010;11(4):388–392.

66. Park BJ, Melfi F, Mussi A, et al. Robotic lobectomy for non-small cell lung cancer (NSCLC): long-term oncologic results. *J Thorac Cardiovasc Surg.* 2012;143(2):383–389.

67. Reinersman JM, Passera E, Rocco G. Overview of uniportal video-assisted thoracic surgery (VATS): past and present. *Ann Cardiothorac Surg.* 2016;5(2):112–117.

68. Song N, Zhao DP, Jiang L, et al. Suxiphoid uniportal video-assisted thoracoscpoc surgery (VATS) for lobectomy: a report of 105 cases. *J Thorac Dis.* 2016;8(s3):251–257.

69. Campione A, Ligabue T, Luzzi L, et al. Comparison between segmentectomy and larger resection of stage IA non-small cell lung carcinoma. *J Cardiovasc Surg (Torino).* 2004;45(1):67–70.

70. Martin-Ucar AE, Nakas A, Pilling JE, West KJ, Waller DA. A case-matched study of anatomical segmentectomy versus lobectomy for stage I lung cancer in high-risk patients. *Eur J Cardiothorac Surg.* 2005;27(4):675–679.

71. El-Sharif A, Gooding WE, Santos R. Outcomes of sublobar resection versus lobectomy for stage I non-small cell lung cancer: a 13-year analysis. *Ann Thorac Surg.* 2006;82:408–415.

72. Kilic A, Schuchert MJ, Pettiford BL. Anatomic segmentectomy for stage I non-small cell lung cancer in the elderly. *Ann Thorac Surg.* 2009;87:1662–1666.

73. Koike T, Yamato Y, Yoshiya K. Intentional limited pulmonary resection for peripheral T1N0M0 small-sized lung cancer. *J Thorac Cardiovasc Surg.* 2003;125:924–928.

74. Iwasaki A, Hamanaka W, Hamada T, et al. Comparison between a case-matched analysis of left upper lobe trisegmentectomy and left upper lobectomy for small size lung cancer located in the upper division. *Thorac Cardiovasc Surg.* 2007;55(7):454–457.

75. Cao C, Gupta S, Chandrakumar D, Tian DH, Black D, Yan TD. Meta-analysis of intentional sublobar resections versus lobectomy for early stage non-small cell lung cancer. *Ann Cardiothorac Surg.* 2014;3:134–141.

76. Okada M, Koike T, Higashiyama M, Yamato Y, Kodama K, Tsubota N. Radical sublobar resection for small-sized non-small cell lung cancer: a multicenter study. *J Thorac Cardiovasc Surg.* 2006;132:769–775.

77. Altorki NK, Yip R, Hanaoka T, et al. Sublobar resection is equivalent to lobectomy for clinical stage 1A lung cancer in solid nodules. *J Thorac Cardiovasc Surg.* 2014;147:62–754; discussion 762–764.

78. Blasberg JD, Harvey IP, Donington JS. Sublobar resection: a movement from the lung cancer study group. *J Thorac Oncol.* 2010;5(10):1583–1593.

79. Guidoccio F, Orsini F, Mariani G. A critical reappraisal of sentinel lymph node biopsy for non-small cell lung cancer. *Clin and Translational Imag.* 2016;4(5):385–394.

80. Wang Y, Darling GE. Complete mediastinal lymph node dissection versus systematic lymph node sampling in surgical treatment of non-small cell lung cancer: do we have the answer? *J Thorac Dis.* 2017;9(11):4169–4170.

FURTHER READING

1. Cerfolio RJ, Maniscalco L, Bryant AS. The treatment of patients with stage IIIA non-small cell lung cancer from N2 disease: who returns to the surgical arena and who survives. *Ann Thorac Surg.* 2008;86(3):912–920.

2. Darling GE, Li F, Patsios D, et al. Neoadjuvant chemoradiation and surgery improves survival outcomes compared with definitive chemoradiation in the treatment of stage IIIA N2 non-small-cell lung cancer. *Eur J Cardiothorac Surg.* 2015;48(5):684–690.

Pulmonary Adenocarcinoma—Pathology and Molecular Testing

PRODIPTO PAL, MD, PHD • MICHAEL CABANERO, MD • MING-SOUND TSAO, MD, FRCPC

INTRODUCTION

Lung cancer is the most common cause and one of the most aggressive human cancers in the world, with 1.8 million new cases (13% of total cancer diagnoses) and 1.59 million deaths estimated to occur worldwide in 2012.[1,2] Pulmonary adenocarcinoma represents approximately 50% of all lung cancers and 60% of non–small cell carcinomas (NSCCs). In the last decade, more accurate histological diagnosis of adenocarcinoma has become essential in selecting patients for testing of molecular alterations with effective targeted therapies. This importance is recognized in the 2015 World Health Organization (WHO) classification of lung tumors, with subtype-specific immunomarkers being integrated into the diagnostic criteria of non–small cell lung cancers (NSCLCs), especially for poorly differentiated tumors in small biopsy samples.[2,3]

HISTOLOGICAL CLASSIFICATION

The first attempt at morphological classification of pulmonary carcinomas was proposed by Marchesani in 1924 and was later incorporated in the WHO histological classification of lung tumors of 1967.[4] Since then, the classification of pulmonary tumors has undergone multiple iterations with significant updates, especially for adenocarcinoma. The major subtypes in the 2015 WHO classification include adenocarcinoma, squamous cell carcinoma, neuroendocrine tumors which include small cell carcinoma and large cell neuroendocrine carcinoma, and large cell carcinoma (Table 2.1). The relatively rarer subtypes include salivary gland type carcinoma (e.g., mucoepidermoid, adenoid cystic) and sarcomatoid carcinoma, which encompass carcinosarcoma, pleomorphic/spindle cell, giant cell carcinomas,

as well as pulmonary blastoma. This chapter will focus on pulmonary adenocarcinoma.

Adenocarcinomas are predominantly located in the lung periphery.[5] However, recent publications suggest that central lung tumors often are histologically adenocarcinomas; specifically 33% of solid predominant, 25% of micropapillary predominant, and 20% of acinar predominant adenocarcinomas can be central tumors.[6,7] On gross examination, most adenocarcinomas appear as irregular-shaped tan-gray to gray-white nodules and are often associated with scarring, anthracotic pigment deposition, and pleural puckering if close to the pleura.[8] The so-called noninvasive tumors with lepidic growth of tumor cells on preexisting alveolar architecture are often difficult to identify on fresh specimens.

Major changes to the classification of lung adenocarcinoma were proposed in 2011 by the International Association for the Study of Lung Cancer (IASLC), American Thoracic Society (ATS), and European Respiratory Society (ERS).[9] For the first time, this proposal recognized lung adenocarcinoma with pure lepidic growth pattern as adenocarcinoma in situ (AIS), and a predominantly AIS tumor with <0.5 cm area of invasion as minimally invasive adenocarcinoma (MIA). AIS and MIA are uncommon, encompassing only 5% of resected adenocarcinomas.

Pulmonary adenocarcinoma is further subclassified according to cell type into nonmucinous and mucinous adenocarcinoma subtypes. A more detailed histological subtyping is rendered in resection specimen. The most common invasive adenocarcinoma is classified based on five histological growth patterns: lepidic, acinar, papillary, micropapillary, or solid (Fig. 2.1). As most adenocarcinomas demonstrate complex and heterogeneous growth patterns, it has been proposed that the

Pulmonary Adenocarcinoma: Approaches to Treatment. https://doi.org/10.1016/B978-0-323-55433-6.00002-X

TABLE 2.1
Major Classification of Pulmonary Non–small Cell Carcinoma[a]

Major Histological Type	Subtype	Diagnostic Histological Features
Squamous cell carcinoma	In situ carcinoma	Full thickness dysplastic change and mitotic figures in bronchial/bronchiolar epithelium
	Keratinizing	Squamous "keratin pearls," intercellular bridges IHC: p40/p63+ (diffuse)
	Nonkeratinizing	No morphological evidence of squamous differentiation IHC: p40/p63+
	Basaloid	Monotonous hyperchromatic tumor cells with palisading; "comedo-type" necrosis common IHC: p40/p63+
Adenocarcinoma		
Nonmucinous adenocarcinoma	Lepidic	Tumor cell growth along preexisting alveolar septa Pure lepidic growth is considered in situ adenocarcinoma
	Acinar	Gland formation with central lumina and lined by tumor cells
	Papillary	Glandular cells with fibrovascular core
	Micropapillary	Tufts of cells lacking fibrovascular cores and often detached
	Solid	Sheets of polygonal cells lacking overt glandular pattern Tumor cells stain positive for TTF-1 by immunohistochemistry or demonstrate presence of intratumoral mucin
Invasive mucinous adenocarcinoma		Columnar or goblet cells with abundant intracytoplasmic mucin Can be TTF-1 negative (85%)
Other variants	Colloid	Alveolar space filled with mucin pools that destroy alveolar wall structures
	Fetal	Complex glands with nonciliated glycogen-rich tumor resembling fetal lung
	Enteric	Resemble colorectal adenocarcinoma with complex glands formed by tall columnar cells, resembling intestinal cells
Adenosquamous carcinoma[a]		Both adenocarcinoma and squamous cell carcinoma components are present At least 10% of any component required
Large cell carcinoma[a]		Undifferentiated non–small cell carcinoma Diagnosis of exclusion and should be reserved for resection specimens
Sarcomatoid carcinoma[a]	Pleomorphic	Poorly differentiated NSCC with at least 10% spindle or giant cells
	Spindle cell	Purely composed of spindle cells
	Giant cell	Purely composed of giant cells
	Carcinosarcoma	Biphasic tumor with non–small cell carcinoma component (adenocarcinoma or squamous cell carcinoma) and sarcomatous heterologous elements
	Pulmonary blastoma	Biphasic tumor with primitive mesenchymal stroma and fetal adenocarcinoma

[a] Adapted from the 2015 WHO Classification.[1]

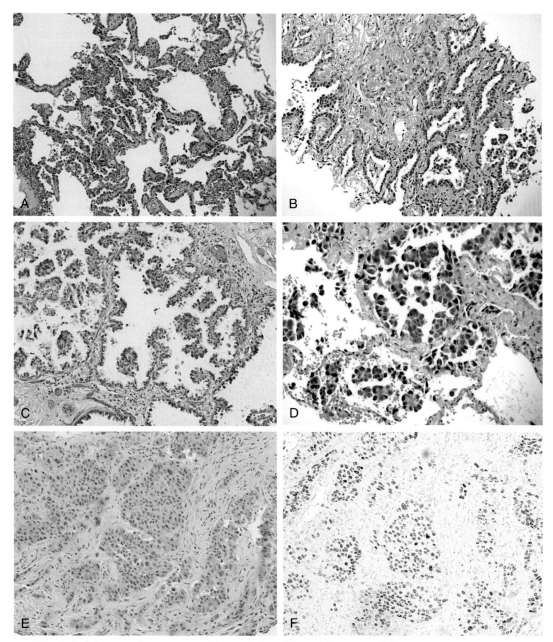

FIG. 2.1 Subtypes of pulmonary adenocarcinoma. **(A)** Lepidic pattern; **(B)** Acinar pattern in a biopsy specimen and focal micropapillary features (bottom right); **(C)** Papillary pattern; **(D)** Micropapillary pattern; **(E)** Solid pattern and corresponding TTF-1 IHC **(F)**. Note: **(A–E)**: Hematoxylin and eosin stains.

breakdown of histological subtypes should be estimated in 5% increments, and the tumor is classified according to its most common or predominant pattern. This subtype classification requires the examination of the entire tumor, thus is mainly applicable to resection specimens. For most diagnostic specimens, which are small biopsy or cytology specimens, subtype classification is not necessary, but there are recommended guidelines to use standardized nomenclature for diagnosis.[1] The accepted terminologies include NSCC, favor adenocarcinoma, squamous cell carcinoma, or not otherwise specified, depending on morphological characteristics or immunohistochemical (IHC) marker expression. The commonly used IHC markers for adenocarcinoma are pneumocyte markers such as thyroid transcription factor 1 (TTF-1), napsin A, and CK7; for squamous cell carcinoma, they include p40 (or p63) and/or CK5/6. With a combination of 2−3 markers (TTF-1, p40/p63, and CK5/6), more than 90% of poorly differentiated NSCLC biopsy specimens can be classified as favoring one of the subtypes. In addition to the above subtypes, several less common variants include invasive mucinous adenocarcinoma (IMA), colloid adenocarcinoma, enteric adenocarcinoma, and fetal adenocarcinoma.

CLINICAL RELEVANCE OF ADENOCARCINOMA SUBTYPE CLASSIFICATION

Lepidic Predominant Adenocarcinoma (Good Prognosis)

In the most recent 2015 WHO tumor classification, the term "lepidic" refers to noninvasive tumor. Tumors such as AIS and MIA are both lepidic tumors and differ primarily on the presence or absence of focal invasion. Invasive tumor is defined as any histology other than lepidic pattern (e.g., acinar, papillary, micropapillary, and solid) and the presence of myofibroblastic stromal reaction in association with tumor cell invasion, vascular, or pleural invasion, and spread through air spaces (STAS). Lepidic growth can also be seen in IMAs, but the latter invariably also include the presence of other growth patterns. However, "lepidic" predominant adenocarcinoma (LPA) essentially refers to nonmucinous adenocarcinoma with predominantly lepidic but also demonstrate invasive patterns.

The distinction between AIS and MIA is primarily on the absence or presence of invasive focus; MIA by definition cannot have an invasive focus more than 0.5 cm and features such as lymphovascular or pleural invasion, STAS, or tumor necrosis.[1] AIS and MIA have close to 100% 5-year disease-free survival (DFS).[10,11] LPA accounts for tumors with >0.5 cm invasive foci. A large number of publications have demonstrated that lepidic predominant adenocarcinoma carries a good prognosis for the patients.

Acinar/Papillary Predominant Adenocarcinoma (Intermediate Prognosis)

Acinar pattern morphologically refers to round- to oval-shaped glands with central lumina. Cribriform architecture, where tumor glands are often fused together, is currently classified under acinar histological pattern. It is important to mention cribriform architecture as it has been reportedly associated with poor prognosis[12] and often associated with the gene-rearranged tumors such as ALK, ROS1.[13] Papillary pattern shows growth of neoplastic cells along a central fibrovascular core. Papillary pattern corresponds to invasive tumor component, even in the absence of myofibroblastic stroma. Across multiple studies, acinar and papillary predominant tumors have been regarded as intermediate risk with a 5-year DFS of ∼80%−85%.[14,15]

Micropapillary and Solid Predominant Adenocarcinoma (Poor Prognosis)

Both micropapillary and solid tumors are considered high-grade adenocarcinoma with poor prognoses. This prognostic association has been reported across multiple series. Micropapillary tumor commonly appears detached; grows in papillary tufts devoid of fibrovascular cores; and has a high rate of lymphovascular invasion, STAS, and recurrence.[14-17] In contrast, solid pattern tumor is composed of sheets of polygonal cells and lack morphologic evidence of glandular architecture. The solid pattern adenocarcinoma shows similar aggressive behavior as micropapillary tumors.[14−16,18]

Invasive Mucinous Adenocarcinoma

The tumor cells have columnar or goblet cell morphology with basally oriented nuclei and abundant intracytoplasmic mucin. IMA has a strong tendency for multicentric bilateral tumor at presentation.[1,2] All the above architectural excluding solid pattern can be seen in IMA. Often times, metastatic mucinous tumors from pancreas, lower gastrointestinal tract, or ovary appear morphologically identical and can be difficult to distinguish. Pulmonary IMA frequently show mutations in *KRAS* (up to 90%)[19−22] and NRG1 fusions.[23,24]

PATHOLOGICAL STAGING OF LUNG ADENOCARCINOMA—UICC/AJCC EIGHTH EDITION

The new (eighth) edition of the lung cancer staging classification system developed by the International Association for the Study of Lung Cancer (IASLC) Staging and Prognostic Factor Committee has been approved by both Union for International Cancer Control (UICC) and American Joint Committee on Cancer (AJCC).[25−29] While UICC activates this new system in 2017, the implementation by AJCC is delayed until January 1, 2018.

The main changes in the AJCC eighth edition corresponds to T-descriptor or tumor size and extent and changes in M-descriptor; there is no formal change in the N-staging. As noted earlier, the in situ carcinoma (AIS or squamous in situ carcinoma [SCIS]) and MIA have been formally introduced as Tis in the AJCC eighth edition of TNM classification. The T-descriptor changes correspond to (1) tumor size, (2) staging of multiple/synchronous lung tumors, and (3) updating tumor spread/extent. The early-stage tumors (previously pT1a and pT1b in AJCC seventh edition) have been expanded to three subcategories in the AJCC eighth edition, i.e., pT1a ($\leq$1 cm), pT1b (>1−2 cm), and pT1c (>2−3 cm). The size criteria for prior pT2 and pT3 tumors from AJCC seventh edition now have been updated. A lung tumor of >3−5 cm now corresponds to pT2 tumor (pT2a: >3−4 cm, pT2b: >4−5 cm), while pT3 tumors are >5−7 cm. Any tumor >7 cm is now classified as pT4.

In the new eighth edition of the UICC/AJCC tumor staging classification, the pathological T stage is also based on the size of the "invasive," nonlepidic histological component of the adenocarcinoma.[30] This has significant implication, as semiquantitative estimation of the "noninvasive" lepidic component and morphologic distinction of other invasive patterns are of utmost importance.

The concept of intrapulmonary metastasis has not been changed: ipsilateral same-lobe tumor nodule (pT3), ipsilateral different-lobe tumor nodule (pT4), and contralateral tumor nodule (M1a). While the staging of multifocal lung cancers has been ambiguous in the AJCC seventh edition, this has been addressed in a series of new publications.[31−33] The critical point is to distinguish synchronous separate primary lung tumors and metastatic tumors. Various criteria have been published to distinguish synchronous versus metastatic tumor. Briefly, if the tumor differs according to cell type (e.g., adenocarcinoma vs. squamous cell carcinoma) or by comprehensive histological patterns, a synchronous but separate primary tumors are favored. While separate primaries should be individually staged, the staging of multiple lung cancers with multiple ground-glass opacities on imaging studies shows low-grade morphology in the lepidic predominant spectrum on pathology (AIS or MIA) is now staged with the tumor with highest stage with the letter "m" in parenthesis.[32−34] Pneumonic type adenocarcinoma, most commonly seen in IMA, is staged based on the size of the tumor and location (pT3 in single lobe, pT4 involving different ipsilateral lobe or M1a involving contralateral lobes). In the eighth edition, tumors involving main bronchus regardless of distance from carina are now staged as pT2 tumors, while

tumors with diaphragm and recurrent laryngeal nerve involvement have been updated to pT4 tumors.

In the M-category, the definition of M1a (separate tumor nodule(s) in a contralateral lobe; tumor with pleural or pericardial nodule(s), or malignant pleural or pericardial effusion) is not changed. However, the M1b category has been expanded to distinguish between extrathoracic oligometastatic (M1b) and tumors with multiple metastatic disease (M1c).

MOLECULAR CLASSIFICATION

The recent coordinated effort by The Cancer Genome Atlas (TCGA) to classify recurrent molecular alterations in multiple cancers has revealed 18 statistically significant altered genes in lung adenocarcinoma.[35] These include TP53 (46%), KRAS (33%), EGFR (14%), BRAF (10%), PIK3CA (7%), MET (7%), RIT1 (2%), STK11 (17%), KEAP1 (17%), NF1 (11%), RB1 (4%), CDKN2A (4%), SETD2 (9%), ARID1A (7%), MARCA4 (6%), RBM10 (8%), U2AF1 (3%), and MGA (8%). Recurrently altered/activated cellular pathways were also identified and include activation of RTK/RAS/RAF pathway, the PI(3)K-mTOR pathway, p53 pathway, cell-cycle regulator pathway, oxidative stress pathways, and mutations in chromatin and RNA splicing factors. Molecular classification from the perspective of targetable oncogene drivers and the various methods for detection will be reviewed later.

TRANSCRIPTOMIC CLASSIFICATIONS

Although gene expression profiles have been used to subclassify a tumor's molecular phenotype and behavior into clinically relevant groups,[36] routine profiling of a tumor's transcriptome has not reached standard clinical practice. Nevertheless, we include a brief discussion on gene expression subclassification to help shed insight into the biology of these tumors.

Over the years, multiple studies have observed three reproducible distinct subtypes of lung adenocarcinoma based on the tumor's transcriptome.[35−40] They were designated with various names, such as bronchioid, squamoid, and magnoid, as they appeared to have similar expression profiles as bronchioalveolar carcinoma (now-termed lepidic adenocarcinoma), squamous cell carcinoma, and large cell carcinoma, respectively.[38] However, these subtype nomenclatures were revised in the TCGA manuscript to synergize the different transcriptional subtypes with tumor histology, anatomic locations, and mutational profile.[35]

Terminal Respiratory Unit Subtype

The terminal respiratory unit (TRU), formerly known as bronchioid, is composed of lung adenocarcinomas that have cell lineage properties linking them to respiratory epithelium of the TRU.[41] Tumors in the TRU transcriptional subunit account for approximately 30% of lung adenocarcinomas[38] and have the highest proportion of tumors that express TTF-1. TRU tumors also maintain morphologic similarity to the benign cells of the TRU. Under the current WHO classification,[3] most nonmucinous adenocarcinomas with lepidic and acinar patterns, as well as some papillary adenocarcinomas, belong to this group. Compared with the other two groups, tumors of the TRU transcriptional subtype have the best clinical outcomes in early-stage disease,[35,38,39] which may be explained by its overall lower rate of distant metastases in early stage. The majority of *EGFR*-mutant tumors, and those harboring kinase-fusion alterations, belong to the TRU,[38] with increased prevalence of younger patients, female gender, and nonsmokers.[41]

Proximal Inflammatory Subtype

The proximal inflammatory (PI) unit, formerly known as squamoid, is enriched for high-grade tumors with solid histomorphology and accounts for approximately 50% of lung adenocarcinomas.[38] Patients tended to be male smokers with tumors that metastasized early and had a higher proportion of central nervous system involvement. In comparison to the TRU subtype, patients with PI subtype tumors had poorer prognosis in early-stage disease but fared better in late-stage disease. Histologically, PI tumors tended to be moderately to poorly differentiated, had a high degree of *TP53* and *NF1* tumor suppressor mutations, and a large degree of *p16* inactivation.[40] Pathways activated in these tumors include WNT signaling, TGF-β signaling, and angiogenesis (HIF1a).

Proximal Proliferative Subtype

The proximal proliferative (PP) unit, formerly known as magnoid, accounts for approximately 20% of lung adenocarcinomas. This subtype was originally termed magnoid as genes expressed in this subtype were most similar to those found in large cell carcinomas.[38,40] These tumors are particularly enriched for *KRAS* mutations. They also included a high degree of *STK11* (aka *LKB1*) inactivation, via chromosomal loss, inactivating mutations, or reduced gene expression.[35] STK11 is a tumor suppressor that regulates growth and metabolism when nutrients are scarce by acting upstream to adenosine monophosphate kinase (AMPK).[42] Germline mutations in the *STK11* gene are associated with

Peutz-Jeghers syndrome,[43,44] and studies have found sporadic *STK11* mutations in lung adenocarcinomas.[45-47] Similar to patients with PI tumors, patients with PP tumors had worse survival than those with TRU tumors.[35,38,39]

ONCOGENIC DRIVER MUTATIONS AND MOLECULAR TESTING IN LUNG ADENOCARCINOMA
Molecular Testing Methods

The various assays used to detect recurrent molecular alterations in NSCLC, including *epidermal growth factor receptor* (*EGFR*) mutations and structural alterations involving the anaplastic lymphoma kinase (*ALK*) and *ROS1* genes, have evolved over the past decade. Starting with single-gene sequencing (i.e., Sanger sequencing) or fluorescence in situ hybridization (FISH), many newer tests use massive parallel sequencing technology, or NGS to target multiple verified and potentially "druggable" genes implicated in oncogenesis. Broadly, these techniques can be categorized into either nontargeted (detect new or known mutations) or targeted (detect only known mutations) assays, and whether single gene/locus (uniplexed) or multiple genes/loci (multiplexed) are interrogated (Table 2.2).

EPIDERMAL GROWTH FACTOR RECEPTOR

The *EGFR* (also known as *HER1* or *ERBB1*) gene, located on chromosome 7, is a transmembrane protein and a member of the epidermal growth factor (EGF) family. The EGF family includes four members (HER1 through HER4) and functions to bind extracellular protein ligands to activate an array of cellular pathways that include differentiation, proliferation, and survival of the cell.[48] Ligand-receptor interaction leads to dimerization of the EGFR with either itself (homodimerization) or with another member of the EGFR family proteins, i.e., HER2, HER3, and HER4 (heterodimerization). Downstream pathways activated include the RAS-RAF-MAPK and the PI3K-AKT-mTOR signaling cascade. Activation of EGFR ultimately leads to transcription of genes that promote cell-cycle progression, proliferation, and survival.

Mutations in the *EGFR* account for approximately 15% in Western countries and up to 50% in Asian countries of lung adenocarcinoma cases, with a higher proportion found in younger age, East Asian, women, and light/never smokers.[49,50] Almost all sensitizing mutations (activating mutations upon which TKI therapy has shown efficacy) occur between exons 18–21. The

TABLE 2.2
Current Actionable Target Genes in Lung Adenocarcinoma and Methods for Detection

Target Gene	Assay	Examples
EGFR	Nontargeted assays—Sanger sequencing, pyrosequencing	
	Targeted assays—allele-specific real-time PCR, PCR amplification with allele-specific base extension	Cobas (Roche, Tucson, AZ), Therascreen (Qiagen, Hilden, Germany), MassARRAY (Agena Bioscience, San Diego, CA)
ALK/ ROS1	Structural alterations—FISH	
Multiple genes	Multiplex RT-PCR	SNaPshot Kit (Applied Biosystems, Foster City, CA)
	Next-generation sequencing panels	Oncomine (Thermofisher, Waltham, MA), FoundationOne (Foundation Medicine, MA), TruSeq Amplicon (Illumina, San Diego, CA)
	Whole exome/ genome sequencing	

most common mutations include a short in-frame deletion at exon 19, which primarily affects amino acid residues 747–750, as well as the missense mutation L858R in exon 21. These two mutations account for approximately 85%–90% of all *EGFR* lung adenocarcinoma mutations, but many other mutations outside these hotspots have shown TKI response.

Despite improved clinical response compared to chemotherapy, acquired resistance to TKI therapy commonly occurs in patients with *EGFR*-sensitizing mutations. These can be broadly classified into four categories: (1) secondary resistance *EGFR* mutations, (2) activation of bypass pathways, (3) activation of downstream pathways, and (4) histologic transformation.

Secondary Resistance Mutations
The most common resistance mechanism is the T790M mutation in exon 20 (kinase domain), and it accounts for approximately 60% of all acquired resistance to EGFR-TKI therapy. Arising in cis with the sensitizing *EGFR* mutation, this "gatekeeper" mutation restores the binding pocket's affinity for adenosine triphosphate (ATP).[51] This effectively renders the competitive inhibition of first- and second-generation TKIs ineffective to ATP.[52,53] Other rare kinase domain secondary *EGFR* mutations have been associated with TKI resistance, including L747S, D761Y, and T854A.[54,55] In 10% of patients with T790M mutations, there is a concomitant amplification of *EGFR* and is thought to outcompete second-generation TKI inhibition by providing stronger kinase domain activation.[56]

Activation of Bypass Pathways
MET amplification accounts for 5% of resistance mechanisms; this amplification allows for excess MET receptors to heterodimerize with HER3 to activate PI(3)K-Akt-mTor signaling despite TKI inhibition.[57] Increased expression of hepatocyte growth factor, the ligand for MET, can also occur.[58] Finally, *HER2* (ErbB2) is found in approximately 8%–13% of those with *EGFR*-sensitizing mutations and leads to parallel signaling of downstream pathways that bypass the effects of EGFR-TKIs.[59]

Activation of Downstream Pathways
BRAF mutations (1%) and *MAPK1* amplifications (<1%) drives continued signaling of the RAS/RAF/MAPK pathway.[60] Similarly, *PTEN* decrease or loss and *PIK3CA* mutations (5%) activate the PI3K-AKT-mTOR pathway even in the presence of EGFR-TKI.[61]

Histologic Transformation
Accounting for 5%–14% of acquired resistance mechanisms, small cell lung carcinoma (SCLC) transformation has been observed since the early days of EGFR targeted therapy.[62] The mechanism for resistance seems to be correlated with decreased EGFR expression in SCLC.[63] Epithelial to mesenchymal transition (EMT) is characterized by histologic change of the epithelial tumor cells to spindle cell morphology and a molecular change of decreased expression of the epithelial marker E-cadherin and increased expression of the mesenchymal marker Vimentin.[64]

Epidermal Growth Factor Receptor Mutation Testing

Nontargeted assays

Sanger sequencing was the standard for *EGFR* testing in the first clinical trials with erlotinib and gefitinib. This method incorporates fluorescent-tagged dideoxy terminators to amplifying DNA strands, which can be sorted by size and the nucleotide sequence read sequentially. A major consideration is the relatively low analytical sensitivity of the assay, which usually requires specimens with high tumor content. As such, this assay is no longer a method of choice for detection of EGFR mutations. Another method, called pyrosequencing, involves measuring the chemiluminescent signal released by pyrophosphate as triphosphate nucleotides are being incorporated into the synthesized DNA strand. Although the fragment length required for pyrosequencing is much shorter than those used for Sanger sequencing, this method offers higher sensitivity and can detect mutations in samples with up to 5% tumor cellularity.

Targeted assays

Targeted assays, often used to detect specific EGFR mutations, offer better sensitivity than nontargeted sequencing assays. Most current platforms require only approximately 5%–10% tumor cellularity and can interrogate multiple hotspot mutations in a single test. The USDA-approved companion diagnostic assay for erlotinib, the Cobas *EGFR* Mutation Test (Roche), uses allele-specific primers to identify the most common *EGFR* mutations, using both tissue and plasma samples, and can interrogate 42 clinically relevant mutations, including T790M. The Therascreen EGFR RCQ PCR kit (Qiagen) is another platform that uses allele-specific primers, in the form of Scorpion primers, or amplification-refractory mutation system (ARMS). Therascreen is able to identify 29 EGFR mutations and was the companion diagnostic in the LUX-Lung 3 trial that led to the approval of afatinib.

ANAPLASTIC LYMPHOMA KINASE

ALK, located on chromosome 2p23, encodes a receptor tyrosine kinase (RTK) and was first described in anaplastic large cell lymphoma.[65] ALK rearrangements were reported in pulmonary adenocarcinoma in 2007.[66,67] The most common fusion partner is *EML4*; however, over 20 different ALK gene partners have been described in recent times.[68–71] The breakpoints on the ALK gene most commonly happen at intron 19, or rarely at exon 20, but preservation of the kinase domain in the resulting fusion gene occurs universally. Typically, the fusion partners contribute coil-coil domains which allows spontaneous dimerization of ALK fusion proteins and subsequently results in constitutive activation of the oncogenic fusion gene products. *ALK*-rearranged pulmonary adenocarcinoma has gained widespread popularity again due to the availability of small molecule TKIs. Several tyrosine kinase inhibitors are now available for the treatment of *ALK*-rearranged lung tumors.

The estimated frequency of NSCLC harboring *ALK* rearrangement is 3%–5%.[72] *ALK*-rearranged tumors are associated with female sex, younger patients, and those with never to light-smoking history.[73–75] As with *EGFR*, *ALK* rearrangements are found in adenocarcinomas and are uncommon in squamous histology or neuroendocrine carcinomas. Pulmonary adenocarcinoma with mucinous features, acinar/cribriform architecture, signet ring cells, and psammomatous calcification are the histologies associated with *ALK*-rearranged tumors[13] (see Fig. 2.2). Thus, both *EGFR*

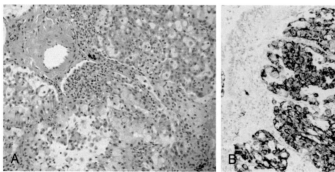

FIG. 2.2 ALK-rearranged pulmonary adenocarcinoma. **(A)** The tumor is arranged in acinar/cribriform architecture, with mucinous features; signet ring morphology is present in lower half (hematoxylin and eosin stain); **(B)** IHC for ALK (5A4 clone) shows diffuse cytoplasmic, often granular ALK expression in tumor cells. *ALK*, anaplastic lymphoma kinase; *IHC*, immunohistochemical.

and *ALK* testing mostly are reserved for patients with adenocarcinoma histology and not recommended for pure squamous cell or neuroendocrine carcinomas.[76] It should be noted, however, that *ALK* rearrangement as well as ALK protein expression by IHC rarely has been reported in squamous cell carcinoma,[77,78] although it has been suggested that this finding may be related to existing challenges in diagnosing NSCLC in small biopsies and limitation of representative tumor sampling.

Much like the case with TKI-treated patients with *EGFR*-sensitizing mutations, patients with *ALK* rearrangements treated with crizotinib almost always develop secondary acquired resistance mutations. These mutations lead to a decrease in binding affinity for crizotinib or an increased binding affinity to ATP.[79] Other resistance mechanisms have also been described and include development of secondary *EGFR* or *KRAS* mutations, and *ALK* and *KIT* gene amplifications.[80–82]

ROS1

ROS1 is an RTK of the insulin receptor family, located on chromosome 6q22 and encodes a transmembrane protein with intracellular C-terminal tyrosine kinase domain and shares marked sequence homology and structural similarities to ALK oncogene.[83] *ROS1* fusion was first described in glioblastoma multiforme,[84,85] later reported in NSCLC by Rikova et al.[67] The first population screening of *ROS1* in NSCLC was reported by Bergethon et al.[86] Subsequently, over 20 *ROS1* fusions have been described in NSCLC as well as in other solid tumors. The precise mechanism of oncogenic activity and constitutive expression of ROS1 fusion products are as yet unclear.

The prevalence of *ROS1* fusion in NSCLC is estimated to be ~1%–2%.[72,86,87] *CD74-ROS1* fusion is the most common fusion variant,[87] followed by other

fusion variants such as *SLC34A2-ROS1*, *TPM3-ROS1*, *SDC4-ROS1*, *EZR-ROS1*, and others. Similar to *ALK*, *ROS1* fusion tumors are enriched in females, never smokers,[88] and with adenocarcinoma histology.[86,89,90] Cribriform/acinar architecture, mucinous features, solid pattern histology, hepatoid morphology, signet ring cell morphology, and tumors with psammomatous calcification are the most common histologic patterns reported in *ROS1* fusion pulmonary adenocarcinoma.[91,92] *ROS1* fusions has not been described in squamous cell carcinoma or lung neuroendocrine carcinoma.

The interest in *ROS1* fusions stems from the availability of targetable small molecular TKI, crizotinib.[93] The published clinical trials corroborate significant clinical activity of crizotinib in *ROS1* fusion tumors.[89,90] Following the clinical trials, multiple acquired resistance mutations have also been reported.[94,95] Fortunately, the second-generation TKIs were developed within short time that were able to target most of the resistance mutations.[96–98]

ALK AND ROS1 TESTING

As a general rule, proper handling and processing of tissue, adequacy of diagnostic material are quintessential steps in assessing and testing for biomarker studies.[99] Tissue fixation with 10% neutral buffered formalin and tissue fixation of 6–72 h are recommended.[72] The main methods to detect both *ALK* and *ROS1* rearrangements are (1) FISH, (2) real-time polymerase chain reaction or RT-PCR, (3) IHC, and (4) NGS.

Break Apart FISH Assay

ALK and *ROS1* rearrangement detection by FISH is achieved by using dual-colored break apart probes that label the 3′ (telomeric) and 5′ (centromeric) part.

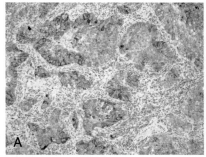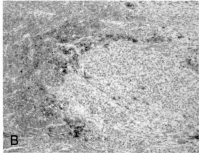

FIG. 2.3 **(A)** PD-L1 (SP263 clone) IHC is evaluated as partial or complete tumor membranous staining. **(B)** Many nonneoplastic cells may also express PD-L1, including lymphocytes (shown here), macrophages, and endothelial cells. Care must be taken to distinguish the cells from tumor cells for appropriate scoring. *PD-L1*, program death ligand 1.

The *ALK* Vysis LSI break apart FISH probe (Abbott Molecular) was approved by Food and Drug Administration (FDA) for the therapy with ALK inhibitors and is commonly used worldwide (US Food and Drug Administration). In contrast, there are several break apart FISH probes for *ROS1*, but none has been FDA approved as companion diagnostics. A minimum of 50 tumor cells are required and a cutoff of 15% is the general recommended guideline. Inaccurate signal interpretation, borderline rates of rearrangement positive cells, erroneous results due to false-positive or false-negative results, and atypical signal profile are the challenges in test interpretation errors.[100]

Reverse Transcription-Polymerase Chain Reaction

Reverse transcription-polymerase chain reaction (RT-PCR) is feasible in clinical laboratories, however, with its own set of challenges. As noted earlier, *ALK* rearrangement has many different candidate fusion partners, even for the *ALK-EML4*, the most common fusion in NSCLC, there are many fusion variants, largely due to different breakpoint regions on *EML4*, thus would require a multiplexed approach. However, with RT-PCR-based methods, a priori knowledge of the candidate fusion genes is needed to identify fusion variants which can later be confirmed by subsequent sequencing[101] and has been used in studies with high level of sensitivity albeit with varying level of specificity (85%–100%) compared with FISH.[102,103] A negative result by RT-PCR requires appropriate caution due to the potential of false-negative results due to the missing unknown fusion variants. In addition, RT-PCR assays are dependent on procuring high-quality RNA from FFPE tissue. Newer RNA-based assays are under active development (assays such as NanoString system) that can simultaneously detect various fusion partners as well as offer the added advantage of detecting other driver fusion-type alterations in a multiplexed setup (such as *ROS1*, *RET*, etc.).[104–106]

Fusion Protein Detection of ALK and ROS1 by IHC

ALK protein expression in NSCLC is generally lower in comparison with ALK expression in anaplastic large cell lymphoma.[107] Therefore, it is important to standardize ALK IHC assay and adequately address various issues pertaining to antigen retrieval, higher affinity primary antibody in higher concentration, and stronger signal amplification steps.[72] There are four commercially available antibodies to date, viz., ALK1 (Dako),

5A4 (Novocastra), D5F3 (Cell Signaling Technology), and anti-ALK (Origene). ALK1 antibody (Dako) is less sensitive and should not be used. The other clones, specifically D5F3 (as companion diagnostic assay) and 5A4 (laboratory-developed test), have been widely studied and have shown to be equally sensitive across multiple large-scale studies.[72] ALK staining is cytoplasmic and granular in character and can occasionally demonstrate membrane accentuation (Fig. 2.2). It is important to be cognizant of various artifacts such as evaluating ALK staining in mucin-producing cells (occasionally in extracellular mucin, as well as cytoplasm of alveolar macrophages and bronchial cells) and nonspecific membranous staining and staining in squamous cell carcinoma (rare instances), large cell neuroendocrine carcinomas, and normal ganglion cells. The reproducibility of ALK IHC results across different laboratories and pathologists is high for standardized/validated procedures.[108]

IHC detection approach for ROS1 and antibody clone D4D6 (Cell Signaling Technology, MA) was introduced by Rimkunas et al.[109] Multiple studies have shown adequate sensitivity of IHC for detecting *ROS1* rearrangements; however, the key problem remains with the specificity of the assay.[87,110] Although there have been several publications on ROS1 IHC, the staining protocol is yet to be standardized. Detailed discussion on ROS1 IHC can be found in the *IASLC Atlas of ALK and ROS1 Testing in Lung Cancer*.[72]

Next-Generation Sequencing

NGS offers the best single platform option to simultaneously detect driver mutations (e.g., mutations in *EGFR*, *KRAS*, etc.), fusion-type structural variants (*ALK*, *ROS1*, *RET*, *NTRK1*, etc.), gene amplification (e.g., *MET*), or deletions. A number of NGS-based approaches have been described recently including multiplexed PCR-based gene panels, hybrid capture–based gene panels, and comprehensive genome/exome sequencing.[111–115]

Specifically, in a large study of NSCLC, 4.4% (47/1070 cases) ALK fusions were detected by NGS approach; however, of these cases, FISH data were available for a subset which revealed a significant percentage of cases were reported as FISH negative (35%).[116] Multiple large-scale and independent studies now have established higher sensitivity/specificity for detection of actionable genomic alterations with NGS-based approaches.[111,114,116,117]

The limitations of NGS, especially in a clinical laboratory setting include cost, high-level complex laboratory setup with in-depth bioinformatics support, and strict adherence to many-faceted quality control matrices. Among preanalytical factors, careful sample assessment, suitable quality and quantities of input DNA/RNA, validation of minimal acceptable sequence depth coverage, and trained personnel for accurate interpretation are of utmost importance.[112] The widespread implementation of NGS technologies in day-to-day clinics remains a work in progress.

OTHERS DRIVER ONCOGENES
MET
MET, the gene encoding hepatocyte growth factor, is amplified in 5%–20% of EGFR-TKI-treated relapsed pulmonary adenocarcinoma. In vitro study hypothesized MET amplification may be present as small subclone in primary pulmonary adenocarcinoma.[118] While MET amplifications are more common in post-treatment NSCLC,[119] the other *MET* mutation is a skipping or splice mutation in exon 14. The exon 14 splice mutation has a reported frequency of ~5% and is enriched in wild-type for known driver gene mutation patients, older age group, female gender, and with never-smoking history.[120–123] Detection for *MET* alterations are dependent on sequencing or NGS-based approaches while MET amplification can be detected by FISH.[124] Multiple targetable molecules including crizotinib, cabozantinib, and others and multiple clinical trials are presently underway.[124]

KRAS
The most commonly mutated driver oncogene in pulmonary adenocarcinoma is *KRAS* (Kirsten rat sarcoma 2 viral oncogene homolog), a member of the RAS family of membrane-associated G-proteins, that exerts its effects on RTKs including *EGFR*. In contrast to EGFR, KRAS mutations are more common in smokers. In larger series, up to 30%–34% of smokers harbored *KRAS* mutation[49,125] as opposed to ~5%–7% in nonsmokers. *KRAS* mutations are more frequent in Caucasians than Asians[126] and are essentially mutually exclusive to *EGFR* mutations or *ALK* fusions.[127] Solid histology pattern, tumor infiltrating leukocytes, and pulmonary mucinous adenocarcinoma are associated with *KRAS* mutations.[20,21] The majority of *KRAS* mutations occurs in codons 12 and 13.[49] The G12A and G12C mutations are more common in nonmucinous adenocarcinoma while G12V, G12D, G13D mutations are seen in mucinous as well as nonmucinous adenocarcinoma histology.[128]

BRAF
BRAF (B-raf proto oncogene, serine/threonine kinase) is a signal transduction protein kinase, lying downstream to *KRAS* signaling pathway and is mutated across multiple tumor type including melanoma, lymphoma/leukemias, and carcinomas. The most widely studied activating *BRAF* mutation, viz., Val600Gly (V600E) is common in melanoma (up to 50%) and colon carcinoma (10%–15%) and is a biomarker of its targetable inhibitor, vemurafenib.[129] *BRAF* mutations are uncommon in NSCLC and has a reported prevalence of up to 4%. The commonly seen mutations in NSCLC are V600E, and other mutations in exon 11 and 15. The *BRAF*-mutated lung tumors, specifically V600E mutation, correlated with micropapillary histology and worse overall survival.[130]

RET
RET rearrangements are rare events in pulmonary adenocarcinoma and has an estimated prevalence of ~1%–2%.[70,131–133] Similar to other RTK fusion tumors such as *ALK* and *ROS1*, *RET*-rearranged tumors are more common in young patients and never smokers to light smokers, and occasionally show poorly differentiated adenocarcinoma morphology.[134] A number of fusion variants have now been described, with *KIF5B-RET* being the most common variant.[135] *RET* fusions are typically detected by FISH or by NGS-based methods. Data regarding IHC-based detection are limited; however, the available antibody clones lack adequate sensitivity for reliable detection in clinical laboratories. Recent clinical trial with RET inhibitor cabozantinib has shown preliminary efficacy,[136,137] multiple clinical trials are presently underway.[138]

NTRK1
NTRK1 (neurotrophic RTK 1) fusions are reported in ~1%–2% of NSCLC. The first reported *NTRK1* fusions in a cohort of pulmonary adenocarcinoma were pan-negative for all known driver mutations; the identified cases were female patients.[139] However, larger and independent studies are needed to assess clinicopathologic characteristics. The availability of targetable drugs (such as crizotinib, entrectenib) and early clinical response data with entrectinib are promising.[97]

HER2
HER2 or *ERBB2* (human *EGFR* 2), located on chromosome 17 is a member of ERBB family encoded by erb-b2 RTK and plays key roles in oncogenesis and progression of several malignancies. HER2 overexpression

is reported in breast, stomach, lung, bladder, ovarian and pancreatic carcinoma. It is a biomarker and therapeutic target in breast and gastric carcinoma and predicts response to targetable molecules trastuzumab and lapatinib. Majority of the reported *HER2* mutations (1%–3% frequency) in NSCLC are small in-frame insertion (exon 20) in its kinase domain, while the transmembrane domain mutation is uncommon (0.18%).[140,141] The clinical efficacy of HER2-targeted therapy in NSCLC is still evolving.[142,143] A recent study showed promising results with Afatinib, a pan-HER2 inhibitor in HER2 transmembrane domain mutation subgroup.[140]

LIQUID BIOPSIES

Management of lung adenocarcinomas stands as a hallmark example of precision oncology. It is now routine to test for *EGFR*-sensitizing mutations and *ALK* rearrangements, with an ever-growing number of actionable targets in the pipeline. Consideration of the tissue material for molecular testing is now more crucial than ever. Initial diagnostic biopsy material can sometimes be very limited, and many patients with advanced disease will not be eligible for surgical treatment and miss the opportunity of acquiring more tissue. An alternative to tissue biopsy is the utilization of circulating tumor cells (CTCs) or circulating tumor DNA (ctDNA) to obtain a "liquid biopsy."

Circulating Tumor Cells

Malignant single cells or aggregates may be found in blood once the tumor has invaded vasculature and entered the circulatory system. These occur at a rate of about 1 in 100 million cells.[144] Elevated levels of these CTCs have shown significant survival differences in multiple cancers,[145,146] including small cell lung cancer[147] and NSCLC.[148,149] The United States Food and Drug Administration has approved one CTC selection platform, the CellSearch System (Janssen Diagnostics, Raritan, New Jersey). However, overall there remains a significant barrier in the clinical implementation of CTC in lung cancer due to the generally low number of detectable tumor cells.

Circulating Tumor DNA

Every living cell secretes small amounts of DNA into the circulation, and its concentration increases in certain conditions such as trauma, inflammation, apoptosis, or necrosis.[150] Patients with malignant disease have been found to have a significant increase in circulating DNA compared with healthy individuals.[151] The fragment lengths of ctDNA are also shorter compared with normal circulating DNA.[152] These, among other observations, have led to the exploitation of using blood samples to detect tumor-specific DNA or ctDNA.

CtDNA is markedly dilute compared with normal circulating DNA and requires highly sensitive methods of detection. These detection methods can be broadly categorized into two ways: targeting specific molecular alterations and targeting all/multiple possible molecular alterations.

Targeting Specific Molecular Alterations

PCR-based detection methods are primarily used to detect specific molecular alterations, such as specific *EGFR*-sensitizing mutations or the T790M resistance mechanism. They obtain specificity by using a sequence-specific primer, such as ARMS,[153,154] or preferentially amplifying mismatched sequences to enrich nontarget sequences of a mixed template, such as PNA-clamping.[155] A new method called digital PCR, greatly improves specificity and sensitivity compared with nondigital methods. This technology involves separating the template mix into tiny individual reaction vessels, most commonly by forming droplets. These individual reaction droplets can then be assessed individually for the presence of the mutation and essentially converts the analog nature of PCR into a linear digital signal that gives way for absolute quantification of variant alleles.[156]

Targeting Multiple Molecular Alterations

Increasing affordability of massive parallel sequencing, or NGS, has led to the implementation of cancer-specific target gene panels in ctDNA. These panels cover a multitude of genes recurrently mutated in cancer. Although still largely used in FFPE tumor tissue, methods that greatly increase its detection sensitivity are beginning to allow its use in liquid biopsies.[157]

Clinical Applications

Liquid biopsies may play important roles in patients with lung cancer. These can be especially helpful in patients with genomically defined tumors, such as those harboring *EGFR*-sensitizing mutations. CTCs and ctDNA containing the specific *EGFR* mutation can persist in the bloodstream after therapy and during relapse. Currently, liquid biopsies serve three purposes in its clinical applicability. They can be used to (1) assess tumor burden, (2) characterize resistance mechanisms, and (3) monitor response to therapy.

Assessing Tumor Burden

Analogous to measuring HIV viral load, quantification of circulating DNA can serve as a surrogate for tumor burden in cancer patients, especially in metastatic disease.[158–160] Its application in early-stage lung adenocarcinoma, however, may not be as noteworthy as in other histologic subtypes. The recent TRACERx study showed that ctDNA in early-stage lung adenocarcinoma was not easily detected compared to non-adenocarcinoma histology.[161] They also showed a correlation between tumor volume and ctDNA variant allele frequencies (VAF), where a primary tumor volume of 10 cm^3 predicted a ctDNA plasma VAF of 0.1%.

Characterizing Resistance Mechanisms

Patients who progress while on TKI therapy may need another biopsy to characterize the tumor's resistance mechanism. If the tumor is inaccessible, conventional methods may possibly carry a significant morbidity risk to the patient. Moreover, limited tissue sampling will not always sample all the subclones present to cover the full spectrum of the tumor's heterogeneity. Plasma detection of resistance mutations, especially T790M, via the significantly less invasive liquid biopsy is a sensible alternative in this regard.[162,163]

Monitoring Response to Therapy

Several groups have demonstrated a role for detecting ctDNA EGFR mutations during treatment with an EGFR-TKI.[162,164] Because of the quantitative nature of the different detection methods, in particular digital PCR, the liquid biopsy is finding utility as a way to monitoring response to therapy.

Although still not ready for routine clinical application, extensive research for more sensitive and specific methods may see liquid biopsy as an essential diagnostic armamentarium in the clinical management of lung cancer patients.

PROGRAM DEATH LIGAND 1

Tumor-associated antigens induce a host immune response which, at least in the early stages of disease, provides a mechanism for control and even destruction of malignant cells. This important process of immunosurveillance is underscored when the immune system is compromised, such as in HIV patients, or when cancer cells evolve acquire various tolerance mechanisms, allowing immune escape. These mechanisms include inhibition of regulatory T-cells, defective antigen presentation, immune suppressive mediators, or dysregulation of costimulatory and coinhibitory molecules.

Much focus on immune checkpoint inhibition, or "releasing the brakes," has been garnered ever since numerous clinical trials have shown remarkably increased efficacy of antiimmune checkpoint inhibitor molecules (e.g., anti-CTLA4, anti-PDL1) in treating various cancers, including lung cancer.[165,166]

Program death ligand 1 (PD-L1), a member of the B7 family, is a major immune checkpoint protein that mediates antitumor immune suppression and response. In lung tissue, it is expressed on a variety of cells, including macrophages, T-cells, epithelial cells, and endothelial cells.[167] Its ligand, programmed death receptor (PD1), is expressed on T-cells and is upregulated after activation by a foreign antigen. The interaction of PD-L1-PD1 serves as an important mediator of the antiinflammatory processes to downregulate inflammatory signals and prevent collateral tissue damage. Some tumors are able to "highjack" this mechanism by expressing PD-L1, escaping destruction of activated T-cells. Fortunately, this also serves as a means for intervention by providing a target for therapy. Many clinical trials have established immune checkpoint inhibition, in particular via the PD1/PD-L1 axis, as a new therapeutic paradigm in the management of cancer, including lung cancer. PD1/PD-L1 axis agents include PD1 inhibitors such as nivolumab and pembrolizumab, and PD-L1 inhibitors such as atezolizumab, durvalumab, and avelumab. Discussion for each clinical trial is beyond the scope of this chapter and details should be sought in the other chapters.

Program Death Ligand 1 Testing

Benefit of anti-PD-L1 immunotherapy is found in only a subset of patients with lung adenocarcinoma. Therefore, testing for tumors for PD-L1 expression via immunohistochemistry serves as an eligibility biomarker used to select patients who might benefit from anti-PD-L1 immunotherapy. It is now a standard clinical practice for lung adenocarcinomas. Different PD-L1 diagnostic antibody clones have been developed that correspond with the different PD1/PD-L1 inhibitors (Table 2.3).

Histologic evaluation of tumor PD-L1 expression requires a few important issues that one needs to be aware of. In lung tissue, PD-L1 expression may be present on dendritic cells, macrophages, mast cells, T-cells, B-cells, and endothelial cells.[168] Examination of the hematoxylin and eosin (H & E)—stained slides should be performed to assess tissue preservation and staining quality. External positive (human tonsils or cell lines) and negative control slides should also be examined. The minimum number for tumor cells needed for adequacy is set by the manufacturer; 50 cells is needed for

TABLE 2.3

Immune Checkpoint Inhibitors, Associated PD-L1 Immunohistochemistry Assays, and Characteristics

Checkpoint Inhibitor	PD-L1 Antibody Clones (Host)	Epitope	Autostainer	Detection System
Nivolumab	28-8 (Rabbit monoclonal)	Extracellular	Dako Link 48	Envision flex
Pembrolizumab	22C3 (Mouse monoclonal)	Extracellular		
Atezolizumab	SP142 (Rabbit monoclonal)	Cytoplasmic	Ventana Benchmark	Optiview + amplification
Durvalumab	SP263 (Rabbit monoclonal)	Cytoplasmic		Optiview
Avulumab	73-10 (Rabbit monoclonal)	Cytoplasmic	Dako	Envision flex

the SP142 assay (Ventana) and 100 cells is needed for the 28-8 and 22C3 pharmDx assays (Agilent Technologies/Dako). Care needs to be taken not to mistake intra-alveolar macrophages for denuded tumor cells. High-magnification examination is necessary to so as not to overlook weak staining (see Figure 2.3).

The availability of various PD-L1/PD1 axis drugs, each accompanied with a corresponding diagnostic antibody clone, not to mention the various cutoffs established for consideration of PD-L1 positivity, has made the field quite complex. Definition of positivity varies depending on the assay used. When assessing for PD-L1 positivity in 28-8, 22C3, SP263, or 73-10 assays, only partial or complete membranous staining of tumor cells should be counted. For the SP142 assay, both tumor cell staining and immune cell staining are considered for the criteria of positivity. These differences make it difficult to standardize one universal IHC test and/or criteria for establishing PD-L1 positivity. It is important to note that PD-L1 positivity for each assay was established individually for the ability to predict response to their corresponding drug. Even so, many studies have been or are currently being undertaken to unify and establish a technical equivalence between the various assays,[169,170] although proving predictive equivalence may be much more difficult. Detailed discussion on PD-L1 immunohistochemistry assays and testing can be found in the *IASLC Atlas on PD-L1 Testing in Lung Cancer.*[171]

CONCLUSIONS

During the last two decades, adenocarcinoma has become the most common type of lung cancers. The 2015 World Health Organization classification system for lung adenocarcinoma is not only based on histological patterns but also highlights prognostic implication.

Furthermore, molecular profiling of lung adenocarcinoma has identified multiple genomic aberrations, including mutations and translocations that are drivers of oncogenicity in these tumors, each of which may be targeted by specific therapy. These have led to increased personalization of the treatment of lung adenocarcinoma patients based on the results of biomarker testing for these target aberrations. With rapid advances in our understanding of the complex genetics of lung adenocarcinoma and technologies to assess them, the classification of lung adenocarcinoma will continue to evolve, with incorporation of novel molecular features that drive the biology and treatment of this tumor.

REFERENCES

1. Travis WDBE, Burke AP, Marx A, Nicholson AG. *WHO Classification of Tumours of Lung, Pleura, Thymus, and Heart.* 4th ed. Lyon: IARC; 2015.
2. Travis WD. The 2015 WHO classification of lung tumors. *Pathologe.* 2014;35(suppl 2):188.
3. Travis WD, Brambilla E, Nicholson AG, et al. The 2015 World Health Organization Classification of Lung Tumors: Impact of Genetic, Clinical and Radiologic Advances Since the 2004 Classification. *J Thorac Oncol.* 2015;10(9):1243−1260.
4. Lamb D. Histological classification of lung cancer. *Thorax.* 1984;39(3):161−165.
5. Shimosato Y, Suzuki A, Hashimoto T, et al. Prognostic implications of fibrotic focus (scar) in small peripheral lung cancers. *Am J Surg Pathol.* 1980;4(4):365−373.
6. Russell PA, Barnett SA, Walkiewicz M, et al. Correlation of mutation status and survival with predominant histologic subtype according to the new IASLC/ATS/ERS lung adenocarcinoma classification in stage III (N2) patients. *J Thorac Oncol.* 2013;8(4):461−468.

7. Russell PA, Wainer Z, Wright GM, Daniels M, Conron M, Williams RA. Does lung adenocarcinoma subtype predict patient survival?: A clinicopathologic study based on the new International Association for the Study of Lung Cancer/American Thoracic Society/European Respiratory Society international multidisciplinary lung adenocarcinoma classification. *J Thorac Oncol.* 2011;6(9):1496−1504.

8. Tsuta K, Kawago M, Inoue E, et al. The utility of the proposed IASLC/ATS/ERS lung adenocarcinoma subtypes for disease prognosis and correlation of driver gene alterations. *Lung Cancer.* 2013;81(3):371−376.

9. Travis WD, Brambilla E, Noguchi M, et al. International association for the study of lung cancer/american thoracic society/european respiratory society international multidisciplinary classification of lung adenocarcinoma. *J Thorac Oncol.* 2011;6(2):244−285.

10. Yoshizawa A, Motoi N, Riely GJ, et al. Impact of proposed IASLC/ATS/ERS classification of lung adenocarcinoma: prognostic subgroups and implications for further revision of staging based on analysis of 514 stage I cases. *Modern pathology : an official journal of the United States and Canadian Academy of Pathology, Inc.* 2011;24(5):653−664.

11. Behera M, Owonikoko TK, Gal AA, et al. Lung Adenocarcinoma Staging Using the 2011 IASLC/ATS/ERS Classification: A Pooled Analysis of Adenocarcinoma In Situ and Minimally Invasive Adenocarcinoma. *Clin Lung Cancer.* 2016;17(5):e57−e64.

12. Warth A, Muley T, Kossakowski C, et al. Prognostic impact and clinicopathological correlations of the cribriform pattern in pulmonary adenocarcinoma. *J Thorac Oncol.* 2015;10(4):638−644.

13. Pan Y, Zhang Y, Li Y, et al. ALK, ROS1 and RET fusions in 1139 lung adenocarcinomas: a comprehensive study of common and fusion pattern-specific clinicopathologic, histologic and cytologic features. *Lung Cancer.* 2014;84(2):121−126.

14. Lee MC, Buitrago DH, Kadota K, Jones DR, Adusumilli PS. Recent advances and clinical implications of the micropapillary histological subtype in lung adenocarcinomas. *Lung Cancer Manag.* 2014;3(3):245−253.

15. Tsao MS, Marguet S, Le Teuff G, et al. Subtype Classification of Lung Adenocarcinoma Predicts Benefit From Adjuvant Chemotherapy in Patients Undergoing Complete Resection. *J Clin Oncol.* 2015;33(30):3439−3446.

16. Kadota K, Nitadori J, Sima CS, et al. Tumor Spread through Air Spaces is an Important Pattern of Invasion and Impacts the Frequency and Location of Recurrences after Limited Resection for Small Stage I Lung Adenocarcinomas. *J Thorac Oncol.* 2015;10(5):806−814.

17. Pyo JS, Kim JH. Clinicopathological Significance of Micropapillary Pattern in Lung Adenocarcinoma. *Pathol Oncol Res.* 2018;24(3):547−555.

18. Morales-Oyarvide V, Mino-Kenudson M. High-grade lung adenocarcinomas with micropapillary and/or solid patterns: a review. *Curr Opin Pulm Med.* 2014;20(4):317−323.

19. Finberg KE, Sequist LV, Joshi VA, et al. Mucinous differentiation correlates with absence of EGFR mutation and presence of KRAS mutation in lung adenocarcinomas with bronchioloalveolar features. *J Mol Diagn.* 2007;9(3):320−326.

20. Rekhtman N, Ang DC, Riely GJ, Ladanyi M, Moreira AL. KRAS mutations are associated with solid growth pattern and tumor-infiltrating leukocytes in lung adenocarcinoma. *Modern pathology : an official journal of the United States and Canadian Academy of Pathology, Inc.* 2013;26(10):1307−1319.

21. Kadota K, Yeh YC, D'Angelo SP, et al. Associations between mutations and histologic patterns of mucin in lung adenocarcinoma: invasive mucinous pattern and extracellular mucin are associated with KRAS mutation. *Am J Surg Pathol.* 2014;38(8):1118−1127.

22. Hwang DH, Sholl LM, Rojas-Rudilla V, et al. KRAS and NKX2-1 Mutations in Invasive Mucinous Adenocarcinoma of the Lung. *J Thorac Oncol.* 2016;11(4):496−503.

23. Duruisseaux M, McLeer-Florin A, Antoine M, et al. NRG1 fusion in a French cohort of invasive mucinous lung adenocarcinoma. *Cancer Med.* 2016;5(12):3579−3585.

24. Fernandez-Cuesta L, Plenker D, Osada H, et al. CD74-NRG1 fusions in lung adenocarcinoma. *Cancer Discov.* 2014;4(4):415−422.

25. Rami-Porta R, Bolejack V, Crowley J, et al. The IASLC Lung Cancer Staging Project: Proposals for the Revisions of the T Descriptors in the Forthcoming Eighth Edition of the TNM Classification for Lung Cancer. *J Thorac Oncol.* 2015;10(7):990−1003.

26. Goldstraw P, Chansky K, Crowley J, et al. The IASLC Lung Cancer Staging Project: Proposals for Revision of the TNM Stage Groupings in the Forthcoming (Eighth) Edition of the TNM Classification for Lung Cancer. *J Thorac Oncol.* 2016;11(1):39−51.

27. Asamura H, Chansky K, Crowley J, et al. The International Association for the Study of Lung Cancer Lung Cancer Staging Project: Proposals for the Revision of the N Descriptors in the Forthcoming 8th Edition of the TNM Classification for Lung Cancer. *J Thorac Oncol.* 2015;10(12):1675−1684.

28. Eberhardt WE, Mitchell A, Crowley J, et al. The IASLC Lung Cancer Staging Project: Proposals for the Revision of the M Descriptors in the Forthcoming Eighth Edition of the TNM Classification of Lung Cancer. *J Thorac Oncol.* 2015;10(11):1515−1522.

29. Nicholson AG, Chansky K, Crowley J, et al. The International Association for the Study of Lung Cancer Lung Cancer Staging Project: Proposals for the Revision of the Clinical and Pathologic Staging of Small Cell Lung Cancer in the Forthcoming Eighth Edition of the TNM Classification for Lung Cancer. *J Thorac Oncol.* 2016;11(3):300−311.

30. Travis WD, Asamura H, Bankier AA, et al. The IASLC Lung Cancer Staging Project: Proposals for Coding T Categories for Subsolid Nodules and Assessment of Tumor Size in Part-Solid Tumors in the Forthcoming Eighth Edition of the TNM Classification of Lung Cancer. *J Thorac Oncol.* 2016;11(8):1204–1223.

31. Detterbeck FC, Franklin WA, Nicholson AG, et al. The IASLC Lung Cancer Staging Project: Background Data and Proposed Criteria to Distinguish Separate Primary Lung Cancers from Metastatic Foci in Patients with Two Lung Tumors in the Forthcoming Eighth Edition of the TNM Classification for Lung Cancer. *J Thorac Oncol.* 2016;11(5):651–665.

32. Detterbeck FC, Bolejack V, Arenberg DA, et al. The IASLC Lung Cancer Staging Project: Background Data and Proposals for the Classification of Lung Cancer with Separate Tumor Nodules in the Forthcoming Eighth Edition of the TNM Classification for Lung Cancer. *J Thorac Oncol.* 2016;11(5):681–692.

33. Detterbeck FC, Marom EM, Arenberg DA, et al. The IASLC Lung Cancer Staging Project: Background Data and Proposals for the Application of TNM Staging Rules to Lung Cancer Presenting as Multiple Nodules with Ground Glass or Lepidic Features or a Pneumonic Type of Involvement in the Forthcoming Eighth Edition of the TNM Classification. *J Thorac Oncol.* 2016;11(5):666–680.

34. Detterbeck FC, Nicholson AG, Franklin WA, et al. The IASLC Lung Cancer Staging Project: Summary of Proposals for Revisions of the Classification of Lung Cancers with Multiple Pulmonary Sites of Involvement in the Forthcoming Eighth Edition of the TNM Classification. *J Thorac Oncol.* 2016;11(5):639–650.

35. Cancer Genome Atlas Research N. Comprehensive molecular profiling of lung adenocarcinoma. *Nature.* 2014;511(7511):543–550.

36. Bhattacharjee A, Richards WG, Staunton J, et al. Classification of human lung carcinomas by mRNA expression profiling reveals distinct adenocarcinoma subclasses. *Proc Natl Acad Sci U S A.* 2001;98(24):13790–13795.

37. Beer DG, Kardia SL, Huang CC, et al. Gene-expression profiles predict survival of patients with lung adenocarcinoma. *Nat Med.* 2002;8(8):816–824.

38. Hayes DN, Monti S, Parmigiani G, et al. Gene expression profiling reveals reproducible human lung adenocarcinoma subtypes in multiple independent patient cohorts. *J Clin Oncol.* 2006;24(31):5079–5090.

39. Wilkerson MD, Yin X, Walter V, et al. Differential pathogenesis of lung adenocarcinoma subtypes involving sequence mutations, copy number, chromosomal instability, and methylation. *PLoS One.* 2012;7(5):e36530.

40. Garber ME, Troyanskaya OG, Schluens K, et al. Diversity of gene expression in adenocarcinoma of the lung. *Proc Natl Acad Sci U S A.* 2001;98(24):13784–13789.

41. Yatabe Y, Mitsudomi T, Takahashi T. TTF-1 expression in pulmonary adenocarcinomas. *Am J Surg Pathol.* 2002;26(6):767–773.

42. Yamada E, Bastie CC. Disruption of Fyn SH3 domain interaction with a proline-rich motif in liver kinase B1 results in activation of AMP-activated protein kinase. *PLoS One.* 2014;9(2):e89604.

43. Hemminki A, Tomlinson I, Markie D, et al. Localization of a susceptibility locus for Peutz-Jeghers syndrome to 19p using comparative genomic hybridization and targeted linkage analysis. *Nat Genet.* 1997;15(1):87–90.

44. Hemminki A, Markie D, Tomlinson I, et al. A serine/threonine kinase gene defective in Peutz-Jeghers syndrome. *Nature.* 1998;391(6663):184–187.

45. Sanchez-Cespedes M, Parrella P, Esteller M, et al. Inactivation of LKB1/STK11 is a common event in adenocarcinomas of the lung. *Cancer Res.* 2002;62(13):3659–3662.

46. Carretero J, Medina PP, Pio R, Montuenga LM, Sanchez-Cespedes M. Novel and natural knockout lung cancer cell lines for the LKB1/STK11 tumor suppressor gene. *Oncogene.* 2004;23(22):4037–4040.

47. Gill RK, Yang SH, Meerzaman D, et al. Frequent homozygous deletion of the LKB1/STK11 gene in non-small cell lung cancer. *Oncogene.* 2011;30(35):3784–3791.

48. Dumstrei K, Nassif C, Abboud G, Aryai A, Aryai A, Hartenstein V. EGFR signaling is required for the differentiation and maintenance of neural progenitors along the dorsal midline of the Drosophila embryonic head. *Development.* 1998;125(17):3417–3426.

49. Dogan S, Shen R, Ang DC, et al. Molecular epidemiology of EGFR and KRAS mutations in 3,026 lung adenocarcinomas: higher susceptibility of women to smoking-related KRAS-mutant cancers. *Clin Cancer Res.* 2012;18(22):6169–6177.

50. Shi Y, Au JS, Thongprasert S, et al. A prospective, molecular epidemiology study of EGFR mutations in Asian patients with advanced non-small-cell lung cancer of adenocarcinoma histology (PIONEER). *J Thorac Oncol.* 2014;9(2):154–162.

51. Yun CH, Mengwasser KE, Toms AV, et al. The T790M mutation in EGFR kinase causes drug resistance by increasing the affinity for ATP. *Proc Natl Acad Sci U S A.* 2008;105(6):2070–2075.

52. Pao W, Miller VA, Politi KA, et al. Acquired resistance of lung adenocarcinomas to gefitinib or erlotinib is associated with a second mutation in the EGFR kinase domain. *PLoS Med.* 2005;2(3):e73.

53. Wu SG, Liu YN, Tsai MF, et al. The mechanism of acquired resistance to irreversible EGFR tyrosine kinase inhibitor-afatinib in lung adenocarcinoma patients. *Oncotarget.* 2016;7(11):12404–12413.

54. Balak MN, Gong Y, Riely GJ, et al. Novel D761Y and common secondary T790M mutations in epidermal growth factor receptor-mutant lung adenocarcinomas with acquired resistance to kinase inhibitors. *Clin Cancer Res.* 2006;12(21):6494–6501.

55. Costa DB, Schumer ST, Tenen DG, Kobayashi S. Differential responses to erlotinib in epidermal growth factor receptor (EGFR)-mutated lung cancers with acquired resistance to gefitinib carrying the L747S or T790M secondary mutations. *J Clin Oncol.* 2008;26(7):1182–1184; author reply 1184-1186.

56. Ercan D, Zejnullahu K, Yonesaka K, et al. Amplification of EGFR T790M causes resistance to an irreversible EGFR inhibitor. *Oncogene.* 2010;29(16):2346–2356.

57. Engelman JA, Zejnullahu K, Mitsudomi T, et al. MET amplification leads to gefitinib resistance in lung cancer by activating ERBB3 signaling. *Science.* 2007;316(5827):1039–1043.

58. Ohashi K, Maruvka YE, Michor F, Pao W. Epidermal growth factor receptor tyrosine kinase inhibitor-resistant disease. *J Clin Oncol.* 2013;31(8):1070–1080.

59. Camidge DR, Pao W, Sequist LV. Acquired resistance to TKIs in solid tumours: learning from lung cancer. *Nat Rev Clin Oncol.* 2014;11(8):473–481.

60. Rosell R, Karachaliou N, Morales-Espinosa D, et al. Adaptive resistance to targeted therapies in cancer. *Transl Lung Cancer Res.* 2013;2(3):152–159.

61. Yu HA, Riely GJ, Lovly CM. Therapeutic strategies utilized in the setting of acquired resistance to EGFR tyrosine kinase inhibitors. *Clin Cancer Res.* 2014;20(23):5898–5907.

62. Oser MG, Niederst MJ, Sequist LV, Engelman JA. Transformation from non-small-cell lung cancer to small-cell lung cancer: molecular drivers and cells of origin. *The Lancet Oncology.* 2015;16(4):e165–e172.

63. Niederst MJ, Sequist LV, Poirier JT, et al. RB loss in resistant EGFR mutant lung adenocarcinomas that transform to small-cell lung cancer. *Nat Commun.* 2015;6:6377.

64. Stewart EL, Tan SZ, Liu G, Tsao MS. Known and putative mechanisms of resistance to EGFR targeted therapies in NSCLC patients with EGFR mutations-a review. *Transl Lung Cancer Res.* 2015;4(1):67–81.

65. Morris SW, Kirstein MN, Valentine MB, et al. Fusion of a kinase gene, ALK, to a nucleolar protein gene, NPM, in non-Hodgkin's lymphoma. *Science.* 1994;263(5151):1281–1284.

66. Soda M, Choi YL, Enomoto M, et al. Identification of the transforming EML4-ALK fusion gene in non-small-cell lung cancer. *Nature.* 2007;448(7153):561–566.

67. Rikova K, Guo A, Zeng Q, et al. Global survey of phosphotyrosine signaling identifies oncogenic kinases in lung cancer. *Cell.* 2007;131(6):1190–1203.

68. Ou SH, Klempner SJ, Greenbowe JR, et al. Identification of a novel HIP1-ALK fusion variant in Non-Small-Cell Lung Cancer (NSCLC) and discovery of ALK I1171 (I1171N/S) mutations in two ALK-rearranged NSCLC patients with resistance to Alectinib. *J Thorac Oncol.* 2014;9(12):1821–1825.

69. Hong S, Fang W, Hu Z, et al. A large-scale cross-sectional study of ALK rearrangements and EGFR mutations in non-small-cell lung cancer in Chinese Han population. *Sci Rep.* 2014;4:7268.

70. Takeuchi K, Soda M, Togashi Y, et al. RET, ROS1 and ALK fusions in lung cancer. *Nat Med.* 2012;18(3):378–381.

71. Takeuchi K, Choi YL, Togashi Y, et al. KIF5B-ALK, a novel fusion oncokinase identified by an immunohistochemistry-based diagnostic system for ALK-positive lung cancer. *Clin Cancer Res.* 2009;15(9):3143–3149.

72. Tsao MS, Hirsch F, Yatabe Y. *IASLC Atlas of ALK and ROS1 Testing in Lung Cancer.* 2nd ed. Editorial Rx Press; 2016.

73. Shaw AT, Yeap BY, Solomon BJ, et al. Effect of crizotinib on overall survival in patients with advanced non-small-cell lung cancer harbouring ALK gene rearrangement: a retrospective analysis. *Lancet Oncol.* 2011;12(11):1004–1012.

74. Shaw AT, Yeap BY, Mino-Kenudson M, et al. Clinical features and outcome of patients with non-small-cell lung cancer who harbor EML4-ALK. *J Clin Oncol.* 2009;27(26):4247–4253.

75. Rodig SJ, Mino-Kenudson M, Dacic S, et al. Unique clinicopathologic features characterize ALK-rearranged lung adenocarcinoma in the western population. *Clin Cancer Res.* 2009;15(16):5216–5223.

76. Lindeman NI, Cagle PT, Beasley MB, et al. Molecular testing guideline for selection of lung cancer patients for EGFR and ALK tyrosine kinase inhibitors: guideline from the College of American Pathologists, International Association for the Study of Lung Cancer, and Association for Molecular Pathology. *J Thorac Oncol.* 2013;8(7):823–859.

77. Alrifai D, Popat S, Ahmed M, et al. A rare case of squamous cell carcinoma of the lung harbouring ALK and BRAF activating mutations. *Lung Cancer.* 2013;80(3):339–340.

78. Ochi N, Yamane H, Yamagishi T, Takigawa N, Monobe Y. Can we eliminate squamous cell carcinoma of the lung from testing of EML4-ALK fusion gene? *Lung Cancer.* 2013;79(1):94–95.

79. Lovly CM, Pao W. Escaping ALK inhibition: mechanisms of and strategies to overcome resistance. *Sci Transl Med.* 2012;4(120):120–122.

80. Lovly CM, Shaw AT. Molecular pathways: resistance to kinase inhibitors and implications for therapeutic strategies. *Clin Cancer Res.* 2014;20(9):2249–2256.

81. van der Wekken AJ, Saber A, Hiltermann TJ, Kok K, van den Berg A, Groen HJ. Resistance mechanisms after tyrosine kinase inhibitors afatinib and crizotinib in non-small cell lung cancer, a review of the literature. *Crit Rev Oncol Hematol.* 2016;100:107–116.

82. Sasaki T, Koivunen J, Ogino A, et al. A novel ALK secondary mutation and EGFR signaling cause resistance to ALK kinase inhibitors. *Cancer Res.* 2011;71(18):6051–6060.

83. Robinson DR, Wu YM, Lin SF. The protein tyrosine kinase family of the human genome. *Oncogene.* 2000;19(49):5548–5557.

84. Birchmeier C, Sharma S, Wigler M. Expression and rearrangement of the ROS1 gene in human glioblastoma cells. *Proc Natl Acad Sci U S A.* 1987;84(24):9270–9274.

85. Charest A, Lane K, McMahon K, et al. Fusion of FIG to the receptor tyrosine kinase ROS in a glioblastoma with an interstitial del(6)(q21q21). *Genes Chromosomes Cancer.* 2003;37(1):58–71.

86. Bergethon K, Shaw AT, Ou SH, et al. ROS1 rearrangements define a unique molecular class of lung cancers. *J Clin Oncol.* 2012;30(8):863–870.

87. Pal P, Khan Z. Ros1-1. *J Clin Pathol.* 2017;70(12):1001–1009.

88. Zhu Q, Zhan P, Zhang X, Lv T, Song Y. Clinicopathologic characteristics of patients with ROS1 fusion gene in non-small cell lung cancer: a meta-analysis. *Transl Lung Cancer Res.* 2015;4(3):300–309.

89. Shaw AT, Ou SH, Bang YJ, et al. Crizotinib in ROS1-rearranged non-small-cell lung cancer. *N Engl J Med.* 2014;371(21):1963–1971.

90. Mazieres J, Zalcman G, Crino L, et al. Crizotinib therapy for advanced lung adenocarcinoma and a ROS1 rearrangement: results from the EUROS1 cohort. *J Clin Oncol.* 2015;33(9):992–999.

91. Zhao J, Zheng J, Kong M, Zhou J, Ding W, Zhou J. Advanced lung adenocarcinomas with ROS1-rearrangement frequently show hepatoid cell. *Oncotarget.* 2016;7(45):74162–74170.

92. Yoshida A, Tsuta K, Wakai S, et al. Immunohistochemical detection of ROS1 is useful for identifying ROS1 rearrangements in lung cancers. *Modern pathology : an official journal of the United States and Canadian Academy of Pathology, Inc.* 2014;27(5):711–720.

93. Shaw AT, Hsu PP, Awad MM, Engelman JA. Tyrosine kinase gene rearrangements in epithelial malignancies. *Nat Rev Cancer.* 2013;13(11):772–787.

94. Awad MM, Katayama R, McTigue M, et al. Acquired resistance to crizotinib from a mutation in CD74-ROS1. *N Engl J Med.* 2013;368(25):2395–2401.

95. Facchinetti F, Loriot Y, Kuo MS, et al. Crizotinib-Resistant ROS1 Mutations Reveal a Predictive Kinase Inhibitor Sensitivity Model for ROS1- and ALK-Rearranged Lung Cancers. *Clin Cancer Res.* 2016;22(24):5983–5991.

96. Dagogo-Jack I, Shaw AT. Expanding the Roster of ROS1 Inhibitors. *J Clin Oncol.* 2017;35(23):2595–2597.

97. Drilon A, Siena S, Ou SI, et al. Safety and Antitumor Activity of the Multitargeted Pan-TRK, ROS1, and ALK Inhibitor Entrectinib: Combined Results from Two Phase I Trials (ALKA-372-001 and STARTRK-1). *Cancer Discov.* 2017;7(4):400–409.

98. Chong CR, Bahcall M, Capelletti M, et al. Identification of Existing Drugs That Effectively Target NTRK1 and ROS1 Rearrangements in Lung Cancer. *Clin Cancer Res.* 2017;23(1):204–213.

99. Thunnissen E, Allen TC, Adam J, et al. Immunohistochemistry of Pulmonary Biomarkers: A Perspective From Members of the Pulmonary Pathology Society. *Archives of pathology & laboratory medicine.* 2018;142(3):408–419.

100. Bubendorf L, Buttner R, Al-Dayel F, et al. Testing for ROS1 in non-small cell lung cancer: a review with recommendations. *Virchows Arch.* 2016;469(5):489–503.

101. Lee SE, Lee B, Hong M, et al. Comprehensive analysis of RET and ROS1 rearrangement in lung adenocarcinoma. *Modern pathology : an official journal of the United States and Canadian Academy of Pathology, Inc.* 2015;28(4):468–479.

102. Shan L, Lian F, Guo L, et al. Detection of ROS1 gene rearrangement in lung adenocarcinoma: comparison of IHC, FISH and real-time RT-PCR. *PLoS One.* 2015;10(3):e0120422.

103. Cao B, Wei P, Liu Z, et al. Detection of lung adenocarcinoma with ROS1 rearrangement by IHC, FISH, and RT-PCR and analysis of its clinicopathologic features. *Onco Targets Ther.* 2016;9:131–138.

104. Suehara Y, Arcila M, Wang L, et al. Identification of KIF5B-RET and GOPC-ROS1 fusions in lung adenocarcinomas through a comprehensive mRNA-based screen for tyrosine kinase fusions. *Clin Cancer Res.* 2012;18(24):6599–6608.

105. Dama E, Tillhon M, Bertalot G, et al. Sensitive and affordable diagnostic assay for the quantitative detection of anaplastic lymphoma kinase (ALK) alterations in patients with non-small cell lung cancer. *Oncotarget.* 2016;7(24):37160–37176.

106. Lira ME, Choi YL, Lim SM, et al. A single-tube multiplexed assay for detecting ALK, ROS1, and RET fusions in lung cancer. *J Mol Diagn.* 2014;16(2):229–243.

107. Mino-Kenudson M, Chirieac LR, Law K, et al. A novel, highly sensitive antibody allows for the routine detection of ALK-rearranged lung adenocarcinomas by standard immunohistochemistry. *Clin Cancer Res.* 2010;16(5):1561–1571.

108. Cutz JC, Craddock KJ, Torlakovic E, et al. Canadian anaplastic lymphoma kinase study: a model for multicenter standardization and optimization of ALK testing in lung cancer. *J Thorac Oncol.* 2014;9(9):1255–1263.

109. Rimkunas VM, Crosby KE, Li D, et al. Analysis of receptor tyrosine kinase ROS1-positive tumors in non-small cell lung cancer: identification of a FIG-ROS1 fusion. *Clin Cancer Res.* 2012;18(16):4449–4457.

110. Sholl LM, Sun H, Butaney M, et al. ROS1 immunohistochemistry for detection of ROS1-rearranged lung adenocarcinomas. *Am J Surg Pathol.* 2013;37(9):1441–1449.

111. Suh JH, Johnson A, Albacker L, et al. Comprehensive Genomic Profiling Facilitates Implementation of the National Comprehensive Cancer Network Guidelines for Lung Cancer Biomarker Testing and Identifies Patients Who May Benefit From Enrollment in Mechanism-Driven Clinical Trials. *Oncologist.* 2016;21(6):684–691.

112. Goswami RS, Luthra R, Singh RR, et al. Identification of Factors Affecting the Success of Next-Generation Sequencing Testing in Solid Tumors. *Am J Clin Pathol.* 2016;145(2):222−237.

113. Hovelson DH, McDaniel AS, Cani AK, et al. Development and validation of a scalable next-generation sequencing system for assessing relevant somatic variants in solid tumors. *Neoplasia.* 2015;17(4):385−399.

114. Drilon A, Wang L, Arcila ME, et al. Broad, Hybrid Capture-Based Next-Generation Sequencing Identifies Actionable Genomic Alterations in Lung Adenocarcinomas Otherwise Negative for Such Alterations by Other Genomic Testing Approaches. *Clin Cancer Res.* 2015; 21(16):3631−3639.

115. Zheng Z, Liebers M, Zhelyazkova B, et al. Anchored multiplex PCR for targeted next-generation sequencing. *Nat Med.* 2014;20(12):1479−1484.

116. Ali SM, Hensing T, Schrock AB, et al. Comprehensive Genomic Profiling Identifies a Subset of Crizotinib-Responsive ALK-Rearranged Non-Small Cell Lung Cancer Not Detected by Fluorescence In Situ Hybridization. *Oncologist.* 2016;21(6):762−770.

117. Cheng DT, Mitchell TN, Zehir A, et al. Memorial Sloan Kettering-Integrated Mutation Profiling of Actionable Cancer Targets (MSK-IMPACT): A Hybridization Capture-Based Next-Generation Sequencing Clinical Assay for Solid Tumor Molecular Oncology. *J Mol Diagn.* 2015;17(3):251−264.

118. Turke AB, Zejnullahu K, Wu YL, et al. Preexistence and clonal selection of MET amplification in EGFR mutant NSCLC. *Cancer cell.* 2010;17(1):77−88.

119. Bean J, Brennan C, Shih JY, et al. MET amplification occurs with or without T790M mutations in EGFR mutant lung tumors with acquired resistance to gefitinib or erlotinib. *Proc Natl Acad Sci U S A.* 2007;104(52): 20932−20937.

120. Zheng D, Wang R, Ye T, et al. MET exon 14 skipping defines a unique molecular class of non-small cell lung cancer. *Oncotarget.* 2016;7(27):41691−41702.

121. Heist RS, Shim HS, Gingipally S, et al. MET Exon 14 Skipping in Non-Small Cell Lung Cancer. *Oncologist.* 2016; 21(4):481−486.

122. Paik PK, Drilon A, Fan PD, et al. Response to MET inhibitors in patients with stage IV lung adenocarcinomas harboring MET mutations causing exon 14 skipping. *Cancer Discov.* 2015;5(8):842−849.

123. Awad MM, Oxnard GR, Jackman DM, et al. MET Exon 14 Mutations in Non-Small-Cell Lung Cancer Are Associated With Advanced Age and Stage-Dependent MET Genomic Amplification and c-Met Overexpression. *J Clin Oncol.* 2016;34(7):721−730.

124. Reungwetwattana T, Liang Y, Zhu V, Ou SI. The race to target MET exon 14 skipping alterations in non-small cell lung cancer: The Why, the How, the Who, the Unknown, and the Inevitable. *Lung Cancer.* 2017;103: 27−37.

125. Slebos RJ, Kibbelaar RE, Dalesio O, et al. K-ras oncogene activation as a prognostic marker in adenocarcinoma of the lung. *N Engl J Med.* 1990;323(9):561−565.

126. Riely GJ, Kris MG, Rosenbaum D, et al. Frequency and distinctive spectrum of KRAS mutations in never smokers with lung adenocarcinoma. *Clin Cancer Res.* 2008;14(18): 5731−5734.

127. Gainor JF, Varghese AM, Ou SH, et al. ALK rearrangements are mutually exclusive with mutations in EGFR or KRAS: an analysis of 1,683 patients with non-small cell lung cancer. *Clin Cancer Res.* 2013;19(15): 4273−4281.

128. Lee B, Lee T, Lee SH, Choi YL, Han J. Clinicopathologic characteristics of EGFR, KRAS, and ALK alterations in 6,595 lung cancers. *Oncotarget.* 2016;7(17):23874−23884.

129. Salama AK, Flaherty KT. BRAF in melanoma: current strategies and future directions. *Clin Cancer Res.* 2013; 19(16):4326−4334.

130. Marchetti A, Felicioni L, Malatesta S, et al. Clinical features and outcome of patients with non-small-cell lung cancer harboring BRAF mutations. *J Clin Oncol.* 2011; 29(26):3574−3579.

131. Michels S, Scheel AH, Scheffler M, et al. Clinicopathological Characteristics of RET Rearranged Lung Cancer in European Patients. *J Thorac Oncol.* 2016;11(1):122−127.

132. Wang R, Hu H, Pan Y, et al. RET fusions define a unique molecular and clinicopathologic subtype of non-small-cell lung cancer. *J Clin Oncol.* 2012;30(35):4352−4359.

133. Tsuta K, Kohno T, Yoshida A, et al. RET-rearranged non-small-cell lung carcinoma: a clinicopathological and molecular analysis. *Br J Cancer.* 2014;110(6):1571−1578.

134. Tsai TH, Wu SG, Hsieh MS, Yu CJ, Yang JC, Shih JY. Clinical and prognostic implications of RET rearrangements in metastatic lung adenocarcinoma patients with malignant pleural effusion. *Lung Cancer.* 2015;88(2):208−214.

135. Dugay F, Llamas-Gutierrez F, Gournay M, et al. Clinico-pathological characteristics of ROS1- and RET-rearranged NSCLC in caucasian patients: Data from a cohort of 713 non-squamous NSCLC lacking KRAS/EGFR/HER2/BRAF/PIK3CA/ALK alterations. *Oncotarget.* 2017;8(32): 53336−53351.

136. Drilon A, Rekhtman N, Arcila M, et al. Cabozantinib in patients with advanced RET-rearranged non-small-cell lung cancer: an open-label, single-centre, phase 2, single-arm trial. *Lancet Oncol.* 2016;17(12):1653−1660.

137. Drilon A, Wang L, Hasanovic A, et al. Response to Cabozantinib in patients with RET fusion-positive lung adenocarcinomas. *Cancer Discov.* 2013;3(6):630−635.

138. Song M, Kim SH, Yoon SK. Cabozantinib for the treatment of non-small cell lung cancer with KIF5B-RET fusion. An example of swift repositioning. *Arch Pharm Res.* 2015;38(12):2120−2123.

139. Vaishnavi A, Capelletti M, Le AT, et al. Oncogenic and drug-sensitive NTRK1 rearrangements in lung cancer. *Nat Med.* 2013;19(11):1469−1472.

140. Ou SI, Schrock AB, Bocharov EV, et al. HER2 Transmembrane Domain (TMD) Mutations (V659/G660) That Stabilize Homo- and Heterodimerization Are Rare Oncogenic Drivers in Lung Adenocarcinoma That Respond to Afatinib. *J Thorac Oncol.* 2017;12(3):446−457.

141. Ettinger DS, Wood DE, Akerley W, et al. Non-Small Cell Lung Cancer, Version 6.2015. *J Natl Compr Canc Netw.* 2015;13(5):515−524.

142. De Greve J, Moran T, Graas MP, et al. Phase II study of afatinib, an irreversible ErbB family blocker, in demographically and genotypically defined lung adenocarcinoma. *Lung Cancer.* 2015;88(1):63−69.

143. De Greve J, Teugels E, Geers C, et al. Clinical activity of afatinib (BIBW 2992) in patients with lung adenocarcinoma with mutations in the kinase domain of HER2/neu. *Lung Cancer.* 2012;76(1):123−127.

144. Kim MY, Oskarsson T, Acharyya S, et al. Tumor self-seeding by circulating cancer cells. *Cell.* 2009;139(7):1315−1326.

145. Cristofanilli M, Budd GT, Ellis MJ, et al. Circulating tumor cells, disease progression, and survival in metastatic breast cancer. *N Engl J Med.* 2004;351(8):781−791.

146. Cohen SJ, Punt CJ, Iannotti N, et al. Relationship of circulating tumor cells to tumor response, progression-free survival, and overall survival in patients with metastatic colorectal cancer. *J Clin Oncol.* 2008;26(19):3213−3221.

147. Hou JM, Krebs MG, Lancashire L, et al. Clinical significance and molecular characteristics of circulating tumor cells and circulating tumor microemboli in patients with small-cell lung cancer. *J Clin Oncol.* 2012;30(5):525−532.

148. Zhou J, Dong F, Cui F, Xu R, Tang X. The role of circulating tumor cells in evaluation of prognosis and treatment response in advanced non-small-cell lung cancer. *Cancer Chemother Pharmacol.* 2017;79(4):825−833.

149. Krebs MG, Sloane R, Priest L, et al. Evaluation and prognostic significance of circulating tumor cells in patients with non-small-cell lung cancer. *J Clin Oncol.* 2011;29(12):1556−1563.

150. Butt AN, Swaminathan R. Overview of circulating nucleic acids in plasma/serum. *Ann N Y Acad Sci.* 2008;1137:236−242.

151. Zaher ER, Anwar MM, Kohail HM, El-Zoghby SM, Abo-El-Eneen MS. Cell-free DNA concentration and integrity as a screening tool for cancer. *Indian J Cancer.* 2013;50(3):175−183.

152. Underhill HR, Kitzman JO, Hellwig S, et al. Fragment Length of Circulating Tumor DNA. *PLoS Genet.* 2016;12(7):e1006162.

153. Whitcombe D, Theaker J, Guy SP, Brown T, Little S. Detection of PCR products using self-probing amplicons and fluorescence. *Nat Biotechnol.* 1999;17(8):804−807.

154. Kimura H, Kasahara K, Kawaishi M, et al. Detection of epidermal growth factor receptor mutations in serum as a predictor of the response to gefitinib in patients with non-small-cell lung cancer. *Clin Cancer Res.* 2006;12(13):3915−3921.

155. Won JK, Keam B, Koh J, et al. Concomitant ALK translocation and EGFR mutation in lung cancer: a comparison of direct sequencing and sensitive assays and the impact on responsiveness to tyrosine kinase inhibitor. *Ann Oncol.* 2015;26(2):348−354.

156. Vogelstein B, Kinzler KW. Digital PCR. *Proc Natl Acad Sci U S A.* 1999;96(16):9236−9241.

157. Newman AM, Lovejoy AF, Klass DM, et al. Integrated digital error suppression for improved detection of circulating tumor DNA. *Nat Biotechnol.* 2016;34(5):547−555.

158. Gautschi O, Bigosch C, Huegli B, et al. Circulating deoxyribonucleic Acid as prognostic marker in non-small-cell lung cancer patients undergoing chemotherapy. *J Clin Oncol.* 2004;22(20):4157−4164.

159. Tissot C, Toffart AC, Villar S, et al. Circulating free DNA concentration is an independent prognostic biomarker in lung cancer. *Eur Respir J.* 2015;46(6):1773−1780.

160. Wei Z, Shah N, Deng C, Xiao X, Zhong T, Li X. Circulating DNA addresses cancer monitoring in non small cell lung cancer patients for detection and capturing the dynamic changes of the disease. *Springerplus.* 2016;5:531.

161. Abbosh C, Birkbak NJ, Wilson GA, et al. Phylogenetic ctDNA analysis depicts early stage lung cancer evolution. *Nature.* 2017;545(7655):446−451.

162. Mok T, Wu YL, Lee JS, et al. Detection and Dynamic Changes of EGFR Mutations from Circulating Tumor DNA as a Predictor of Survival Outcomes in NSCLC Patients Treated with First-line Intercalated Erlotinib and Chemotherapy. *Clin Cancer Res.* 2015;21(14):3196−3203.

163. Thress KS, Brant R, Carr TH, et al. EGFR mutation detection in ctDNA from NSCLC patient plasma: A cross-platform comparison of leading technologies to support the clinical development of AZD9291. *Lung Cancer.* 2015;90(3):509−515.

164. Lee JY, Qing X, Xiumin W, et al. Longitudinal monitoring of EGFR mutations in plasma predicts outcomes of NSCLC patients treated with EGFR TKIs: Korean Lung Cancer Consortium (KLCC-12-02). *Oncotarget.* 2016;7(6):6984−6993.

165. Pardoll DM. The blockade of immune checkpoints in cancer immunotherapy. *Nat Rev Cancer.* 2012;12(4):252−264.

166. Ott PA, Hodi FS, Robert C. CTLA-4 and PD-1/PD-L1 blockade: new immunotherapeutic modalities with durable clinical benefit in melanoma patients. *Clin Cancer Res.* 2013;19(19):5300−5309.

167. Yu H, Boyle TA, Zhou C, Rimm DL, Hirsch FR. PD-L1 Expression in Lung Cancer. *J Thorac Oncol.* 2016;11(7):964−975.

168. Ai B, Liu H, Huang Y, Peng P. Circulating cell-free DNA as a prognostic and predictive biomarker in non-small cell lung cancer. *Oncotarget.* 2016;7(28):44583−44595.

169. Hirsch FR, McElhinny A, Stanforth D, et al. PD-L1 Immunohistochemistry Assays for Lung Cancer: Results from Phase 1 of the Blueprint PD-L1 IHC Assay Comparison Project. *J Thorac Oncol*. 2017;12(2):208−222.

170. Parra ER, Villalobos P, Mino B, Rodriguez-Canales J. Comparison of Different Antibody Clones for Immunohistochemistry Detection of Programmed Cell Death Ligand 1 (PD-L1) on Non-Small Cell Lung Carcinoma. *Appl Immunohistochem Mol Morphol*. 2018;26(2):83−93.

171. Tsao MS, Kerr KM, Dacic S, Yatabe Y, Hirsch F. *IASLC Atlas of PD-L1 Immunohistochemistry Testing in Lung Cancer*. Editorial Rx Press; 2017.

CHAPTER 3

Adjuvant and Neoadjuvant Therapy in Non–Small-Cell Lung Cancer

JEFFREY R. ZWEIG, MD • HEATHER A. WAKELEE, MD

INTRODUCTION

The use of adjuvant therapy in patients with non–small-cell lung cancer (NSCLC) applies to patients with surgically resected stage IB, II, and IIIA disease as based on the Tumor, Node, Metastasis staging system. While the majority of those with stage IB and II NSCLC are cured, 30%–40% still relapse. The use of adjuvant platinum-based chemotherapy in these patient groups results in an absolute survival benefit at 5 years of approximately 5%, with the greatest benefit seen in patients with stage II and IIIA disease.[1] This is the only treatment that has been proven to improve cure rates after resection, albeit with a modest benefit. Complete surgical resection remains the standard of care in early-stage NSCLC.[2] With more advanced stage disease, 5-year survival rates decrease significantly, with around 66% of patients with stage IB disease alive at 5 years versus 36% of patients with stage IIIA disease.[3] Therefore there remains an important need to improve on these outcomes and identify better postsurgical therapies for individual patients.

Most research to date in the adjuvant setting has focused on the use of chemotherapy. However, interest in the last years has grown significantly in the use of molecularly targeted agents and immunotherapies in early-stage disease, given the significant benefit seen with these drugs in the unresectable and/or metastatic setting. Herein, the current landscape of adjuvant and neoadjuvant therapy will be discussed, with attention to established data regarding the use of chemotherapy and radiation, along with the evolving data regarding the use of targeted agents, immunotherapy, and improved diagnostics such as circulating tumor DNA (ctDNA).

ADJUVANT CHEMOTHERAPY

Up until 1995, most clinical trials of adjuvant chemotherapy in operable NSCLC were inconclusive with regard to survival benefit, with small sample size and selection bias playing a large role. A 1991 national consensus report drew the conclusion that based on available data, there was an unproven benefit of postoperative chemotherapy and any use of it was considered experimental.[4] In 1995 the Non-small Cell Lung Cancer Collaborative Group published a large metaanalysis on 9387 patients from 52 randomized clinical trials.[5] In the 14 trials comparing surgery alone to surgery plus adjuvant chemotherapy, they found that cisplatin-based chemotherapy regimens (cisplatin, doxorubicin, cyclophosphamide [CAP], or cisplatin plus vindesine) as compared with older long-term alkylating agents (mainly CAP and nitrosourea) in combination with surgery, showed a nonstatistically significant absolute survival benefit of 5% at 5 years (hazard ratio [HR] 0.87, 95% confidence interval [CI] 0.74–1.02, $P = .08$). Long-term alkylating regimens, however, actually showed chemotherapy in combination with surgery to be detrimental compared with surgery alone, with a 15% increase in the risk of death.[5] Although not statistically significant, this trend toward improved overall survival (OS) with a cisplatin-based chemotherapy regimen after surgery was encouraging and paved the way for larger randomized phase III trials to further investigate the role of adjuvant cisplatin-based treatment.

The results of the first several randomized phase III trials trying to validate these findings with adjuvant platinum-based regimens were negative. The Eastern Cooperative Oncology Group (ECOG) 3590 study (Intergroup 0115) was a randomized phase III trial of 488 patients after resection of stage II or IIIA NSCLC, assessing the use of adjuvant radiation versus concurrent chemoradiation with cisplatin and etoposide for 4 planned cycles.[6] The primary endpoint was OS. The results were published in 2000 and failed to show a difference between these two groups. The median OS was

Pulmonary Adenocarcinoma: Approaches to Treatment. https://doi.org/10.1016/B978-0-323-55433-6.00003-1

39 months (95% CI 30–52) in the radiation alone group versus 38 months (95% CI 31–42) in the chemoradiation group ($P = .56$). There was also no difference in treatment effect when subgroups were compared according to age (younger than 60 years or older than 60 years), sex, race, stage (II vs. IIIA), ECOG performance status (PS; 0 vs. 1), and the number of operations performed (1 vs. greater than 2). Notably, 31% of patients in the combined chemotherapy plus radiation group were unable to complete all 4 cycles of chemotherapy, with patient refusal and excessive toxicity being the most common reasons. A treatment effect, thus, may have been harder to establish. The authors concluded that there was no evidence of superiority of either regimen and adjuvant chemotherapy should be restricted to clinical trials.[6]

In 2003, the results of the Adjuvant Lung Project Italy (ALPI) study were published.[7] Between 1994 and 1999, 1209 patients with stage I, II, or IIIA resected NSCLC were randomized to chemotherapy with 3 cycles of mitomycin C, vindesine, and cisplatin (MVP) versus no treatment. The primary endpoint was OS, with secondary endpoints being progression-free survival (PFS) and toxicity. The results showed no statistically significant OS difference between the two groups after a follow-up of 64.5 months (HR 0.96, 95% CI 0.81–1.13, $P = .589$). Similarly, there was no difference in PFS (HR = 0.89, 95% CI 0.76–1.03, $P = .128$). However, similar to the ECOG 3590 study, only 69% of patients received the full 3 cycles of MVP, thus poor compliance and toxicity with the treatment regimen were a drawback of the study and likely contributed to the results.[7]

The European Big Lung Trial, published in 2004, was a third negative randomized trial.[8] A total of 381 patients with stage I, II, or III NSCLC were randomized to either 3 cycles of weekly chemotherapy with 4 separate cisplatin-based chemotherapy regimens (cisplatin/vindesine, mitomycin/ifosfamide/cisplatin, mitomycin/vinblastine/cisplatin, or vinorelbine/cisplatin) or observation. Ninety-five percent of patients had a prior complete surgical resection. OS was the primary endpoint. Owing to toxicity, only 60% of patients in the chemotherapy arm were given all 3 cycles of treatment without delay or modifications, and 30% of patients in the chemotherapy arm experienced grade 3 or 4 toxicity. The study failed to show an OS benefit between the arms with a median survival of 33.9 months in the chemotherapy arm and 32.6 months in the observation arm (HR 1.02, 95% CI 0.77–1.35, $P = .90$).[8]

The first large randomized positive adjuvant trial was the International Adjuvant Lung Cancer Trial (IALT),

published in 2004.[9] Here 1867 patients with resected stage I, II, and III NSCLC were randomized to either 3 or 4 cycles of cisplatin-based chemotherapy or observation. At randomization, 36.5% had stage I disease, 24.2% had stage II disease, and 39.3% had stage III disease. Chemotherapy regimens included cisplatin plus either etoposide, vinorelbine, vinblastine or vindesine, with etoposide and vinorelbine given to the majority of patients (56.5% and 26.8%, respectively). A quarter of the patients also received postoperative radiotherapy (27.7% in the control group vs. 22.3% in the chemotherapy group). The primary endpoint was OS, with secondary endpoints being disease-free survival (DFS), second primary cancers, and adverse effects. After a median follow-up of 56 months, 44.5% of patients in the chemotherapy arm versus 40.4% in the observation arm were alive at 5 years (HR for death 0.86, 95% CI 0.76–0.98, $P < .03$). In terms of DFS rate, 39.4% of patients in the chemotherapy arm versus 34.3% in the observation arm were disease free at 5 years (HR 0.83, 95% CI 0.74–0.94, $P < .003$). Higher than previous trials, 73.4% of patients in the chemotherapy arm were compliant with the planned cumulative dosage of cisplatin. The absolute 5-year benefit in survival was 4.1%, consistent with that predicted by the 1995 Nonsmall Cell Lung Cancer Collaborative Group metaanalysis. Subgroup differences between treatment and stage showed that patients receiving etoposide with cisplatin and those with stage III disease appeared to benefit most.[9] Long-term follow-up of this trial, however, showed that patients treated with an adjuvant cisplatin-based regimen had a nonstatistically significant absolute survival benefit at 5 years of 3.9% (HR 0.91, 95% CI 0.81–1.02, $P = .1$), whereas the DFS effect persisted with a significant absolute benefit of 4.3% at 5 years (HR 0.88, 95% CI 0.78–0.98, $P = .02$).[10]

After the IALT trial results, both the National Cancer Institute of Canada (NCIC) JBR.10 and the Adjuvant Navelbine International Trialist Association (ANITA) trial were able to also demonstrate a positive effect of adjuvant cisplatin-based chemotherapy. The JBR.10 trial, published in 2005, enrolled 482 patients, with stage IB or II resected NSCLC, from the United States and Canada and randomized them to adjuvant cisplatin plus vinorelbine for 4 cycles versus observation with a primary endpoint of OS and secondary endpoints of recurrence-free survival (RFS), safety, toxicity, and quality of life.[11] Contrary to previous studies, no patients received any radiation during the course of their therapy. After a median follow-up of 5.1 years (range 1.5–9.3 years) in the chemotherapy group and

5.3 years (range 0.4–9 years) in the observation group, the results showed an OS benefit of 94 months in the chemotherapy arm versus 73 months in the observation arm (HR 0.69, 95% CI 0.52–0.91, $P = .009$). Five-year survival rates were 69% and 54% in the chemotherapy arm and observation arm, respectively, ($P = .03$). The median RFS was not reached in the chemotherapy group versus 46.7 months in the observation group (HR 0.60, 95% CI 0.45–0.79, $P < .001$). Subgroup analysis showed that survival advantage was limited to patients with stage II disease with a 20% 5-year survival benefit (HR 0.59, 95% CI 0.42–0.85, $P = .004$) versus 7% in those with stage IB disease ($P = .79$), although this represented a smaller number of patients. Furthermore, those with RAS mutations also did not appear to benefit from adjuvant chemotherapy (HR 0.95, 95% CI 0.53 to 1.71, $P = .87$).[11]

The long-term follow-up of JBR.10 published in 2010, showed that OS persisted after a median follow-up of 9.3 years (HR 0.78, 95% CI 0.61–0.99, $P = .04$), with an absolute survival benefit at 5 years of 11%.[12] The benefit again appeared to be most pronounced in those patients with stage II disease. As a whole, patients with stage IB disease did not have a statistically significant benefit from chemotherapy (HR 1.03, 95% CI 0.7 to 1.52, $P = 0.87$); however, when stratified according to tumors greater than 4 cm versus those less than 4 cm, there was a trend toward improved survival in patients with larger tumors receiving adjuvant chemotherapy (HR 0.66, 95% CI 0.39–1.14, $P = .113$).[12]

Similar to JBR.10, the ANITA trial was a phase III study that randomized NSCLC patients to 4 cycles of adjuvant cisplatin plus vinorelbine or observation after complete surgical resection.[13] This was an international study from 14 countries with 840 patients randomized with stage IB (36%), II (24%), and IIIA (39%) disease. Postoperative radiotherapy was optional and left to each participating center to decide, although frequently recommended to patients with node-positive disease. OS was the primary endpoint, with secondary endpoints being DFS and safety. After a median follow-up of 76 months, median OS in the chemotherapy arm was 65.7 and 43.7 months in the observation arm (HR 0.80, 95% CI 0.66–0.96, $P = .017$). The absolute OS benefit at 5 years with chemotherapy was 8.6% which was also still evident at 7 years (8.4%). Median DFS was 36.3 months in the chemotherapy arm versus 20.7 months in the observation group (HR 0.76, 95% CI 0.64–0.91, $P = .002$). At 5 years, the absolute DFS benefit of chemotherapy was 8.7%.[13]

Similar to the JBR.10 trial, in patients with stage IB disease there was no difference in 5-year survival, with 62% of patients in the chemotherapy arm alive versus 64% in the control group (HR 1.10, 95% CI 0.76–1.57). However, the test used for survival interaction between tumor stage and chemotherapy was not significant ($P = .07$). With regard to radiation, the decision to give radiation was not randomized, even though patients with N2 disease had a survival benefit in the subgroup descriptive analysis. Adverse events in the chemotherapy arm were similar to those reported previously using vinorelbine, although 2% patients died from treatment toxicity, possibly explained by higher doses used of cisplatin and vinorelbine. The authors concluded a positive survival difference of adjuvant chemotherapy, specifically in those patients with stage II and IIIA disease deriving the most benefit from adjuvant chemotherapy.[13]

Given both the positive and negative OS results of the aforementioned phase III trials, the Lung Adjuvant Cisplatin Evaluation (LACE) trial was a metaanalysis designed to summate these overall effects, specifically identifying treatment options and groups of patients most likely to benefit from adjuvant chemotherapy.[1] The LACE analysis pooled the results of the five largest trials in completely resected patients conducted after the 1995 NSCLC metaanalysis. This included 4584 patients from the ALPI, European Big Lung, IALT, JBR.10, and ANITA trials. Published in 2008, the results confirmed a positive survival benefit of cisplatin-based adjuvant chemotherapy, with a 5-year absolute benefit of 5.4% after a median follow-up of 5.2 years (HR 0.89, 95% CI 0.82–0.96, $P = .005$). DFS was also favored in those who received adjuvant chemotherapy with an absolute benefit of 5.8% at 5 years (HR 0.84, 95% CI 0.78–0.91, $P = .001$).[1]

When assessed by stage, both patients with stage IA (HR 1.41, 95% CI 0.96–2.09) and IB (HR 0.93, 95% CI 0.78–1.10) disease did not derive benefit from adjuvant chemotherapy, whereas those with node-positive or stage II-IIIA disease had a significant positive survival benefit (HR 0.83, 95% CI 0.73–0.95). Comparisons among the different cisplatin-based chemotherapy regimens (cisplatin plus vinorelbine, cisplatin plus etoposide or vinca alkaloid, or cisplatin plus other) overall showed no difference ($P = .11$), although there was a trend towards improved OS with cisplatin plus vinorelbine (HR 0.80, 95% CI 0.70–0.91), but these patients also received higher doses of cisplatin in comparison. There was no change of chemotherapy effect with planned or given radiotherapy for either OS or DFS.[1] The authors concluded that cisplatin-based chemotherapy is of benefit in patients with completely resected early-stage NSCLC.

In 2011, a similar conclusion of survival benefit from adjuvant chemotherapy was made, based on the results of the Non-small Cell Lung Cancer Collaborative Group postoperative chemotherapy metaanalysis.[14] There were two metaanalyses presented. With the primary endpoint being OS, the first metaanalysis assessed 8447 patients from 34 randomized trials starting on or after Jan. 1, 1965 comparing surgery alone to surgery plus adjuvant chemotherapy. The second metaanalysis assessed 2660 patients from 13 trials comparing surgery plus adjuvant chemotherapy and radiotherapy versus surgery plus adjuvant radiotherapy. In the first metaanalysis, an absolute survival increase of 4% at 5 years was found (from 60% to 64%) when chemotherapy was given after surgery (HR 0.86, 95% CI 0.81–0.92, $P < .0001$). The same survival benefit of 4% was also found (from 29% to 33%) in the second metaanalysis when chemotherapy was added to radiotherapy after surgery (HR 0.88, 95% CI 0.81–0.97, $P = .009$). The lower survival rates in the second metaanalysis were thought attributable to inclusion of predominately stage III patients with a higher rate of incomplete resection.[14]

In these metaanalyses, there was no difference among chemotherapy regimens, although the most reliable evidence of benefit came from trials using a combination of cisplatin plus vinorelbine in comparison to the use of older vinca alkaloids (vinblastine, vindesine, and vincristine) or etoposide. The use of tegafur and uracil or tegafur alone in older Asian studies appeared to result in similar benefit to platinum-based regimens, even though it is difficult to apply these data to non-Asian populations.[14] Interestingly, there was no difference in the effect of platinum-based chemotherapy by stage in contrast to previous studies showing a trend toward poorer survival in patients getting adjuvant chemotherapy with stage IA disease and no significant difference in those with stage IB disease.[1]

STAGE I DISEASE

Based on the LACE and Non-small Cell Lung Cancer Collaborative Group metaanalysis, adjuvant chemotherapy remains a recommended postsurgical approach for patients with stage II and IIIA disease, with around a 5% OS benefit. The decision to treat patients with adjuvant chemotherapy for stage I disease is less concrete. Based on the aforementioned data, and the likely detrimental effect of adjuvant chemotherapy on patients with stage IA (T1N0) disease,[1] it is not recommended that these patients receive adjuvant chemotherapy and should proceed with standard surveillance after a complete surgical resection. In patients with stage IB disease

(T2aN0), however, the NCCN guidelines recommend chemotherapy for patients with high-risk disease after a complete or R0 resection (category 2A recommendation). High-risk features include poorly differentiated tumors, use of wedge resection, vascular invasion or visceral pleural involvement, unknown node status, or tumors greater than 4 cm.[2] Data supporting tumor size greater than 4 cm came initially from the Cancer and Leukemia Group B (CALGB) 9633 trial, published in 2008.[15] In this trial, 344 patients with T2N0 NSCLC with complete resection were randomized to 4 cycles of carboplatin plus paclitaxel versus observation, with OS being the primary endpoint. After a median follow-up of 74 months the results showed that survival was not statistically different between the two groups, with a median OS of 95 months in the chemotherapy arm and 78 months in the observation arm (HR 0.83, 95% CI 0.64–1.08, $P = .12$). In the exploratory analysis, however, when patients were divided into those with tumors greater than 4 cm in diameter and less than 4 cm, they found that patients with tumors greater than 4 cm had a statistically significant survival difference in favor of adjuvant chemotherapy over observation, with a 31% reduction in the risk of death and a median survival of 99 months versus 77 months, respectively (HR 0.69, 95% CI 0.48–0.99, $P = .043$).[15]

In the Japan Lung Cancer Research Group (JLCRG) study, 979 patients with resected stage IA and IB NSCLC were randomized to adjuvant oral uracil and tegafur (UFT) for 2 years or observation with the primary endpoint of OS.[16] After a median follow-up of 72 months, the results showed that the 5-year OS was 88% in the UFT group versus 85% in the control group, a statistically significant difference (HR 0.71, 95% CI 0.52–0.98, $P = .04$). This difference was driven by the 27% of patients with stage IB disease where the subgroup analysis showed a significant survival benefit in this group (HR 0.48, 95% CI 0.29–0.81, $P = .005$) versus no survival benefit in the larger subset of patients with stage IA disease (HR 0.97, 95% CI 0.64–1.46, $P = .87$). In addition, they found that patients with tumors greater than 3 cm in size also derived a significant survival benefit in contrast to those less than 3 cm.[16] Based on these data, UFT remains an adjuvant treatment option in Japan, although is not available in Europe and North America.

The results of a smaller third randomized trial in Italy published in 2006 also supported the use of adjuvant chemotherapy in patients with stage IB disease.[17] Here 140 patients with stage IB NSCLC, after surgical resection, were randomized to observation or 6 cycles of chemotherapy with cisplatin and etoposide, with the primary endpoint being OS and secondary endpoint being DFS. The results showed a significant OS difference between the groups, with a median OS of 84.8 months in the chemotherapy arm versus 41.6 months in the control arm ($P = .02$). The 5-year OS rate was 62% versus 42%, with the 10-year OS rate of 44% versus 20% in the chemotherapy and observation arms, respectively. DFS was also significant, with a median difference of 78.4 months in the chemotherapy arm versus 25.6 months in the observation arm ($P = .0001$).[17]

Taken together, these three randomized trials suggest that the subset of stage I patients with larger tumors appear to benefit most from adjuvant chemotherapy. The subgroup analyses of OS benefit in CALGB 9633 and JBR.10 in patients with stage IB tumors greater than 4 cm, and in the JLCRG study of patients with tumors greater than 3 cm, lend support to this [11,15,16]. In clinical practice, a 4-cm cutoff of when to consider adjuvant chemotherapy in stage IB disease is often used. Other factors should be taken into account if the tumor is less than 4 cm as few reproducible and internationally randomized data exist to support the use of adjuvant therapy otherwise in this patient population. The major aforementioned adjuvant phase III trials are reviewed in Table 3.1.

CHOICE OF CHEMOTHERAPY

It is generally agreed on that in North America and Europe, the use of a cisplatin-based doublet regimen is the standard of care when giving adjuvant chemotherapy. Previously mentioned studies have varied greatly in not only the dosage of cisplatin used in their trials but also what chemotherapy agent cisplatin has been paired with. In the LACE metaanalysis there was a trend toward improved OS with cisplatin plus vinorelbine, and this difference was significant when the other combinations in the study were pooled ($P = .04$).[1] However, it still remained unclear what the optimal regimen was, and no conclusion could be drawn regarding the effect of the various cisplatin doses and OS differences.

The E1505 trial was a randomized trial assessing the effect of the addition of bevacizumab to a cisplatin-based doublet on 1501 patients with completely resected NSCLC.[18] Investigators could choose from 4 chemotherapy options to pair with cisplatin: vinorelbine, gemcitabine, and docetaxel in those patients with squamous histology, or any of these agents or pemetrexed for patients with nonsquamous histology. The primary endpoint was OS. Results, first presented

as an abstract in 2016, showed that there was no difference in survival among those patients who got bevacizumab and those who did not. There was also no difference in DFS. Furthermore, there was no OS or DFS difference detected among the 4 different doublet combinations in both squamous and nonsquamous histology. With regard to tolerance, in those patients with nonsquamous histology administered with pemetrexed, it was associated with less grade 3–5 toxicity in comparison to other regimens. The cisplatin plus pemetrexed regimen was also preferred among practitioners when given the opportunity to choose.[18]

A small phase II trial also showed improved tolerability with pemetrexed as a pairing agent with cisplatin in early-stage resected NSCLC. The TREAT study, published in 2013, randomized 132 patients with completely resected stage IB to IIIA NSCLC to 4 cycles of adjuvant cisplatin plus pemetrexed or 4 cycles of cisplatin plus vinorelbine.[19] Forty-three percent had squamous histology and 57%, nonsquamous histology. The primary objective was clinical feasibility rate defined as no grade 4 neutropenia or thrombocytopenia, no thrombocytopenia with bleeding, no grade 3 or 4 febrile neutropenia or nonhematologic toxicity, and no premature withdrawal or death. Feasibility rates were 95.5% in the cisplatin plus pemetrexed arm versus 75.4% in the cisplatin plus vinorelbine arm ($P = .001$). There was also significantly less hematological grade 3 or 4 toxicity in the cisplatin plus pemetrexed arm ($P < .001$), as well as greater delivery of total mean doses of drug given ($P < .0001$). To answer the question of which regimen is superior, the JIPANG study is an ongoing randomized phase III trial in Japan comparing cisplatin plus vinorelbine with cisplatin plus pemetrexed in completed resected nonsquamous NSCLC, with OS being the primary endpoint.[20]

With regard to the use of cisplatin or carboplatin, in a retrospective comparison of adjuvant carboplatin plus paclitaxel to cisplatin plus vinorelbine, 438 patients with completely resected NSCLC were evaluated.[21] Results showed that median OS was not different between the two groups with 5-year OS rates of 73% in those who received carboplatin plus paclitaxel and 71% in those who received cisplatin plus vinorelbine ($P = .71$). There was also no difference in RFS ($P = .68$). The two different regimens brought different toxicities, with myalgias, sensory neuropathy, and alopecia more common in the carboplatin plus paclitaxel group versus vomiting, anemia, neutropenia, and fatigue more common in the cisplatin plus vinorelbine group. There was also more discontinuation of treatment and dose reduction in the cisplatin plus

TABLE 3.1
Phase III Adjuvant Trials

Trial	Included Stage	Adjuvant Comparison	Radiation Given	N	Primary Endpoint	Result	*P*-value
ECOG 3590[6]	II and IIIA	Concurrent cisplatin/etoposide x4 cycles + XRT vs. XRT alone	Yes	488	OS	No significant difference in survival	0.56
ALPI[7]	I, II, and IIIA	Mitomycin C/vindesine/ cisplatin x3 cycles vs. observation	Optional	1209	OS	5-year 1% OS benefit in the chemo arm	0.589
European Big Lung Trial[8]	I, II, and III	Cisplatin + either vindesine, mitomycin/ ifosfamide, mitocycin/ vinblastine or vinorelbine x3 cycles vs. observation	Optional	381	OS	2-year OS rate of 58% in the chemo arm versus 60% in the obs arm	0.90
IALT[9]	I, II, and III	Cisplatin + either etoposide, vinorelbine, vinblastine or vindesine x3-4 cycles vs. observation	Optional	1867	OS	5-year OS rate of 44.5% in the chemo arm versus 40.4% in the obs arm	<0.03
JBR.10[11]	IB and II	Cisplatin/vinorelbine x4 cycles vs. observation	No	482	OS	5-year OS rate of 69% in the chemo arm versus 54% in the obs arm	0.03
ANITA[13]	IB, II, and IIIA	Cisplatin/vinorelbine x4 cycles vs. observation	Optional	840	OS	5-year 8.6% OS benefit in the chemo arm	0.017
CALGB 9633[15]	IB	Carboplatin/ paclitaxel x4 cycles vs. observation	No	344	OS	5-year OS rate of 60% in the chemo arm versus 58% in the obs arm	0.125
JLCRG[16]	IA and IB	Uracil/tegafur x2 years vs. observation	No	979	OS	5-year OS rate of 88% in the chemo arm versus 85% in the obs arm	0.04

ALPI, Adjuvant Lung Project Italy; *ANITA*, Adjuvant Navelbine International Trialist Association; *chemo*, chemotherapy; *IALT*, International Adjuvant Lung Cancer Trial; *JLCRG*, Japan Lung Cancer Research Group; *N*, number of patients enrolled; *obs*, observation; *versus*, versus; *OS*, overall survival; *XRT*, radiation therapy.

vinorelbine arm. The authors concluded that despite this not being prospective data, carboplatin plus paclitaxel can be considered as an effective and well tolerated adjuvant therapy regimen.

Although retrospective data suggest potential equivalency between cisplatin and carboplatin, cisplatin remains the preferred platinum agent of choice in the adjuvant setting. The CALGB 9633 trial is the only randomized reported study using carboplatin, with long-term follow-up not confirming an OS benefit in the stage IB patient population as a whole.[15] Carboplatin may be considered on an individual basis, specifically in patients with contraindications to getting cisplatin, such as significant baseline hearing loss, neuropathy, or those less likely to tolerate the higher emetogenic profile of cisplatin. Depending on how one defines elderly, it is reasonable to extrapolate that carboplatin may also be a better tolerated agent in the elderly. Not enough data in the adjuvant setting exist though for direct comparison between cisplatin and carboplatin in this subpopulation. In the LACE metaanalysis, 9% of patients who were at least 70 years old had no increase in severe toxicity rates of cisplatin-based therapy, although they also did not have a significant OS benefit (HR 0.90, 95% CI 0.70—1.16, $P = .29$). Also in the LACE metaanalysis, a significant increase of chemotherapy benefit was observed in patients with better PS as the use of chemotherapy in those patients with a PS of 2 appeared detrimental.[1] Cisplatin can be considered in the elderly, although with significant caution and particular attention to comorbidities and PS.

Overall, it still remains inconclusive which chemotherapy agent is best paired with cisplatin and the ideal dosage of cisplatin in the adjuvant setting. The NCCN guidelines recommend 4 cycles of a cisplatin-based doublet after complete surgical resection, with cisplatin doses used being 50 mg/m^2 on days 1 and 8 every 28 days 75—100 mg/m^2 on day 1 every 21 days depending on the doublet combination used.[2] In nonsquamous histology, pemetrexed appears to have the least toxicity and is most preferred by practitioners, with the E1505 trial showing no apparent OS or DFS difference between doublet regimens, although this was not the primary aim of the study. The JIPANG study is ongoing,[20] directly comparing vinorelbine to pemetrexed, and will be informative when results are available. Historically, the most experience and survival data are known with vinorelbine. In squamous histology, vinorelbine, gemcitabine, docetaxel, and etoposide are all feasible options and present various toxicity profiles. In patients unable to tolerate cisplatin, carboplatin remains an appropriate substitute.

ADJUVANT RADIATION THERAPY

The role of postoperative radiation therapy (PORT) remains a controversial topic in early-stage NSCLC, specifically in stage IIIA disease. Many of the aforementioned large adjuvant trials included radiotherapy as part of the treatment algorithm along with chemotherapy after complete resection but were not randomized and underpowered to deliberately ask the question of added benefit of PORT versus surgery alone. In 1998, the PORT Meta-analysis Trialists Group

published a metaanalysis of data on 2128 patients from nine randomized trials assessing the effect of patients assigned to PORT versus surgery alone.[22] Radiation doses ranged from 30 to 60 Gy and delivered more than 10—30 fractions on varying schedules with most of the patients being male with stage II-III squamous cell carcinoma.

At a median follow-up of 3.9 years, there was an overall significant adverse effect of PORT on survival (HR 1.21, 95% CI 1.08—1.34, $P = .001$), with a 21% relative increase in the risk of death and 7% drop in survival at 2 years from 55% to 48%. Local RFS favored surgery alone (HR 1.16, 95% CI 1.05—1.29, $P = .005$) and distant RFS as well (HR 1.16, 95% CI 1.04—1.29, $P = .007$). In the subgroup analysis, there was no difference between PORT and surgery alone in terms of age, sex, or tumor histology. When stratified according to the stage and nodal status, patients with stage I and II or N0—N1 disease receiving PORT had worsened survival in comparison to those with stage III or N2 disease, where PORT had no clear detrimental effect (HR 0.97 and 0.96 for stage III and N2 disease, respectively). The authors concluded that no subgroup showed evidence of benefit from PORT and that it should not be routinely recommended in early-stage NSCLC.[22]

An updated systemic Cochrane review was published in 2016 on PORT in NSCLC by the PORT Meta-analysis Trialists Group, confirming the previous 1998 report.[23] Fourteen adjuvant trials were identified evaluating surgery versus surgery plus radiotherapy with data from 11 of the 14 trials available with 2343 total patients analyzed. The results again showed a significant adverse effect of PORT on survival (HR 1.18, 95% CI 1.07—1.31, $P = .001$) with an 18% relative increase in the risk of death and absolute detriment of 5% at 2 years from 58% to 52%. In subgroup analyses, there was no differential effect of PORT based on age ($P = .67$), sex ($P = .49$), histology ($P = .38$), nodal status ($P = .39$), or stage ($P = .12$).

When looking at modern radiotherapy techniques with linear accelerators versus older cobalt machines, for those trials with only linear accelerators, there was no difference in survival (HR 1.02, 95% CI 0.80—1.31, $P = .85$).[23] In contrast, a review of three randomized controlled trials and eight retrospective trials suggested an OS benefit of PORT when radiotherapy was given only with the use of linear accelerators in patients with N2 disease (HR 0.77, 95% CI 0.62—0.92, $P = .02$). An improvement in local regional RFS was also seen (HR 0.51, 95% CI 0.41—0.65, $P < .001$).[24] A separate metaanalysis of 2387 patients from 11 phase III trials investigated the effect of modern techniques of PORT on OS and local recurrence (LR).[25] All 11 trials were included for OS analysis, and eight trials were included for LR analysis. As a whole, there was no improvement in OS with PORT (relative risk [RR] 1.02, 95% CI 0.84–1.24, $P = .84$), although PORT did significantly improve OS and decrease LR when given with only linear accelerators (RR 0.76, 95% CI 0.61–0.95, $P = .02$ and RR 0.31, 95% CI 0.12–0.79, $P = .01$, respectively). In the four trials of patients with N2 disease primarily treated with induction chemotherapy and surgery, the mean LR rate at first relapse at 5 years was 29.4%. The authors estimated that in patients with stage IIIA or N2 disease, linear accelerator–based PORT could increase OS by 13%, which parallels that seen in the subset analysis of the ANITA trial with patients with N2 disease, where PORT after complete resection and adjuvant chemotherapy resulted in a 5-year increase in OS of 13% (from 34% to 47%).[13]

In summary, PORT still has no standard role in early-stage NSCLC and is likely detrimental in those with stage I and II disease. In patients with stage IIIA or pathological N2 disease the added value of PORT is less clear, with some retrospective and nonrandomized studies suggesting a survival benefit in this patient subgroup. To help definitively answer the question of PORT benefit, the randomized phase III Lung Adjuvant Radiotherapy Trial is ongoing, comparing modern three-dimensional conformal PORT with no PORT in patients with resected pathological N2 NSCLC.[26] It should be noted that in most patients with clinical N2 disease without prior treatment, the recommended therapeutic approach remains definitive concurrent chemoradiation.[2]

NEOADJUVANT CHEMOTHERAPY

The data on the use of neoadjuvant chemotherapy in early-stage NSCLC as compared with adjuvant chemotherapy are less robust as larger trials were stopped when the benefit of adjuvant chemotherapy emerged. Nonetheless, several trials completed to date have shown a positive OS benefit of neoadjuvant therapy. In general, the potential advantages of neoadjuvant therapy include increased compliance, treatment of micrometastatic disease, and downstaging of tumors to enhance the possibility of an R0 resection. Potential disadvantages include delaying surgery and the possibility of increased morbidity before and after surgery.

In the 1990s there were two smaller randomized trials both terminated early based on a significant benefit of neoadjuvant chemotherapy. In 1994 the results of a

randomized trial comparing perioperative chemotherapy and surgery with surgery alone in resectable stage IIIA NSCLC were reported.[27] Sixty patients were randomized to receive 6 cycles of cisplatin/CAP/etoposide and surgery or surgery alone. Results showed that patients undergoing perioperative chemotherapy and surgery had an estimated median OS of 64 months versus 11 months in those who had surgery alone ($P < .008$). There was a 3-year survival rate of 56% in those getting perioperative chemotherapy versus 15% in those undergoing surgery alone.[27] In 1999 the 7-year follow-up of 60 patients randomized to three cycles of neoadjuvant cisplatin/mitomycin/isofamide followed by surgery or surgery alone reported a median OS of 22 months in the chemotherapy arm versus 10 months in the surgery alone arm ($P = .005$). This translated into a 5-year OS rate of 17% in the chemotherapy arm versus 0% in the surgery alone arm.[28]

In 2006, a systemic review and metaanalysis of seven randomized trials and 988 patients showed a 6% absolute OS benefit of neoadjuvant chemotherapy in operable NSCLC (HR 0.82, 95% CI 0.69–0.97, $P = .02$).[29] This was seen across all stages of disease, increasing survival from 14% to 20% at 5 years. All chemotherapy regimens were platinum based and included cisplatin or carboplatin plus either a vinca alkaloid, etoposide, taxane or other. There was no difference seen between chemotherapy regimens ($P = .99$).[29]

As most of the trials included in the systemic review were smaller trials, two of the larger trials, Southwest Oncology Group (SWOG) trial S990 and Chemotherapy for Early Stages Trial (CHEST), would later publish updated results in 2010 and 2012, respectively, which held clinical significance. The SWOG S990 trial included 354 patients with stage IB-IIIA NSCLC randomized to 3 cycles of neoadjuvant carboplatin/paclitaxel followed by surgery or surgery alone.[30] The primary endpoint was OS. The trial was closed early as reports of the survival benefit of adjuvant chemotherapy began surfacing and changing the landscape of treatment of early-stage NSCLC. The results, nonetheless, showed a nonstatistically significant survival benefit of 62 months in the neoadjuvant chemotherapy arm versus 41 months in the surgery alone arm (HR 0.79, 95% CI 0.60–1.06, $P = .11$). The median PFS was also not significant (HR 0.80, 95% CI 0.61–1.04, $P = .10$).[30]

In CHEST, 270 patients with stages IB, II, or IIIA NSCLC were randomized to 3 cycles of preoperative cisplatin plus gemcitabine followed by surgery or surgery alone.[31] The primary endpoint was PFS. Cisplatin plus gemcitabine was chosen based on encouraging phase II data in patients with stage IIIA NSCLC, showing around a 70% response rate with this platinum-based doublet, a median OS of 18.9 months, and 1-year estimated survival of 69%.[32] The results favored the chemotherapy arm with a median PFS of 4 years in the neoadjuvant chemotherapy plus surgery arm versus 2.9 years in the surgery alone arm (adjusted HR 0.70, 95% CI 0.50–0.97, $P = .03$). OS was also significantly longer for those getting neoadjuvant chemotherapy with a median OS of 7.8 years versus 4.8 years for surgery alone (adjusted HR 0.63, 95% CI 0.43–0.92, $P = .02$). Subgroup analysis by stage showed a significant PFS and OS benefit in those patients with stage IIB/IIIA disease, but not stage IB/IIA, thought to be attributed to a lack of power.[31]

Two large metaanalyses maintained a significant positive benefit of neoadjuvant chemotherapy. In 2010 an updated metaanalysis of 13 randomized trials reported an overall significant survival benefit of neoadjuvant chemotherapy over surgery alone (HR 0.84, 95% CI 0.77–0.92, $P = .0001$).[33] A subgroup analysis of eight of the trials with survival data on patients with stage III disease also showed a significant benefit of neoadjuvant chemotherapy (HR 0.84, 95% CI 0.75–0.95, $P = .005$).[33] The largest metaanalysis to date was published in 2014 by the NSCLC Meta-Analysis Collaborative Group.[34] Here data from 2385 patients and 15 randomized studies reported a 5-year absolute survival benefit of 5% in patients receiving neoadjuvant chemotherapy from 40% to 45% (HR 0.87, 95% CI 0.78–0.96, $P = .007$). Neoadjuvant chemotherapy also had a significant benefit on time to distant recurrence (HR 0.69, 95% CI 0.58–0.82, $P < .0001$) and RFS (HR 0.85, 95% CI 0.76–0.94, $P = .002$). There was no clear difference between subgroups according to age, sex, histology, clinical stage, or chemotherapy regimen.[34]

Given the presented data on both adjuvant and neoadjuvant chemotherapy in early-stage NSCLC and the similar 5% OS benefit derived from either approach, it has been debated whether preoperative or postoperative chemotherapy is clinically more appropriate. The Neoadjuvant vs. Adjuvant Taxol/Carbo Hope (NATCH) trial was designed to try to help answer this question.[35] The NATCH trial enrolled 624 patients with stage IA (tumor size > 2 cm), IB, II, or T3N1 disease and randomized them to one of the three arms: surgery alone, 3 cycles of neoadjuvant carboplatin/paclitaxel followed by surgery, or surgery followed by 3 cycles of adjuvant carboplatin/paclitaxel. The primary endpoint was DFS. The results showed no significant difference among the three arms with 5-year DFS rates of 34.1% in the surgery arm, 38.3% in the preoperative chemotherapy arm,

and 36.6% in the postoperative chemotherapy arm. There was a nonsignificant trend toward improved DFS when preoperative chemotherapy was compared with surgery alone (HR 0.92, 95% CI 0.81–1.04, $P = .17$) and no significant benefit when adjuvant chemotherapy was compared with surgery alone (HR 0.96, 95% CI 0.75–1.22, $P = .74$). No difference in OS was seen across the arms. Of note, 90% of patients in the preoperative arm completed 3 cycles of chemotherapy compared with 61% of patients in the postoperative arm. The authors noted that the negative results of the study may partly be explained by the high rate of stage I patients enrolled in each arm who are less likely as a group to benefit from chemotherapy. The study as a whole may also have been underpowered to detect small clinically meaningful differences among the arms.[35]

A second randomized trial assessing 528 patients with stage I-II NSCLC compared a planned 4 cycles of preoperative chemotherapy (PRE group) with either cisplatin/gemcitabine or carboplatin/paclitaxel with 2 cycles of preoperative chemotherapy with the same regimens followed by 2 cycles of postoperative chemotherapy (PERI group).[36] The third and fourth cycles were given only to responders in each case. The results failed to show a difference between the two approaches, with a 3-year OS of 67.4% in the PRE group versus 67.7% in the PERI group (HR 1.01, 95% CI 0.79–1.30, $P = .92$). There was also no difference in response rates, DFS, toxicity, or postoperative mortality between the two chemotherapy regimens.[36]

In conclusion, despite there being positive OS data on giving neoadjuvant chemotherapy in early-stage NSCLC, this has been mostly replaced by the aforementioned adjuvant chemotherapy data, for which there have been a greater number of larger randomized trials. There is no clear clinical survival benefit of one approach over the other, but adjuvant chemotherapy with 4 cycles of cisplatin-based chemotherapy after complete surgical resection continues to be the preferred clinical algorithm in patients with stage IIB and IIIA NSCLC and in patients with stage IB disease with tumors greater than 4 cm. Neoadjuvant therapy remains a consideration though, particularly in patients with single-station N2 disease as a means of downstaging the tumor to enhance complete surgical resection or in those patients where there is increased concern regarding compliance of chemotherapy after surgery. The timing of when to start adjuvant therapy is not definite, but most experts agree that treatment should start within 8 weeks after surgery as this was the general timeframe used in most adjuvant trials.

MOLECULARLY TARGETED THERAPY

Interest in the use of molecularly targeted therapies in the adjuvant setting of early-stage NSCLC was inspired by the success of these agents in patients with advanced NSCLC, whereby the identification of specific driver mutations in these patients has changed the algorithm of how advanced NSCLC is treated. Studies have shown that more than 60% of NSCLC patients have at least one oncogenic driver with around a quarter of those tumors having actionable mutations. Mutations in the epidermal growth factor receptor (EGFR) and translocations in the echinoderm microtubule–associated protein–like 4 anaplastic lymphoma kinase (EML4-ALK) domain represent the most notable targetable mutations, occurring in approximately 15%–17% and 4%–8%, respectively, of patients with NSCLC in the United States.[37,38] In Asian countries, however, EGFR mutations occur much more frequently, and in one prospective study of 1482 patients from seven Asian regions with advanced adenocarcinoma of the lung, an EGFR mutation was identified in 51.4% of tumors.[39] With the use of gefitinib, erlotinib, and afatinib in patients harboring an EGFR exon 21 missense (L858 R) or exon 19 deletion mutation, compared with first-line platinum-based chemotherapy, the use of these EGFR inhibitors in treatment-naïve advanced NSCLC patients has shown both an improved response rate and PFS benefit in several randomized phase III trials.[40–44] In addition, results of the phase III FLAURA trial that found the third-generation EGFR inhibitor osimertinib to have superior PFS benefit when compared directly with older generation gefitinib or erlotinib in EGFR TKI–naïve advanced NSCLC patients, has led to an additional new standard of care option in the frontline setting.[45]

Similarly, the ALK inhibitors crizotinib and ceritinib have also shown a substantial improved response rate and PFS benefit over chemotherapy in patients with treatment-naïve advanced NSCLC that found to have an ALK translocation.[46,47] Furthermore, when the newer second-generation ALK inhibitor alectinib was directly compared with the older generation first-in-class crizotinib in the frontline in advanced ALK rearranged NSCLC, a significant PFS benefit and longer time to central nervous system progression were seen.[48] Significant crossover in frontline trials with EGFR and ALK inhibitors compared with standard chemotherapy likely explains the lack of OS benefit seen in these trials. However, as a whole these agents have undoubtedly prolonged survival and widened the treatment options in EGFR- and ALK-mutated patients with advanced disease.

With significant data existing in the unresectable/metastatic setting, the concept of applying these agents to the adjuvant setting became relevant. Most data at present exist regarding the adjuvant use of EGFR inhibitors, with the earliest data on adjuvant EGFR TKI treatment in early-stage resected NSCLC coming from retrospective and nonrandomized trials. In a retrospective impact on DFS analysis published by Memorial Sloan-Kettering in 2011 of 167 patients with EGFR mutated completely resected stage I to III NSCLC, patient outcomes in those receiving adjuvant EFGR TKI therapy were reviewed using a prospectively maintained surgical database.[49] In the patient cohort of 167 patients 56% had an exon 19 deletion, 44% had an exon 21 (L858R) missense mutation, and 33% of patients received a perioperative TKI with erlotinib or gefitinib. Seventy percent of patients had stage I resected disease, whereas the adjuvant group who received erlotinib or gefitinib had a higher proportion of stage III patients. Thirty-nine percent in the adjuvant group received cisplatin-based chemotherapy versus 21% in the group not given a TKI. The results showed that patients treated with a perioperative TKI had a trend toward improved DFS, with a 2-year DFS rate of 89% compared with 72% for patients who were not treated with a perioperative TKI (HR 0.53, 95% CI 0.28–1.03, $P = .06$). The 2-year OS rate was 96% in the TKI-treated group versus 90% in the group not receiving a TKI (HR 0.62, 95% CI 0.26–1.51, $P = .296$).[49] This analysis provided a framework for future trials to further investigate the effect of adjuvant TKI therapy in patients with resected EGFR-mutated NSCLC.

The SELECT study presented for the first time in 2012 was a multicenter phase II nonrandomized prospective study evaluating adjuvant erlotinib in 100 patients with resected stage IA-IIIA EGFR-mutated NSCLC.[50] Enrolled patients received erlotinib 150 mg daily for 2 years after completion of any standard adjuvant chemotherapy and/or radiation treatment. The preliminary results after a median follow-up of 3.4 years showed that the 2-year DFS was 89%, consistent with prior reported DFS data. Although this represented phase II data without a comparator arm and did include patients with stage IA disease, these were the first prospective data to suggest that adjuvant targeted therapy may be of benefit.

Another small Chinese phase II trial published in 2014 randomized 60 patients with EGFR-mutated, resected stage IIIA NSCLC receiving 4 cycles of adjuvant carboplatin/pemetrexed to additionally receive gefitinib or placebo for 6 months after chemotherapy.[51]

The primary endpoint was DFS. The results showed a significant 2-year DFS of 39.8 months in those patients receiving the addition of gefitinib to chemotherapy versus 27 months in those who did not receive TKI (HR 0.37, 95% CI 0.16–0.85, $P = .014$). At 2 years, the OS data were immature, with 92% alive in the chemotherapy plus gefitinib arm versus 77% in the chemotherapy arm alone (HR 0.37, 95% CI 0.12–1.11, $P = .076$). The trial was not powered to assess an OS benefit.

With encouraging phase II data, phase III trials were already underway assessing for adjuvant EGFR TKI therapy benefit. The NCIC BR.19 trial was the first randomized double-blind phase III trial assessing adjuvant EGFR TKI therapy in patients with resected stage IB-IIIA NSCLC.[52] However, the trial was terminated early due to safety concerns after the Iressa Survival Evaluation in Lung Cancer trial comparing gefitinib with placebo in patients with refractory advanced NSCLC showed no survival benefit with gefitinib, and the SWOG S0023 trial assessing maintenance gefitinib after chemoradiation in unresectable stage III NSCLC failed to improve OS and appeared potentially harmful.[53,54] A total of 503 of the planned 1242 patients were randomized to 2 years of adjuvant gefitinib or placebo after surgical resection and optional adjuvant chemotherapy of which only 17% of patients received. The primary endpoints were OS, DFS, and toxicity. Patients were not selected for EGFR mutations, and only 15 patients were found to have EGFR-mutated tumors. In this small subgroup, exploratory analysis showed that there was no significant benefit seen on DFS (HR 1.84, 95% CI 0.44–7.73, $P = .40$) or OS (HR 3.16, 95% CI 0.61–16.45; $P = .15$). The trial overall was also negative, and owing to several limitations, most notably small sample size of EGFR-mutated patients, no definitive conclusion on adjuvant EGFR therapy could be drawn.[52]

In contrast to the BR.19 trial the RADIANT trial was a randomized double-blind phase III trial that selected patients with stage IB-IIIA NSCLC who were EGFR positive by overexpression of EGFR protein by immunohistochemistry (IHC) or EGFR gene amplified by fluorescence in situ hybridization (FISH) and randomized them to adjuvant erlotinib 150 mg daily for 2 years or placebo after surgical resection and optional adjuvant chemotherapy.[55] Evaluating EGFR status by IHC and FISH is no longer considered significant biomarkers, and the trial included only 161 patients of the 973 patients randomized with deletion exon 19 or L858 R activating EGFR mutations, which are known to predict response to EGFR TKIs. More than half of the total patients got adjuvant chemotherapy. The primary endpoint was DFS.

In the overall group, there was no difference in DFS (HR 0.90, 95% CI 0.74–1.10, $P = .324$). In the subgroup of EGFR-mutated patients, DFS favored erlotinib, with a median DFS of 46.4 months in the erlotinib group versus 28.5 months in the placebo group (HR 0.61, 95% CI 0.38–0.98, $P = .039$). This was not statistically significant due to the trial's hierarchical design, making no subgroup analysis significant if the primary endpoint in the overall analysis was negative. Of note, of the EGFR-mutated patients, there was a significantly higher percentage of stage IIIA patients in the placebo arm (30.5%) versus the erlotinib arm (17.6%), which may account for the DFS difference seen. The OS data, although remain immature, thus far do not favor the erlotinib arm in the EGFR-mutant subgroup.[55]

In patients with EGFR-mutated NSCLC in the aforementioned trials, none of the trials was designed to ask the question of whether an EGFR TKI should be used in addition to or in replacement of platinum-based chemotherapy. The ADJUVANT trial (CTONG 1104) was designed to answer the question of whether patients with EGFR-activating mutations (exon 19 deletion or exon 21 L858R mutation) had superior DFS with targeted EGFR TKI therapy or chemotherapy. A total of 222 Asian patients with completely resected stage II-IIIA NSCLC with an EGFR-activating mutation were randomized 1:1 to gefitinib 250 mg daily for 2 years or cisplatin plus vinorelbine for up to 4 cycles.[56] The primary endpoint was DFS, with secondary endpoints being OS, safety, and quality of life measures. Nearly two-thirds of patients in each arm had stage IIIA disease. After a median follow-up of 36.5 months, those randomized to gefitinib had a significantly longer DFS of 28.7 months versus 18 months in those getting chemotherapy (HR 0.60, 95% CI 0.42–0.87, $P = .005$). Grade 3 or higher adverse events were less common in those getting gefitinib, and quality of life measures were also improved compared with chemotherapy. OS data remain immature, although the trial investigators concluded that in those patients with stage II-IIIA NSCLC undergoing adjuvant therapy after resected disease, if an activating EGFR mutation is present, gefitinib should be considered an important treatment option.[56]

The ADJUVANT trial was the first trial directly comparing chemotherapy with EGFR-targeted therapy. Compared with the BR.19 and RADIANT trials that had several limitations and lacked conclusive evidence of adjuvant EGFR TKI benefit, this trial design is the most informative to date for patient care in patients with resected early-stage EGFR-mutated NSCLC. As the trial took place exclusively in Asia and there are yet any mature OS data, the question remains whether the data are generalizable to the larger international population and also whether this should replace standard of care chemotherapy in the adjuvant setting which has a known approximately 5% OS benefit. If DFS does not translate into an OS benefit, one may question the utility of EGFR TKI therapy as cure is the goal in the adjuvant setting, and OS is a paramount endpoint. The adjuvant EGFR TKI phase III trials are summarized in Table 3.2.

There still remain several questions about whether to randomize patients after chemotherapy to TKI treatment or to use TKI treatment in replace of chemotherapy, what the optimal duration of TKI treatment should be, whether a first-generation EGFR TKI or subsequent generation TKI is better, and whether stage IB patients should be included in the trials or just stage II-IIIA. Future trials are working to answer some of these questions with several ongoing phase III adjuvant EGFR trials underway and detailed in Table 3.3. The IMPACT (WJOG6401 L) trial in Japan is similar in design to the ADJUVANT trial, comparing the use of 2 years of gefitinib with 4 cycles of cisplatin/vinorelbine in stage II-IIIA resected NSCLC. In both the ICTAN (NCT01996098) and ICWIP (NCT02125240) trials the use of icotonib versus observation is being evaluated after resection and adjuvant chemotherapy. To address the question

of the optimal duration of therapy with an adjuvant EGFR TKI, in the United States, a phase II study is assessing the use of afatinib for 3 months or 2 years in patients with resected stage I-III EGFR-mutated NSCLC (NCT01746251).

The most pivotal of these trials is likely the Adjuvant Lung Cancer Enrichment Marker Identification and Sequencing Trial (ALCHEMIST) that is a three-trial integrated study of adjuvant treatment in stage IB-IIIA resected non-squamous NSCLC. After surgery and optional chemotherapy, patients are undergoing randomization to 2 years of erlotinib or placebo if they carry an EGFR mutation, 2 years of crizotinib or placebo if they carry an ALK rearrangement, or 1 year of nivolumab or observation if they are wildtype for both EGFR and ALK, with OS being the primary endpoint. With a target enrollment of several thousand patients, results of this trial will not be available for many years.[57]

Regarding patients with ALK-positive resected NSCLC, there have been no prospective trials reported to date using ALK inhibitors in the adjuvant setting. Interestingly, it has been reported that patients with early-stage resected ALK-positive NSCLC may have inferior outcomes compared with those that are wildtype. In a study of 300 patients identified from the Mayo Clinic Lung Cancer Cohort, patients with ALK-positive disease by IHC and FISH had higher histologic-grade

TABLE 3.2
Phase III Adjuvant EKGF TKI Trials

Trial	Included Stage	N	Selected for EGFR Mutation	Adjuvant Treatment	Primary Endpoint	Primary Result	P-value
BR.19[52]	IB-IIIA	503 (15 with EGFR mutations)	No	Gefitinib x2 years vs. placebo after optional chemo	OS and DFS	OS 5.1 years (gefitinib) vs. NR (placebo); DFS 4.2 years (gefitinib) vs. NR (placebo)	0.14 (OS) and 0.15 (DFS)
Radiant[55]	IB-IIIA	973 (161 with EGFR mutation)	No, selected by positive EGFR overexpression	Erlotinib x2 years vs. placebo after optional chemo	DFS	50.5 mo (erlotinib) vs. 48.2 mo (chemo)	0.324
Adjuvant[56]	II-IIIA	222	Yes	Gefitinib x2 years vs. cisplatin/ vinorelbine x4 cycles	DFS	28.7 mo (gefitinib) vs. 18 mo (chemo)	0.005

chemo, chemotherapy; *DFS*, disease-free survival; *EGFR*, epidermal growth factor receptor; *mo*; months; *N*, number of patients enrolled; *NR*, not reached; *OS*, overall survival.

TABLE 3.3
Ongoing Phase III Adjuvant EGFR TKI Trials in EGFR-Mutated NSCLC

Trial	Included Stage	Adjuvant Treatment	N	Primary Endpoint
IMPACT WJOG6401 L	II-IIIA	Gefitinib x2 years vs. cisplatin/ vinorelbine x4 cycles	230	DFS
ICTAN NCT01996098	IIA-IIIA	Icotinib x6 months or 12 months vs. placebo after 4 cycles of adjuvant platinum-based chemo	477	DFS
ICWIP NCT02125240	II-IIIA	Icotinib vs. placebo after 4 cycles of adjuvant platinum-based chemo	300	DFS
EVIDENCE NCT02448797	II-IIIA	Icotinib until progression vs. cisplatin/ vinorelbine x4 cycles	320	DFS
ADAURA NCT02511106	IB-IIIA	Osimertinib vs. placebo (adjuvant chemo optional)	700	DFS
ALCHEMIST A081105	IB-IIIA	Erlotinib vs. placebo x2 years (adjuvant chemo optional)	450	OS

ALCHEMIST, Adjuvant Lung Cancer Enrichment Marker Identification and Sequencing Trial; *chemo*, chemotherapy; *DFS*, disease-free survival; *N*, estimated patient enrollment; *OS*, overall survival.

tumors, a doubling of their 5-year risk of progression ($P = .0071$), and an increased rate of brain and liver metastasis compared with those who had ALK-negative tumors.[58] Although several newer ALK inhibitors have been approved in the metastatic setting since this study was published, further investigation of ALK inhibitors in the adjuvant setting remains a significant unmet need. The phase III ALCHEMIST trial randomizing patients with an ALK rearrangement after surgery to crizotinib or placebo for 2 years (adjuvant chemotherapy optional) is ongoing. It is anticipated that other ALK TKIs will also be explored in the adjuvant setting.

Further attempts at adjuvant targeted therapy with vascular endothelial growth factor blockers such as bevacizumab have not been shown to be beneficial. As mentioned previously, the E1505 study showed no DFS benefit or OS benefit when bevacizumab was added to standard platinum-based chemotherapy.[18] Although interest has grown significantly in the use of molecularly targeted therapy in NSCLC, no data thus far have been shown to induce an OS benefit. The ADJUVANT trial in EGFR-mutated NSCLC appears potentially promising with a DFS benefit of gefitinib over chemotherapy, with OS data immature at this time. Several other phase III trials are currently underway, thus testing patient tumors for EGFR mutations, and the EML4-ALK translocation in the adjuvant setting has value to enhance trial enrollment and further enrich the field of adjuvant targeted therapy options for patients with driver mutations.

IMMUNOTHERAPY

Much is still to be learned about the use of adjuvant and neoadjuvant immunotherapy in NSCLC. While initially being an exciting potential treatment avenue, the use of cancer vaccines has not been shown to be of benefit in patients with resected early-stage NSCLC. The melanoma-associated antigen-A3 (MAGE-A3) is known to be expressed in 30%–50% of NSCLC patients, with higher expression in squamous than non-squamous NSCLC. It is a tumor-specific antigen, only expressed in the testis and placenta of normal adult tissue, thus has represented a good target for the creation of a tumor vaccine. In the randomized, double-blind phase III MAGRIT trial, 2312 patients with completely resected stage IB-IIIA MAGE-A3–positive NSCLC were randomized 2:1 to receive a MAGE-A3–directed tumor vaccine for 13 injections versus placebo during 27 months.[59] Fifty-two percent of patients who enrolled received adjuvant chemotherapy initially. After a median follow-up of 38.1 months in the MAGE-A3 group and 39.5 months in the placebo group, there was no difference in the median DFS (HR 1.02, 95% CI 0.89–1.18, $P = .74$). The median DFS in the vaccine-treated group was 60.5 months versus 57.9 months in the control group. In the subgroup analysis there was also no difference in DFS between those patients that additionally received chemotherapy (HR 1.10, 95% CI 0.90–1.34, $P = .36$) and those who just received the vaccine after resection (HR 0.97, 95% CI 0.80–1.18, $P = .76$). As a result of the trial, further development of the vaccine was halted, and no further adjuvant vaccine trials are currently underway.[59]

Part of the rationale for the use of immunotherapy in the adjuvant treatment of postoperative NSCLC came from a metaanalysis of four randomized controlled trials comparing adoptive immunotherapy (AI) with control therapies in postoperative NSCLC patients.[60] A total of 472 patients, the majority of whom had stage IIIA disease, were evaluated. Control arms of the trials included patients treated with chemotherapy alone, chemotherapy or radiation therapy, or chemotherapy plus or minus radiotherapy. Those in the AI arm were treated with activated killer T-cells and dendritic cells (AKT-DC), DCs and cytokine-induced killer cells (DC-CIK), lymphokine-activated killer cells and interleukin-2 (LAK-IL-2), and tumor-infiltrating lymphocytes and recombinant IL-2 (TIL-rIL-2). The OS analysis showed that patients receiving an AI treatment had a 39% reduction in the RR of death compared with those in the control arm (HR 0.61, 95% CI 0.45−0.84, $P = .002$). Although there were significant limitations to the study including different AI protocols some of which included the addition of chemotherapy, a lack of reported HRs, and the inclusion of stage IV non-curative resection cases, the results were, nonetheless, encouraging and provided rationale to conduct larger prospective randomized trials.[60]

Studying the use of checkpoint inhibition with programmed death-1 (PD-1) and programmed death ligand 1 (PD-L1) inhibitors in the adjuvant setting has been fueled by the proven OS benefit of these agents over standard chemotherapy in patients with advanced NSCLC. In the frontline setting, pembrolizumab is approved as a monotherapy in patients with greater than 50% PD-L1 expression based on the KEYNOTE-024 trial, showing both a PFS and OS benefit when compared with standard platinum-based chemotherapy.[61] It is also approved frontline in combination with carboplatin/pemetrexed chemotherapy irrespective of PD-L1 expression based on the phase II KEYNOTE-021 data showing a PFS benefit when compared with chemotherapy alone.[62] Pembrolizumab, nivolumab, and atezolizumab remain viable options in the second-line setting after initial platinum-based chemotherapy for patients with advanced NSCLC, all showing an OS benefit when compared with docetaxel.[63−66]

Furthermore, the use of immunotherapy in unresectable stage III disease has been shown to be of benefit after definitive chemoradiation and has led to anticipation of results from immunotherapy studies in the adjuvant setting in resected disease. The PACIFIC trial was a randomized phase III study of 709 patients with locally advanced stage III NSCLC treated with definitive platinum-based chemoradiation without progression, then randomized in a 2:1 ratio to receive 1 year of the PD-L1 inhibitor durvalumab every 2 weeks or placebo.[67] The coprimary endpoints were PFS and OS. The results showed a significant PFS benefit in the durvalumab arm of 16.8 months compared with 5.6 months in the placebo arm (HR 0.52, 95% CI 0.42−0.65, $P < .001$). This benefit was consistent across all subgroups and observed irrespective of PD-L1 expression. OS data were immature at the time of analysis,[67] but durvalumab gained FDA approved in February 2018 for use in patients with unresectable stage III NSCLC that has not progressed after prior chemoradiation treatment, and is now incorporated into the NCCN treatment algorithm.[2]

In the adjuvant setting, however, most trials with the use of checkpoint inhibitors are ongoing with eventual results anticipated over the next several years. Several of these trials are listed in Table 3.4. Additionally, there has been interest in understanding the role of PD-1 expression as assessed by IHC to determine whether it is prognostic in early-stage NSCLC and whether it is predictive of response to adjuvant chemotherapy. In the advanced setting, high PD-L1 expression has been correlated with improved response and survival benefit from checkpoint inhibitor therapies. In a retrospective analysis of 982 patients pooled from the IALT, JBR.10, and CALGB 9633 adjuvant trials, tumor sections using the E1L3N antibody were studied with PD-L1 staining intensity and percentage in tumor cells (TCs) and immune cells (ICs) evaluated.[68] Among the patients, 32%, 20.8%, and 14.3% had TC expression of greater than or equal to 1%, 25%, and 50%, respectively. With regard to ICs, 38.7%, 31.4%, and 15.1% had PD-L1 expression greater than or equal to 1%, 25%, and 50%, respectively.

The results failed to show a DFS or OS benefit from adjuvant platinum-based chemotherapy based on PD-L1 expression in TCs ($P = .78$ for DFS and $P = .83$ for OS) and ICs ($P = .13$ for DFS and 0.12 for OS). The level of expression was neither prognostic nor predictive of response to adjuvant treatment after complete resection in early-stage NSCLC. There was a correlation between positive PD-L1 expression and squamous histology, KRAS, and intense lymphocyte infiltrate but not with TP53. Those patients with EGFR-mutated tumors showed an overall non-significant lower PD-L1 expression.[68] These data may be helpful in the future when evaluating ongoing checkpoint trials.

TABLE 3.4
Ongoing Phase III Adjuvant Immunotherapy Trials

Trial	Included Stage	Adjuvant Treatment	N	Primary Endpoint
ALCHEMIST(ANVIL) NCT02595944	IB-IIIA	Nivolumab x1 year vs. observation (adjuvant chemo optional)	714	OS
Impower010 NCT02486718	IB-IIIA	Atezolizumab x16 cycles vs. BSC after adjuvant cisplatin-based chemo x4 cycles	1127	DFS
NCT02273375	IB-IIIA	Durvalumab or placebo x1 year after optional adjuvant platinum-based chemo	1100	DFS
KEYNOTE-091(PEARLS) NCT02504372	IB-IIIA	Pembrolizumab or placebo x1 year after optional adjuvant platinum-based chemo	1380	DFS

ALCHEMIST, Adjuvant Lung Cancer Enrichment Marker Identification and Sequencing Trial; *BSC*, best supportive care; *chemo*, chemotherapy; *DFS*, disease-free survival; *N*, estimated patient enrollment; *OS*, overall survival.

NEOADJUVANT IMMUNOTHERAPY

Interest in neoadjuvant immunotherapy came from seeing the benefit of neoadjuvant chemotherapy previously discussed, with approximately a 5% absolute improvement in survival over 5 years in the NSCLC Meta-Analysis Collaborative Group trial.[34] Neoadjuvant treatment has also proven effective in breast cancer, where neoadjuvant chemotherapy and a resultant pathologic complete response has been shown to improve OS and DFS as compared with patients who have residual disease at the time of surgery.[69] It should be noted, however, that there has been no proven OS or DFS benefit of neoadjuvant treatment compared with adjuvant treatment in breast cancer based on a large 2007 metaanalysis.[70] Neoadjuvant immunotherapy trials allow for the early calculation of primary endpoints, the ability to evaluate tissue before and after surgery for biomarker analysis, and the heightened possibility to downstage a tumor to reach an R0 resection and increase cure rates. Immunotherapy can produce deep and durable responses and when used in the neoadjuvant setting, there is the potential for inducing early immunity to fight micrometastases.

Most of the data on neoadjuvant immunotherapy in NSCLC remain in early phase, although there have been some encouraging data reported. At ASCO 2017, preliminary results of a phase I neoadjuvant trial with nivolumab were presented.[71] Twenty-two patients with stage IB-IIIA NSCLC received 2 doses of nivolumab on day minus 28 and day minus 14 before surgery. Twenty patients proceeded with resection. The primary endpoint was safety, and using objective pathologic

response criteria, efficacy was evaluated. Pretreatment and posttreatment biomarker analysis was also performed. The results showed a 43% major pathologic response (MPR) defined as less than 10% viable TCs in the resected specimen. Pretreatment PD-L1 positivity did not correlate with the MPR. After a median follow-up of 9 months, 86% of patients remained recurrence free and alive. Nivolumab administration did not delay the timing of or interfere with surgery. The correlative studies using multiplexed immunofluorescence showed a posttreatment influx of CD8+ T-cells. Of the 11 patients with increased sequence alterations and mutation-associated neoantigens (MANAs), this was significantly correlated with pathologic response ($P = .001$). Additionally, T-cell functional assays were performed on peripheral blood and tumors, and there was found to be T-cell specific clones for dominant MANAs, suggesting a potential biomarker of nivolumab response.[71]

Although early and with a small sample size, these data suggest that in selected patients getting neoadjuvant immunotherapy, early tumor specific immunity can be induced, potentially correlating with prolonged responses. In the metastatic setting the concept of using tumor mutation burden (TMB) as a predictor of response to immunotherapy has been of significant interest. In an exploratory subset analysis of 58% of patients in the CheckMate-026 trial, which was a negative phase III trial evaluating the use of nivolumab versus platinum-based chemotherapy as frontline treatment in unresectable/metastatic NSCLC patients with PD-L1 expression greater than 5%,[72] patients with high TMB (defined as greater than or equal to 243 somatic mutations) treated with nivolumab had an improved median PFS of 9.7 months versus 5.8 months in those patients with high TMB randomized to chemotherapy (HR 0.62, 95% CI 0.38−1.00). The opposite was true for those patients with low or median TMB, where nivolumab treatment showed a worse PFS compared with chemotherapy (HR 1.82, 95% CI 1.30−2.55).[73] Applying this same concept to neoadjuvant treatment as a means of selecting patients who may be high responders to immunotherapy has significant potential relevance.

Several larger phase II trials are now ongoing using immunotherapy in the neoadjuvant setting. These trials are listed in Table 3.5. The largest of these trials is the Lung Cancer Mutation Consortium 3 phase II study of atezolizumab (NCT02927301), whereby patients with stage IB-IIIA NSCLC eligible for resection with curative intent will undergo neoadjuvant atezolizumab with two 21-day cycles. After surgery, in patients who derived a clinical benefit from neoadjuvant therapy, they will go on to receive up to 12 months of adjuvant atezolizumab. Pretumor and posttumor blood samples will be collected for biomarker evaluation. The primary outcome will be the percentage of patients with an MPR. Data are not anticipated until 2023. Many questions do remain on how best to evaluate immunotherapy in the neoadjuvant setting. Some of these include the following: What is the optimal number of neoadjuvant cycles that should be given? Should treatment be combined with chemotherapy to enhance response? Is combining neoadjuvant and adjuvant immunotherapy necessary? If so, how long should adjuvant treatment be given? What are the optimal biomarkers that should be evaluated? Trials over the next many years will hopefully help answer some of these questions.

CONCLUSIONS AND FUTURE DIRECTIONS
The standard treatment for resected stage IB-IIIA NSCLC remains adjuvant chemotherapy with 4 cycles of a cisplatin-based regimen. Sadly, many of these patients will recur, and there is a significant need for improved therapies to enhance cure rates. Neoadjuvant chemotherapy appears equivalent to adjuvant therapy, even though larger randomized trials in the adjuvant setting have led to its preferred use over neoadjuvant treatment. In patients with molecular mutations in EGFR, there still remains no conclusive OS benefit of adjuvant

---

TABLE 3.5
Ongoing Phase II Neoadjuvant Immunotherapy Trials

Trial	Included Stage	Neoadjuvant/Adjuvant Treatment	N	Primary Outcome
NCT02572843	IIIA	Neo cisplatin/docetaxel x3 cycles followed by 2 cycles of durvalumab then adj durvalumab given 1 year after an R0 resection	68	EFS
NCT02818920	IB-IIIA	Neo pembrolizumab x2 cycles then +/− adj chemo and XRT followed by adj pembrolizumab x4 cycles	32	Surgical feasibility rate
NCT02716038	IB-IIIA	Neo atezolizumab plus carboplatin/nab-paclitaxel x up to 3 months before surgery	30	MPR
NCT02994576	IB-IIIA	Neo atezolizumab x1 cycles	60	Safety
NCT02927301	IB-IIIA	Neo atezolizumab x2 cycles then adj atezolizumab x1 year	180	MPR
NCT02259621	IB-IIIA	Neo nivolumab x3 cycles +/− ipilimumab x1 cycle	20	Safety
NCT03081689	IIIA	Neo nivolumab plus carboplatin/paclitaxel x3 cycles then adj nivolumab x1 year	46	PFS

adj, adjuvant; *chemo*, chemotherapy; *EFS*, event-free survival; *MPR*, major pathologic response; *N*, estimated patient enrollment; *neo*, neoadjuvant; *PFS*, progression-free survival; *XRT*, radiation therapy.

EGFR TKIs, although results of the ADJUVANT trial showing improved DFS are encouraging, and further randomized trials are underway. Given the significant response of patients with an ALK translocation to ALK TKI therapy in the metastatic setting, there is a major need for prospective adjuvant trials in this patient subgroup. The ALCHEMIST trial is ongoing, although accrual will take years and preliminary results even longer to obtain. Although not standardized, consideration should be given to testing patient tumors for EGFR and ALK at the time of surgery to enhance clinical trial enrollment if a molecular mutation in EGFR or ALK translocation is found.

Immunotherapy has transformed the treatment algorithm in advanced NSCLC, and trials are ongoing in both the adjuvant and neoadjuvant setting to investigate checkpoint inhibitor efficacy. The use of the MAGE-A3 cancer vaccine did not improve DFS in the adjuvant setting, although preliminary data of small numbers of patients receiving neoadjuvant nivolumab suggest the feasibility of obtaining MPRs after just 2 doses with potentially prolonged responses after surgery. Response to immunotherapy appears linked to TMB, with increased sequence alterations and MANAs correlating with improved pathologic response. More data are needed, but evaluation of mutational burden may ultimately prove to serve as a better biomarker for response to immunotherapy treatment than PD-L1 expression.

A final thought-provoking concept in the treatment of early-stage NSCLC is the use of ctDNA to better identify and select patients for adjuvant therapy. The ongoing TRACERx study is monitoring the clonal evolution of NSCLC through tumor sampling and genetic analysis from the time of diagnosis through death to understand the importance of clonal heterogeneity on clinical outcomes.[74] In a prospective study of 100 patients from the TRACERx cohort, ctDNA in early-stage NSCLC was evaluated using constructed multiregion exome sequencing—derived tumor phylogenetic trees.[75] The multiplex PCR next-generation sequencing (NGS) platform showed a sensitivity and specificity of 99% and 99.6%, respectively, for detecting single nucleotide variants (SNVs). A threshold of two SNVs detected was used to call a sample ctDNA positive.

Ninety-six preoperative plasma samples were able to be analyzed and 48% (46/96) were found to be positive for ctDNA. Clonal SNVs were detected in all 46 positive samples, and 27 of 40 evaluated samples (68%) had subclonal SNVs. Multivariate analysis showed nonadenocarcinoma histology, a high Ki67 proliferation index, and the presence of lymphovascular invasion to be independent predictors of ctDNA detection. Avidity of tumors on PET scans was also predictive of ctDNA (area under the curve = 0.84, $P < .001$). Pathologic tumor size and tumor volume from CT analyses correlated with the mean plasma variant allele frequency of clonal SNVs. Using these data, presurgical and postsurgical plasma ctDNA profiling was completed in a subgroup of 24 patients, 14 of whom had confirmed relapses. Interestingly, at least two SNVs were detected in 93% (13 of 14) of patients with confirmed NSCLC relapse before or at the time relapse was detected, with a lead-time interval of 10—346 days (median 70 days) from positive ctDNA detection to recurrence by imaging. Furthermore, in patients who had detectible ctDNA after adjuvant chemotherapy, disease recurrence occurred within 1 year after surgery. In contrast, one of the evaluated patients with no detectable ctDNA after adjuvant chemotherapy remained relapse free 688 days after surgery.[75]

A separate study from Stanford University using a novel NGS technology to analyze ctDNA called cancer personalized profiling by deep sequencing retrospectively assessed 255 samples from 40 patients with stage IB-III NSCLC treated with curative intent for the presence of molecular residual disease (MRD).[76] Eighty-two percent of patients had stage II or III disease. Plasma samples were collected both before treatment and at every 2—6 month follow-up visits, mostly coinciding with surveillance imaging. The authors found that ctDNA was detected in 54% of patients during at least one posttreatment follow-up time point, and all of these patients ultimately recurred. Those patients with detectable ctDNA at any follow-up time point had lower freedom from progression and survival than those patients in whom no ctDNA was detected ($P < .001$). Furthermore, the detection of ctDNA preceded by a median of 5.2 months progression as evidenced radiographically using radiographically using response evaluation criteria in solid tumor (RECIST) 1.1 criteria in 72% of patients. Using 36 months before treatment as a prespecified MRD landmark, they found that 100% of patients progressed at this timeframe if they had detectable ctDNA versus only 7% of patients if they had undetectable ctDNA.[76]

Although at present, cost may limit the viability of NGS technology for detecting ctDNA, there is the potential for significant utility in evaluating which patients will likely derive the most benefit from adjuvant treatment and identifying which patients are most at risk for recurrence. Certainly more prospective research awaits, but given the applications of ctDNA, its accuracy as a tumor detection tool and the highly prognostic value of its use, there is great optimism that this will eventually make its way into surveillance and treatment algorithms. There is a clear need for improved cure rates in early-stage NSCLC, and much work remains to be performed. However, the future remains bright. Among the many ongoing adjuvant and neoadjuvant clinical trials, a better understanding of the role of targeted therapy, immunotherapy, and ctDNA is expected, with the hope that this will translate over time into more cures and prolonged patient survival.

DISCLOSURE STATEMENT

Consulting or Advisory Role: ACEA Biosciences, Novartis, Clovis Oncology (uncompensated), Genentech/Roche (uncompensated). Research Funding: Genentech/Roche, Novartis, Exelixis, Celgene, BMS, AstraZeneca/Medimmmune, Gilead, Pfizer, Xcovery, Pharmacyclics.

REFERENCES

1. Pignon JP, Tribodet H, Scagliotti GV, et al. Lung adjuvant cisplatin evaluation: a pooled analysis by the LACE collaborative group. *J Clin Oncol*. 2008;26(21):3552.
2. National Comprehensive Cancer Network. Non-Small Cell Lung Cancer (Version 9.2017). nccn.org/professionals/physician_gls/pdf/nscl.pdf.
3. Goldstraw P, Chansky K, Crowley J, et al. The IASLC lung cancer staging project: proposals for revision of the TNM stage groupings in the forthcoming (eighth) edition of the TNM classification for lung cancer. *J Thorac Oncol*. 2016;11:39.
4. Holmes EC, Bleehen NM, Le Chevalier T, et al. Postoperative adjuvant treatments for non-small cell lung cancers: a consensus report. *Lung Cancer*. 1991;7(1):1–3.
5. Chemotherapy in non-small cell lung cancer: a meta-analysis using updated data on individual patients from 52 randomised clinical trials. Non-small Cell Lung Cancer Collaborative Group. *BMJ*. 1995;311(7010):899–909.
6. Keller SM, Adak S, Wagner H, et al. A randomized trial of postoperative adjuvant therapy in patients with completely resected stage II or IIIA non-small-cell lung cancer. Eastern Cooperative Oncology Group. *N Engl J Med*. 2000;343(17):1217–1222.
7. Scagliotti GV, Fossati R, Torri V, et al. Randomized study of adjuvant chemotherapy for completely resected stage I, II, or IIIA non-small-cell Lung cancer. *J Natl Cancer Inst*. 2003;95:1453–1461.
8. Waller D, Peake MD, Stephens RJ, et al. Chemotherapy for patients with non-small cell lung cancer: the surgical setting of the Big Lung Trial. *Eur J Cardiothorac Surg*. 2004;26(1):173–182.
9. Arriagada R, Bergman B, Dunant A, et al. Cisplatin-based adjuvant chemotherapy in patients with completely resected non-small-cell lung cancer. *N Engl J Med*. 2004;350(4):351–360.
10. Arriagada R, Dunant A, Pignon JP, et al. Long-term results of the international adjuvant lung cancer trial evaluating adjuvant Cisplatin-based chemotherapy in resected lung cancer. *J Clin Oncol*. 2010;28:35–42.
11. Winton T, Livingston R, Johnson D, et al. Vinorelbine plus cisplatin vs. observation in resected non-small-cell lung cancer. *N Engl J Med*. 2005;352(25):2589–2597.
12. Butts CA, Ding K, Seymour L, et al. Randomized phase III trial of vinorelbine plus cisplatin compared with observation in completely resected stage IB and II non-small-cell lung cancer: updated survival analysis of JBR-10. *J Clin Oncol*. 2010;28(1):29–34.
13. Douillard JY, Rosell R, De Lena M, et al. Adjuvant vinorelbine plus cisplatin versus observation in patients with completely resected stage IB-IIIA non-small-cell lung cancer (Adjuvant Navelbine International Trialist Association [ANITA]): a randomised controlled trial. *Lancet Oncol*. 2006;7:719–727.
14. NSCLC Meta-analyses Collaborative Group, Arriagada R, Auperin A, et al. Adjuvant chemotherapy, with or without postoperative radiotherapy, in operable non-small-cell lung cancer: two meta-analyses of individual patient data. *Lancet*. 2010;375(9722):1267–1277.
15. Strauss GM, Herndon JE, Maddaus MA, et al. Adjuvant paclitaxel plus carboplatin compared with observation in stage IB non-small-cell lung cancer: CALGB 9633 with the cancer and Leukemia group B, radiation therapy oncology group, and North central cancer treatment group study groups. *J Clin Oncol*. 2008;26(31):5043–5051.
16. Kato H, Ichinose Y, Ohta M, et al. A randomized trial of adjuvant chemotherapy with Uracil-Tegafur for adenocarcinoma of the lung. *N Engl J Med*. 2004;350(17):1713–1721.
17. Roselli M, Mariotti S, Ferroni P, et al. Postsurgical chemotherapy in stage IB non-small-cell lung cancer: long-term survival in a randomized study. *Int J Cancer*. 2006;119(4):955–960.
18. Wakelee HA, Dahlberg SE, Keller SM, et al. Adjuvant chemotherapy with or without bevacizumab in patients with resected non-small cell lung cancer (E1505): an open-label, multicentre, randomised, phase 3 trial. *Lancet Oncol*. 2017;18(12):1610–1623.
19. Kreuter M, Vansteenkiste J, Fischer JR, et al. Randomized phase 2 trial on refinement of early-stage NSCLC adjuvant chemotherapy with cisplatin and pemetrexed versus cisplatin and vinorelbine: the TREAT study. *Ann Oncol*. 2013;24:986–992.
20. Yamamoto N, Kenmotsu H, Yamanaka T, et al. Randomized phase III study of cisplatin with pemetrexed and cisplatin with vinorelbine for completely resected nonsquamous non-small-cell lung cancer: the JIPANG study protocol. *Clin Lung Cancer*. 2018;19(1):e1–e3.

21. Chang WJ, Sun JM, Lee JY, et al. A retrospective comparison of adjuvant chemotherapeutic regimens for non-small cell lung cancer (NSCLC): paclitaxel plus carboplatin versus vinorelbine plus cisplatin. *Lung Cancer*. 2014;84(1): 51—55.

22. PORT Meta-Analysis Trialists Group. Postoperative radiotherapy in non-small cell lung cancer: systematic review and meta-analysis of individual patient data from nine randomised controlled trials. *Lancet*. 1998;352:257—263.

23. Burdett S, Rydzewska L, Tierney J, et al. Postoperative radiotherapy for non-small cell lung cancer. *Cochrane Database Syst Rev*. 2016;10:CD002142.

24. Patel SH, Ma Y, Wernicke AG, et al. Evidence supporting contemporary post-operative radiation therapy (PORT) using linear accelerators in N2 lung cancer. *Lung Cancer*. 2014;84:156—160.

25. Billiet C, Dealuwe H, Peeters S, et al. Corrigendum to "Modern post-operative radiotherapy for stage III non-small cell lung cancer may improve local control and survival: a meta-analysis". *Radiotherapy Oncol*. 2014;113(2):300—301.

26. LUNG ART-IGR 2006/1202 (ongoing). Phase III study comparing post-operative conformal radiotherapy to no post-operative radiotherapy in patients with completely resected non-small cell lung cancer and mediastinal N2 involvement. NCT00410683.

27. Roth JA, Fossella F, Komaki R, et al. A randomized trial comparing perioperative chemotherapy and surgery with surgery alone in resectable stage IIIA non-small-cell lung cancer. *J Natl Cancer Inst*. 1994;86:673—680.

28. Rosell R, Gomez-Codina J, Camps C, et al. Preresectional chemotherapy in stage IIIA non-small-cell lung cancer: a 7-year assessment of a randomized controlled trial. *Lung Cancer*. 1999;26:7—14.

29. Burdett S, Stewart LA, Rydzewska L. A systematic review and meta-analysis of the literature: chemotherapy and surgery versus surgery alone in non-small cell lung cancer. *J Thorac Oncol*. 2006;1(7):611—621.

30. Pisters KM, Valliere E, Crowley JJ, et al. Surgery with or without preoperative paclitaxel and carboplatin in early-stage non-small-cell lung cancer: Southwest Oncology Group Trial S9900, an intergroup, randomized, phase III trial. *J Clin Oncol*. 2010;28(11):1843—1849.

31. Scagliotti GV, Pastorino U, Vansteenkiste JF, et al. Randomized phase III study of surgery alone or surgery plus preoperative cisplatin and gemcitabine in stages IB to IIIA non-small-cell lung cancer. *J Clin Oncol*. 2012;30(2): 172—178.

32. Van Zandwijk N, Smit EF, Kramer GW, et al. Gemcitabine and cisplatin as induction regimen for patients with biopsy-proven stage IIIA N2 non-small-cell lung cancer: a phase II study of the European Organization for Research and Treatment of Cancer Lung Cancer Cooperative Group (EORTC 08955). *J Clin Oncol*. 2000;18:2658—2664.

33. Song WA, Zhou NK, Wang W, et al. Survival benefit of neoadjuvant chemotherapy in non-small cell lung cancer: an updated meta-analysis of 13 randomized control trials. *J Thorac Oncol*. 2010;5(4):510—516.

34. NSCLC Meta-analysis Collaborative Group. Preoperative chemotherapy for non-small-cell lung cancer: a systematic review and meta-analysis of individual participant data. *Lancet*. 2014;383(9928):1561—1571.

35. Felip E, Rosell R, Maestre JA, et al. And the Spanish Lung Cancer Group. Preoperative chemotherapy plus surgery versus surgery plus adjuvant chemotherapy versus surgery alone in early-stage non-small-cell lung cancer. *J Clin Oncol*. 2010;28:3138—3145.

36. Westeel V, Quoix E, Puyraveau M, et al. A randomised trial comparing preoperative to perioperative chemotherapy in early-stage non-small-cell lung cancer (IFCT 0002 trial). *Eur J Cancer*. 2013;49(12):2654—2664.

37. Kris MG, Johnson BE, Berry LD, et al. Using multiplexed assays of oncogenic drivers in lung cancers to select targeted drugs. *JAMA*. 2014;311(19):1998—2006.

38. Cheng DT, Mitchell TN, Zehir A, et al. Memorial Sloan Kettering-integrated mutation profiling of actionable cancer targets (MSK-IMPACT): a hybridization capture-based next-generation sequencing clinical assay for solid tumor molecular Oncology. *J Mol Diagn*. 2015;17(3): 251—264.

39. Shi Y, Au JS, Thongprasert S, et al. A prospective, molecular epidemiology study of EGFR mutations in Asian patients with advanced non-small-cell lung cancer of adenocarcinoma histology (PIONEER). *J Thorac Oncol*. 2014;9(2): 154—162.

40. Fukuoka M, Wu YL, Thongprasert S, et al. Biomarker analyses and final overall survival results from a phase III, randomized, open-label, first-line study of gefitinib versus carboplatin/paclitaxel in clinically selected patients with advanced non-small-cell lung cancer in Asia (IPASS). *J Clin Oncol*. 2011;29(21):2866—2874.

41. Zhou C, Wu YL, Chen G, et al. Erlotinib versus chemotherapy as first-line treatment for patients with advanced EGFR mutation-positive non-small-cell lung cancer (OPTIMAL, CTONG-0802): a multicentre, open-label, randomised, phase 3 study. *Lancet Oncol*. 2011;12(8): 735—742.

42. Rosell R, Carcereny E, Gervais R, et al. Erlotinib versus standard chemotherapy as first-line treatment for European patients with advanced EGFR mutation-positive non-small-cell lung cancer (EURTAC): a multicentre, open-label, randomised phase 3 trial. *Lancet Oncol*. 2012; 13(3):239—246.

43. Sequist LV, Yang JC, Yamamoto N, et al. Phase III study of afatinib or cisplatin plus pemetrexed in patients with metastatic lung adenocarcinoma with EGFR mutations. *J Clin Oncol*. 2013;31(27):3327—3334.

44. Wu YL, Zhou C, Liam CK, et al. First-line erlotinib versus gemcitabine/cisplatin in patients with advanced EGFR mutation-positive non-small-cell lung cancer: analyses from the phase III, randomized, open-label, ENSURE study. *Ann Oncol*. 2015;26(9):1883—1889.

45. Soria JC, Ohe Y, Vansteenkiste J, et al. Osimertinib in untreated EGFR-Mutated advanced non-small-cell lung cancer. *N Engl J Med*. 2018;378(2):113—125.

46. Solomon BJ, Mok T, Kim DW, et al. First-line crizotinib versus chemotherapy in ALK-positive lung cancer. *N Engl J Med.* 2014;371(23):2167−2177.

47. Soria JC, Tan DS, Chiari R, et al. First-line ceritinib versus platinum-based chemotherapy in advanced ALK-rearranged non-small-cell lung cancer (ASCEND-4): a randomised, open-label, phase 3 study. *Lancet.* 2017; 389(10072):917−929.

48. Peters S, Camidge DR, Shaw AT, et al. Alectinib versus crizotinib in untreated ALK-positive non-small-cell lung cancer. *N Engl J Med.* 2017;377(9):829−838.

49. Janjigian YY, Park BJ, Zakowski MF, et al. Impact on disease-free survival of adjuvant erlotinib or gefitinib in patients with resected lung adenocarcinomas that harbor EGFR mutations. *J Thorac Oncol.* 2011;6(3):569−575.

50. Pennell NA, Neal JW, Chaft JE, et al. SELECT: a multicenter phase II trial of adjuvant erlotinib in resected early-stage EGFR mutation-positive NSCLC. *J Clin Oncol.* 2014; 32(15 suppl):abstr 7514.

51. Li N, Ou W, Ye X, et al. Pemetrexed-carboplatin adjuvant chemotherapy with or without gefitinib in resected stage IIIA-N2 non-small cell lung cancer harbouring EGFR mutations: a randomized, phase II study. *Ann Surg Oncol.* 2014;21(6):2091−2096.

52. Goss GD, O'Callaghan C, Lorimer I, et al. Gefitinib versus placebo in completely resected non-small-cell lung cancer: results of the NCIC CTG BR.19 study. *J Clin Oncol.* 2013; 31(27):3320−3326.

53. Thatcher N, Chang A, Parikh P, et al. Gefitinib plus best supportive care in previously treated patients with refractory advanced non-small-cell lung cancer: results from a randomised, placebo-controlled, multicentre study (Iressa Survival Evaluation in Lung Cancer). *Lancet.* 2005; 366(9496):1527−1537.

54. Kelly K, Chansky K, Gaspar LE, et al. Phase III trial of maintenance gefitinib or placebo after concurrent chemoradiotherapy and docetaxel consolidation in inoperable stage III non-small-cell lung cancer: SWOG S0023. *J Clin Oncol.* 2008;26(15):2450−2456.

55. Kelly K, Altorki NK, Eberhardt WE, et al. Adjuvant erlotinib versus placebo in patients with stage IB-IIIA non-small-cell lung cancer (RADIANT): a randomized, double-blind, phase III trial. *J Clin Oncol.* 2015;33(34):4007−4014.

56. Zhong WZ, Wang Q, Mao WM, et al. Gefitinib versus vinorelbine plus cisplatin as adjuvant treatment for stage II-IIIA (N1-N2) EGFR-mutant NSCLC (ADJUVANT/CTONG1104): a randomised, open-label, phase 3 study. *Lancet Oncol.* 2018;19(1):139−148.

57. Govindan R, Mandrekar SJ, Gerber DE, et al. ALCHEMIST trials: a golden opportunity to transform outcomes in early stage non−small cell lung cancer. *Clin Cancer Res.* 2015; 21(24):5439−5444.

58. Yang P, Kulig K, Boland JM, et al. Worse disease-free survival in never-smokers with ALK+ lung adenocarcinoma. *J Thorac Oncol.* 2012;7(1):90−97.

59. Vansteenkiste JF, Cho BC, Vanakesa T, et al. Efficacy of the MAGE-A3 cancer immunotherapeutic as adjuvant therapy in patients with resected MAGE-A3-positive non-small-cell lung cancer (MAGRIT): a randomised, double-blind, placebo-controlled, phase 3 trial. *Lancet Oncol.* 2016; 17(6):822−835.

60. Zeng Y, Ruan W, He J, et al. Adoptive immunotherapy in postoperative non-small-cell lung cancer: a systematic review and meta-analysis. *PLoS One.* 2016;11(9):e0162630.

61. Reck M, Rodríguez-Abreu D, Robinson AG, et al. Pembrolizumab versus chemotherapy for PD-L1-positive non-small-cell lung cancer. *N Engl J Med.* 2016;375(19): 1823−1833.

62. Langer CJ, Gadgeel SM, Borghaei H, et al. Carboplatin and pemetrexed with or without pembrolizumab for advanced, non-squamous non-small-cell lung cancer: a randomised, phase 2 cohort of the open-label KEYNOTE-021 study. *Lancet Oncol.* 2016;17(11):1497−1508.

63. Herbst RS, Baas P, Kim DW, et al. Pembrolizumab versus docetaxel for previously treated, PD-L1-positive, advanced non-small-cell lung cancer (KEYNOTE-010): a randomised controlled trial. *Lancet.* 2016;387(10027): 1540−1550.

64. Brahmer J, Reckamp KL, Baas P, et al. Nivolumab versus docetaxel in advanced squamous-cell non-small-cell lung cancer. *N Engl J Med.* 2015;373(2):123−135.

65. Borghaei H, Paz-Ares L, Horn L, et al. Nivolumab versus docetaxel in advanced Nonsquamous non-small-cell lung cancer. *N Engl J Med.* 2015;373(17):1627−1639.

66. Rittmeyer A, Barlesi F, Waterkamp D, et al. Atezolizumab versus docetaxel in patients with previously treated non-small-cell lung cancer (OAK): a phase 3, open-label, multicentre randomised controlled trial. *Lancet.* 2017; 389(10066):255−265.

67. Antonia SJ, Villegas A, Daniel D, et al. Durvalumab after chemoradiotherapy in stage III non-small-cell lung cancer. *N Engl J Med.* 2017;377(20):1919−1929.

68. Tsao MS, Le Teuff G, Shepherd FA, et al. PD-L1 protein expression assessed by immunohistochemistry is neither prognostic nor predictive of benefit from adjuvant chemotherapy in resected non-small cell lung cancer. *Ann Oncol.* 2017;28(4):882−889.

69. Cortazar P, Zhang L, Untch M, et al. Pathological complete response and long-term clinical benefit in breast cancer: the CTNeoBC pooled analysis. *Lancet.* 2014;384(9938): 164−172.

70. Mieog JS, van der Hage JA, van de Velde CJ. Preoperative chemotherapy for women with operable breast cancer. *Cochrane Database Syst Rev.* 2007;(2):CD005002.

71. Chaft JE, Forde PM, Smith KN, et al. Neoadjuvant nivolumab in early-stage, resectable non-small cell lung cancers. *J Clin Oncol.* 2017;35(suppl):abstr 8508.

72. Carbone DP, Reck M, Paz-Ares L, et al. First-line nivolumab in stage IV or recurrent non-small-cell lung cancer. *N Engl J Med.* 2017;376(25):2415−2426.

73. Peters S, Creelan B, Hellmann MD, et al. Impact of tumor mutation burden on the efficacy of first-line nivolumab in stage IV or recurrent non-small cell lung cancer: an exploratory analysis of CheckMate 026. *AACR.* 2017; Abstract #CT082.

74. Jamal-Hanjani M, Hackshaw A, Ngai Y, et al. Tracking genomic cancer evolution for precision medicine: the lung TRACERx study. *PLoS Biol.* 2014;12(7):e1001906.

75. Abbosh C, Birkbak NJ, Wilson GA, et al. Phylogenetic ctDNA analysis depicts early-stage lung cancer evolution. *Nature.* 2017;545(7655):446–451.

76. Chaudhuri AA, Chabon JJ, Lovejoy AF, et al. Early detection of molecular residual disease in localized lung cancer by circulating tumor DNA profiling. *Cancer Discov.* 2017; 7(12):1394–1403.

CHAPTER 4

Management of Locally Advanced Lung Cancer

HAK CHOY, MD • JAMESON TRAVIS MENDEL, MD

INTRODUCTION

In the United States approximately 222,500 patients are estimated to be diagnosed with lung cancer per year.[1] The 5-year relative survival rate of lung cancer has increased from 12.2% in 1960–63 to 19.5% in 2007–13, undoubtedly secondary to improvements in local treatment and systemic therapy.[2] Smoking remains the leading cause of lung cancer in the United States, resulting in a 20-fold increase in the lung cancer risk in patients who are active smokers. Additional risk factors include secondhand smoke exposure, ionizing radiation, occupational exposures (e.g., arsenic, chromium, nickel, asbestos, tar, soot, and silica dust), indoor/outdoor pollution, older age, male sex (especially African Americans), acquired lung diseases, and HIV infection.[3]

Efforts in smoking cessation have not been in vain as the prevalence of high-intensity smoking in the United states has decreased, likely contributing to the persistent decrease in lung cancer incidence from the early 2000s (Fig. 4.1 below).[3,4] Interestingly lung cancer incidence continues to decrease, despite publication of the National Lung Screening Trial in 2011.[5]

Lung cancer in nonsmokers is not uncommon, with approximately 40,000 cases per year in the United States.[6] Unfortunately lung cancer remains the leading cause of cancer death, accounting for one-quarter (26%) of all cancer deaths per year.[1] Although surgical approaches and radiotherapeutic techniques have changed over time, evolution of targeted and immunomodulatory systemic treatment options is expected to play an essential future role in the treatment of locally advanced non–small-cell lung cancer (LA-NSCLC).

ANATOMY

Nodal Stations (adapted from Rami-Porta et al. AJCC eighth edition update[7])

1. *Low cervical, supraclavicular, and sternal notch nodes* extend from the lower margin of the cricoid cartilage to the cranial edge of the manubrium.
2. *Upper paratracheal nodes* begin at the upper border of the manubrium and lung apex to the intersection of the innominate vein with the trachea on the right or the superior border of the aortic arch on the left.
3. *Prevascular* (between the sternum and posterior aspect border of the superior vena cava or left carotid artery) and *retrotracheal nodes* extend from the apex of the chest to the carina.
4. *Lower paratracheal nodes* start at the lower border of station 3 and end at the lower border of the azygos vein on the right and superior aspect of the left main pulmonary artery.
5. *Subaortic (aortopulmonary window) nodes* reside between the lower border of the aortic arch and the upper rim of the left main pulmonary artery.
6. *Para-aortic nodes* are found on the lateral margin of the aortic arch.
7. *Subcarinal nodes* encompass the space below the carina to the lower lobe bronchus on the left and the lower border of the bronchus intermedius on the right.
8. *Paraesophageal nodes* include the nodes adjacent to the wall of the esophagus from the lower lobe bronchus on the left and the bronchus intermedius on the right to the diaphragm.
9. *Pulmonary ligament nodes* are found within the pulmonary ligament.

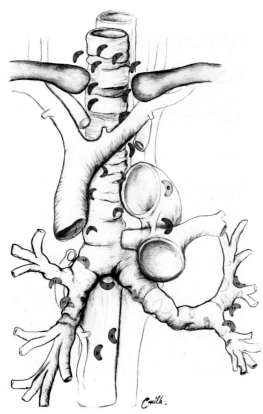

FIG. 4.1 Lymph node stations in lung cancer.

10. *Hilar nodes* are located adjacent to the mainstem bronchus and hilar vessels.
11. *Interlobar nodes* are between the origins of the lobar bronchi.
12. *Lobar nodes* are adjacent to the lobar bronchi.
13. *Segmental nodes* are adjacent to the segmental bronchi.
14. *Subsegmental nodes* are adjacent to the subsegmental bronchi.

SCREENING

Given the relatively asymptomatic nature of developing lung cancers, about 40% of patients are initially diagnosed with advanced stage disease.[8] As LA-NSCLC is associated with poor prognosis, substantial interest exists surrounding screening options for patients at high-risk for developing lung cancer. Unfortunately, early screening trials by the National Cancer Institute[9] and Memorial Sloan-Kettering[10] were unable to show significant reduction in lung cancer deaths with

annual chest roentgenogram and sputum cytology. However, as computed tomography (CT) has become more available and inexpensive, screening with annual CT of the chest is now economically feasible and practical.

Between 2002 and 2004 the National Lung Screening Trial enrolled 53,454 patients at high risk for lung cancer in 33 separate US medical centers. Patients were randomly assigned to three annual low-dose CT scans or annual chest X-rays. Eligible patients were aged between 55 and 74 years with greater than 30 pack-year smoking history (currently smoking or quit within 15 years), no recent unexplained weight loss >15 pounds, and no hemoptysis. Adherence to screening was phenomenal at 90%. Although the majority of positive results were false positives (96.4% in low-dose CT arm and 94.5% chest X-ray arm), screening with annual low-dose CT scans reduced relative lung cancer mortality by 20% and relative all-cause mortality by 6.7%.[5] As a result the US Preventive Services Task Force now recommends annual low-dose CT screening in patients at high risk for developing lung cancer.[11] However, not all lung cancers are detected with CT screening and can potentially develop between scans. In an attempt to assess the effect of increasing screening intervals on lung cancer mortality, the European NELSON trial randomized patients to low-dose CT screening with increasing screening intervals of 1, 2, and 2.5 years versus no screening. Eligible patients were aged 50–75 years, with smoking history of >15 cigarettes per day for more than 25 years or >10 cigarettes per day for more than 30 years. Patients were either currently smoking or quit less than 10 years before enrollment. Three percent of the 7155 participants were diagnosed with lung cancer, and 34 participants were diagnosed with interval lung cancers. As compared with cancers detected at initial screening, interval cancers were more likely to be advanced stage and more often small-cell carcinomas. Interestingly an abnormality was identified in approximately 2/3 of the interval cancers on a retrospective imaging review, missed due to detection, interpretation, and human error.[12,13]

As with most disease sites, lung cancer screening in high-risk populations does decrease mortality. However, further workup of radiographically suspicious lesions can come at the cost of increased morbidity. In the future, lung cancer screening and screening for various other malignancies may be drastically improved with the advent of liquid biopsy and assessment of circulating tumor DNA.[14]

MANIFESTATIONS

Symptoms

- General-fatigue, weight loss, anorexia, cough, shortness of breath
- Central tumors-partial/complete airway obstruction, hemoptysis, postobstructive pneumonia
- Peripheral tumors-chest wall pain (often asymptomatic)
- Superior sulcus-pain, upper extremity weakness (brachial plexus involvement), Horner syndrome (ptosis, miosis, and anhidrosis), SVC syndrome
- Metastasis-bone pain, headache, neurologic deficits, abdominal pain

Paraneoplastic Syndromes

- Hypercalcemia-squamous cell; parathyroid-related protein
- Hyponatremia-small cell; SIADH
- Pulmonary hypertrophic osteoarthropathy-adenocarcinoma
- Coagulopathy-adenocarcinoma
- Gynecomastia-large cell
- Paraneoplastic cerebellar degeneration-small cell
- VIP syndrome-carcinoid tumors; flushing/diarrhea

WORKUP

Basic workup begins with history and physical examination, with focus on smoking history, history of unexplained weight loss, and overall performance status (PS). Laboratories should include CBC, CMP, alkaline phosphatase, and LDH. Pulmonary function tests are typically obtained and reviewed before definitive therapy as pulmonary function may preclude patients from certain definitive treatment options. Patients under consideration for pneumonectomy should have FEV1 >2L (>80% expected). Risk factors for increased mortality after pneumonectomy include the following: right-sided tumor, age >70 years, and low-volume surgical centers.[15] Lobectomy candidates should have FEV1 and DLCO >40% of expected. Quantitative lung perfusion scans are another useful technique to assess pretreatment pulmonary function.[16]

Imaging

Initial imaging usually consists of a CT scan of the chest. Contrast is highly encouraged if tolerated to aid in anatomic delineation of thoracic structures and hilar/mediastinal nodes. FDG-positron emission tomography (PET) is superior to CT and bone scan for staging, with sensitivity and specificity of approximately 0.80 and 0.90, respectively.[17–20] ACOSOG Z0050 evaluated the utility of PET imaging after routine staging with CT chest/abdomen/pelvis, bone scan, and brain magnetic resonance imaging (MRI)/CT in 303 resectable stage I-IIIA NSCLC patients. Detection of N1 and N2/3 disease was superior using PET with a negative predictive value of 87% for N2 and N3 disease.[21] In this study, positive predictive value was relatively poor at 56%—possibly due to the numerous conditions causing false positives, such as tuberculosis, aspergillomas, rheumatoid nodules, Wegener's granulomatosis, and amyloidosis.[22] While PET avoids unnecessary thoracotomy in 20% of patients,[20] pathologic mediastinal assessment is recommended in patients with negative PET[21] as sensitivity and specificity drastically decreases with lesions <1–1.5 cm.[23,24] MRI of the brain is recommended for stage IIB and above or those eliciting symptoms concerning for brain metastasis. Additionally, MRI of the spine may help to delineate disease extension in patients with superior sulcus tumors.

Sputum Cytology

Although rarely used, sputum cytology can establish a cancer diagnosis in patients who cannot, for whatever reason, undergo biopsy. The sensitivity and specificity of this test can be up to 66% and 99%, respectively.[25] However, this varies widely depending on the location and size of the tumor. To ensure adequate sampling, representative samples should have alveolar macrophages and bronchial epithelial cells.

Mediastinoscopy

Pathologic evaluation of the mediastinum is generally recommended in patients with stage ≥ IB disease. Several surgical approaches exist to sample mediastinal lymph nodes. In a central or cervical mediastinoscopy, an incision is made approximately 1 cm above the suprasternal notch of the sternum, allowing for dissection and sampling of nodal stations 1–4R and 7. A central mediastinoscopy is considered gold standard at some institutions, with reported false-negative rates of 5.5% and mortality rates <1%.[26] Left-sided tumors often exhibit lymphatic drainage to para-aortic and aortopulmonary window nodes (stations 5–6) that are typically not safely accessible with central mediastinoscopy. In these cases, nodes can be sampled via an anterior (Chamberlain) approach. An incision is made in the medial left second intercostal space, allowing for careful dissection and access to stations 4L, 5, 6, and 7. An extended cervical mediastinoscopy is another specialized approach used to assess the aortopulmonary window but is not commonly used.

Endobronchial Ultrasound–Guided Transbronchial Needle Aspiration

Less invasive techniques, such as endobronchial ultrasound–guided transbronchial needle aspiration (EBUS-TBNA) or transesophageal endoscopic ultrasound–guided fine needle aspiration (EUS-FNA), are commonly used to assess mediastinal lymph nodes. However, concerns do exist regarding sampling accuracy with these techniques as retrospective studies have shown that 28% of patients (N2) with negative TBNA had positive nodes on central mediastinoscopy.[27] However, the ASTER trial prospectively randomized 241 patients to either surgical staging or endosonography with combined EBUS-TBNA and EUS-FNA and showed similar sensitivities between mediastinoscopy (85%) and endosonography (79%).[28]

Fiberoptic Bronchoscopy with Bronchoalveolar Lavage

Fiberoptic bronchoscopy with bronchoalveolar lavage is considered the standard for determining the endobronchial extent of disease. Washings and brushings can be performed to histologically confirm involvement with sensitivities of 43% and 54%, respectively.[25]

HISTOLOGY
Adenocarcinoma

The most common lung cancer histology, adenocarcinoma, makes up 38% of all lung cancers.[29] As epithelial tumors with glandular differentiation, adenocarcinomas are generally located peripherally, and immunohistochemistry (IHC) can be positive for mucicarmine, napsin A, and/or thyroid transcription factor 1 (TTF-1).[31] TTF-1 is expressed in 75% of adenocarcinomas and correlates with better prognosis.[32]

Squamous Cell Carcinoma

Squamous cell carcinomas make up 20% of lung cancers[29] and are typically located centrally. Histologic diagnosis is established by microscopic visualization of an epithelial tumor with keratinization or IHC markers consistent with squamous cell carcinoma, such as p40, p60, and cytokeratins 5/6.[31] p40 is a marker for squamous differentiation and is present almost 100% of the time.[33] Basaloid squamous cell carcinomas can be microscopically confused with squamous cell carcinomas; however, these can be differentiated with IHC staining.

Large-Cell Lung Carcinoma

Large-cell carcinomas make up only 3% of lung cancer diagnoses.[29] This is an undifferentiated NSCLC that does not have squamous, glandular, or small-cell differentiation and usually a diagnosis of exclusion. Typically, large cell carcinomas cannot be diagnosed on core biopsy and are always TTF-1 negative (Table 4.1).[31]

Molecular Analysis

As in other disease sites, molecular analysis of NSCLC over the years has revolutionized treatment options and strategies. Common mutations and associated characteristics are described in Table 4.2.

STAGING (EIGHTH EDITION) (TABLES 4.3 AND 4.4)
Pleural Invasion

- PL0—tumor within the subpleural lung parenchyma or invading superficially into the pleural connective tissue
- PL1—tumor invades beyond the elastic layer
- PL2—tumor invades the pleura surface
- PL3—tumor invades any component of the parietal pleura

TABLE 4.1 Histologic Characteristics of Lung Cancer				
Histology	**Frequency**	**Location**	**Differentiation**	**IHC**
Adenocarcinoma	38%	Peripheral	Glandular	Mucicarmine, napsin A, TTF-1[a]
Squamous cell carcinoma	20%	Central	Keratinization	p40[b], p60, cytokeratins 5and 6
Large-cell lung carcinoma	3%	Central or peripheral	Undifferentiated	TTF-1 negative

IHC, immunohistochemistry.

[a] Thyroid transcription factor (TTF-1)—expressed in 75% of adenocarcinomas and correlates with better prognosis.

[b] p40 is a marker for squamous differentiation and present ~100% of the time.

TABLE 4.2
Molecular Analysis of NSCLC

Mutation	Frequency	Location	Function	Clinical Associations
Rat sarcoma viral oncogene homolog (RAS)[a]	15%–20%	Chromosome 12 at position 12.1	Membrane-associated proteins that mediate signal transduction from binding ligands via the Ras/MAPK pathway[34]	More common in patients with adenocarcinomas and patients with a history of smoking[35] and associated with resistance to EGFR inhibitors[b,36]
Epidermal growth factor receptor (EGFR)	20%	Chromosome 7 at position 12	Mutated transmembrane tyrosine kinase, resulting in increased kinase activity and hyperactivation of downstream pathways[37]	Mutations are found more frequently in nonsmokers, Asian women, and patients with adenocarcinoma histology.[38] Resistance to TKIs associated with KRAS mutation, acquired T790M mutation in kinase domain, and amplification of alternative kinases.[39]
Human epidermal growth factor receptor 2 (HER2)	<5%	Chromosome 17 at position 12	Forms heterodimers with other EGF receptors, enhancing kinase activation[40]	More common in Asian females, nonsmokers, and patients with adenocarcinoma with lepidic pattern.[41] Targeted antibodies in unselected NSCLC have shown little activity.[42]
Proto-oncogene tyrosine-protein kinase ROS (ROS-1)	1%–2%	Chromosome 6 at position 22	RTK in insulin receptor gene family; related to ALK	More common in patients with adenocarcinoma and nonsmokers.[43]. Responds to crizotinib.[44]
Anaplastic lymphoma kinase (ALK)	3%–7%	Chromosome 2	Cytoplasmic protein with constitutive kinase activity	More common in young patients who have never smoked and mutually exclusive with EGFR and KRAS mutations.[45,46]
MET	2%–20%	Chromosome 7 at position 31	RTK for hepatocyte growth factor/HGF ligand[47, 48]	Associated with worse prognosis[49,50]
RET	<2%	Chromosome 10 at position 11.2	RTK	Smokers, youngsters, patients with poorly differentiated adenocarcinoma.[51]
BRAF	<4%	Chromosome 7 at position 34	Serine/threonine kinase involved in the Ras/MAPK pathway[52]	More common in patients with adenocarcinoma and a smoking history.[53]

NSCLC, non–small-cell lung cancer.

[a] HRAS, KRAS (most common in lung), NRAS.

[b] Overlapping EGFR and KRAS mutations occur infrequently (<1%).[54]

TABLE 4.3
Primary Tumor (T)

Category	Criteria	Subcriteria
TX	Cannot be assessed, or malignant cells in sputum/washings but tumor not clinically visualized	
T0	No evidence of tumor	
Tis	Carcinoma in situ	
T1	<3 cm, surrounded by lung or visceral pleura, no invasion of main bronchus	1. ≤1 cm 2. >1 −2 cm 3. >2 −3 cm
T2	>3 cm but <5 cm or involvement of the main bronchus (not carina), visceral pleura invasion, and/or obstructive atelectasis/pneumonitis extending to the hila	1. >3 −4 cm 2. >4 −5 cm
T3	>5 cm but ≤7 cm or invading parietal pleura, chest wall, phrenic nerve, parietal pericardium, or separate tumor nodules in the same lobe as the primary tumor	
T4	>7 cm or invasion of the diaphragm, mediastinum, heart, great vessels, trachea, recurrent laryngeal nerve, esophagus, vertebral body, and/or carina	

TABLE 4.4
Regional Lymph Node (N)

Category	Criteria	Subcriteria
NX	Regional nodes not assessed	
N0	No regional nodal metastasis	
N1	Involvement of ipsilateral peribronchial and/or ipsilateral hilar lymph nodes and intrapulmonary nodes	
N2	Ipsilateral mediastinal and/or subcarinal nodal involvement	
N3	Contralateral mediastinal/hilar or supraclavicular nodal involvement	
M0	No distant metastasis	
MI	Distant metastasis	1. Tumor nodules in contralateral lobe, pleura, or pericardium and/or malignant effusion (pleural or pericardial) 2. Single extrathoracic metastasis 3. Multiple extrathoracic metastasis

MANAGEMENT
Smoking Cessation

Smoking is associated with increased mortality and the risk for second primary cancers.[55] In patients with NSCLC, smoking is associated with worse overall survival (OS) in those undergoing definitive treatment with surgery, radiation, or chemoradiation.[56−58] Consequently smoking cessation should be highly encouraged. Several agents, such as, nicotine replacement, bupropion, and varenicline, can be used to support smoking cessation.

With the legalization of recreational marijuana in several North American states and widespread medical legalization, we are likely to see a significant rise in daily cannabis users. Therefore questions regarding its effects on cancer risk and treatment outcomes are likely to become more commonplace in clinical practice. Although epidemiologic studies attempting to analyze lung cancer risk with marijuana use are conflicting,[59−61] marijuana smoke does contain known carcinogens and other chemicals implicated in respiratory diseases[62]; therefore continued use should not be encouraged in patients with lung cancer. However, oral ingestion of prescription cannabinoids, such as dronabinol, may help appetite stimulation.[63,64]

RESECTABLE LA-NSCLC

Although patients with stage III (N1) NSCLC are thought to benefit from surgical resection, patients with obvious clinical N2 disease do not, with a survival of <10% at 3 years.[65] These findings, along with multiple other series, prompted the initiation of multiple trials attempting to address the role of multimodality treatment, which has ultimately led to the controversy in management of locally advanced disease we see today.

Induction Chemotherapy

Induction chemotherapy is thought to help promote complete surgical resection and eradication of micrometastatic disease. Several initial phase II and III trials identified the advantages of neoadjuvant chemotherapy before surgical resection in stage III patients.[66-71] In an early feasibility study of 41 patients with N2 disease a 75% clinical response rate to preoperative chemotherapy and high rates of complete resection in patients who demonstrated significant response radiographically were reported.[68]

To further clarify the role of induction chemotherapy in operable stage IIIA NSCLC, Roth et al. randomized 60 patients to induction chemotherapy (cyclophosphamide, etoposide, and cisplatin) and surgery or surgery alone. Those who exhibited a response to chemotherapy received an additional three cycles of chemotherapy postoperatively. The trial was terminated early because of the magnitude of treatment effect on unplanned interim analysis, demonstrating a median survival benefit of 64 months compared with 11 months in patients treated with surgery alone.[69] A similar trial conducted by Rosell et al. verified the benefits of induction chemotherapy in patients with stage IIIA NSCLC.[70] In a large phase III trial the French randomized 355 patients with stage I-IIIA NSCLC to neoadjuvant chemotherapy followed by surgery or surgery alone. Chemotherapy consisted of two preoperative cycles of mitomycin 6 mg/m^2, ifosfamide 1.5 g/m^2, and cisplatin 30 mg/m^2 plus two adjuvant cycles for patients with at least a clinical partial response. Patients with pT3 or N2 disease and/or incomplete surgery received postoperative radiation therapy (PORT). The study was surprisingly negative at the primary endpoint, OS. Median OS was 26 months for surgery alone versus 37 months in the preoperative chemotherapy arm ($P = .15$). On subset analysis there was a survival benefit for preoperative chemotherapy in patients with N0 and N1 disease but not N2 disease. Remarkably 82% of patients underwent pneumonectomy, which may confound the results. However, reported postoperative mortality was only 5.6% between arms.[67]

As patients with N2 disease did not seem to derive significant benefit from surgery, the EORTC conducted a large randomized trial to compare surgery versus radiotherapy alone in unresectable stage IIIA-N2 NSCLC with response to induction chemotherapy. Induction chemotherapy consisted of three cycles of cisplatin 80 mg/m^2 or carboplatin AUC 5 in combination with at least one other chemotherapy drug. PORT was recommended for patients with incomplete surgical resection. Forty percent of patients received PORT. Of those who underwent resection, 42% had pathologic downstaging and 5% had a pathologic complete response. In the radiation arm only half (55%) of the patients received the prescribed dose. The trial was negative with no difference in OS at 5 years (~15%).[72] Based on these results it is felt that patients with N2 disease do not derive a significant benefit with the addition of surgical resection.

Regardless of the definitive treatment modality, response to induction therapy and mediastinal downstaging is prognostic. In a Swiss phase II trial, 90 potentially operable patients with stage IIIA (pN2) NSCLC received three cycles of docetaxel 85 mg/m^2 and cisplatin 40 mg/m^2, then underwent surgical resection. Patients received adjuvant radiotherapy if there were positive margins and/or involvement of the uppermost mediastinal lymph nodes. Nineteen percent of patients were noted to have a pathologic complete response to induction therapy on resection and 31% were downstaged to ypN0. As expected, patients with pathologic mediastinal downstaging had superior 3-year OS of 61% versus 11% without.[73]

Unfortunately translating these trials to the modern era can be difficult as N2 disease represents a heterogeneous group of patients. In surgical series with 702 patients from six French surgical centers, involvement of ≥2 mediastinal nodal levels was a poor prognostic factor for survival on multivariate analysis.[74] This has been reflected in the most recent IASLC lung cancer staging, where curves separate between N2 single versus N2 multiple.[75] Regardless, it is important to understand that neoadjuvant therapy can be used to promote complete surgical resection in patients with borderline resectable disease.

Trimodality

Given the encouraging survival for patients with N2 disease who achieve complete pathologic response, the treatment paradigm for stage III NSCLC shifted toward escalating induction therapy. In patients unsuitable for upfront surgical resection the Southwest Oncology Group (SWOG) conducted a phase II study with 126 stage IIIA(N2) or stage IIIB patients to assess the feasibility of induction chemoradiotherapy followed by surgical resection in stable or responding disease. Induction therapy consisted of two cycles of cisplatin 50 mg/m^2 and etoposide 50 mg/m^2 with concurrent radiotherapy to 45 Gy. Although a highly selected group of surgically fit patients, OS for the cohort was ~25% at 3 years—twice what would be expected with radiation alone. No significant difference between patients with IIIA(N2) or IIIB disease was identified, and majority of patients were noted to fail distally. Pathologic complete response in the mediastinum was the strongest predictor of survival after thoracotomy with a 3-year survival of 44% versus 18% without. Of note, 2-year OS in patients with contralateral lymph nodes was 0%.[76] Similar results were demonstrated in an earlier phase II trial from Rush Medical College.[77]

To further assess the risk-benefit of preoperative chemoradiotherapy, the intergroup 0139 trial randomized 396 stage IIIA(N2) NSCLC patients with no evidence of progression after induction chemoradiotherapy to surgery or continued chemoradiation to a definitive dose (61 Gy). Induction therapy consisted of two cycles of cisplatin 50 mg/m^2 on days 1, 8, 29, and 36 and etoposide 50 mg/m^2 on days 1, 5, 29, and 33 plus concurrent radiotherapy to 45 Gy. Both groups received two cycles of adjuvant cisplatin and etoposide. The primary endpoint was OS. Median survival was 23.6 months in the surgery group versus 22.2 months in the definitive chemoradiotherapy group (hazard ratio [HR] 0.87; $P = .24$). However, progression-free survival (PFS) was improved from 10.5 to 12.8 months with surgical resection ($P = .017$). Patients with a pN0 resection had a median survival of 34 months. Not surprisingly, pneumonectomy was associated with high perioperative mortality as 14 of 16 treatment-related deaths were attributed to pneumonectomy—5/23 with simple and 9/31 with complex pneumonectomy. Those who underwent lobectomy had an excellent median survival of 33.6 months.[78,79] As there is concern regarding the utility of pneumonectomy, several retrospective studies have attempted to address the safety of pneumonectomy after induction chemotherapy or chemoradiotherapy, suggesting increased postoperative mortality rates (6%–20%) in patients older than 70 years and those with a right-sided pneumonectomy.[80–84]

More recently the Swiss conducted a randomized trial comparing induction sequential chemoradiotherapy or induction chemotherapy alone followed by surgical resection in 232 patients with stage IIIA(N2) NSCLC. Patients received three cycles of 100 mg/m^2 cisplatin and 85 mg/m^2 docetaxel. This was followed by radiotherapy to 44 Gy over 3 weeks for patients in the chemoradiotherapy group. The study was closed early due to futility and showed no difference in the primary endpoint, event-free survival, advocating for the omission of induction radiation. However, results of this study should be interpreted with caution as the patient population had a seemingly low burden of mediastinal nodal disease; chemoradiation was not given concurrently; and despite known morbidity/mortality rate of pneumonectomy, ~24% of patients received pneumonectomy.[85]

Despite multiple phase III trials, management of patients with stage III NSCLC remains highly controversial. The NCCN conducted a member questionnaire for resectable NSCLC to determine current practice patterns in stage III NSCLC patients with N2 disease. They found that 90.5% of surveyed surgeons would consider surgery in patients with one N2 station with lymph node <3 cm and 47.6% would consider surgery with more than one N2 station, as long as no lymph nodes were >3 cm.[86] At most institutions if complete resection is theoretically achievable in an operable patient, then resection is generally recommended after some form of induction therapy—preferably chemoradiation as performed in the intergroup 0139 trial.

SUPERIOR SULCUS TUMORS

Superior sulcus tumors, also known as Pancost tumors, are named after Dr. Henry Pancoast who first described this clinical syndrome (shoulder pain, Horner syndrome, and upper extremity weakness) in the early 1900s. Shoulder pain usually presents as the initial symptom, commonly with radiation down the ipsilateral extremity in the ulnar distribution, and with time leading to extremity weakness. If the stellate ganglion is involved, Horner syndrome (ptosis, papillary miosis, and facial anhidrosis) can develop. Workup and staging follows a similar pattern as other NSCLCs, with the exception of the inclusion of a thoracic inlet MRI to visualize vascular, vertebral, brachial plexus, and/or nerve root involvement.

If medically operable, management typically follows a trimodality approach. These recommendations are based on the results of the SWOG 9416/intergroup 0160 trial. In this phase II trial, 110 patients with T3–4 N0–1 superior sulcus tumors underwent induction therapy with two cycles of cisplatin 50 mg/m^2 and etoposide 50 mg/m^2 with concurrent radiotherapy (45 Gy in 25 fractions). Of note the mediastinum and hilum were not included in the radiation field. If no progression, patients underwent resection followed by two additional cycles of chemotherapy. In this study 95% of patients completed induction therapy, 80%

proceeded to surgery, and 76% had complete resection. OS was 44% at 5 years, which appeared to have improved over historical controls (~30%). Remarkably 56% of patients had a pathologic complete response and 75% had R0 resection. In those with complete resection, 5-year survival was 54%.[87] Similar results have been demonstrated in Japanese and French series.[88,89]

Additionally, upfront surgical resection has been explored. In a phase II study from MDACC, 32 patients with superior sulcus tumors underwent segmentectomy or lobectomy with en bloc resection of the involved chest wall followed by radiation therapy to a dose of 60 Gy in twice-daily fractionation if there were negative surgical margins or 64.8 Gy if positive with concurrent cisplatin and etoposide. Three cycles of adjuvant cisplatin and etoposide were given after completion of definitive therapy. Seventy-eight percent of patients were able to complete the prescribed treatment, and there was no operative mortality. Local control at 10 years was 76%, and OS was 45%. The brain was the most common site of distant failure. However, of the 11 patients who received prophylactic cranial irradiation, none experienced failure in the brain.[90] Although either approach has similar outcomes, most institutions advocate for neoadjuvant chemoradiation in appropriate patients.

Postoperative Radiation Therapy

After surgical resection alone, local recurrence can occur in ≥50% of patients with stage II/III disease.[91,92] The most common site of local failure is the bronchial stump/staple line. However, recurrence in mediastinal lymph nodes often occurs, especially in patients with known nodal metastasis. Interestingly right lung segments tend to drain into the ipsilateral mediastinum, whereas drainage of the left lung can often pass into the contralateral mediastinum.[93] Radiotherapy is often used in select patients to reduce recurrence in these high-risk regions.

Radiation Alone

Early retrospective studies identified a local control and survival benefit with addition of PORT in NSCLC patients with mediastinal nodal metastasis.[94-97] These thought-provoking results initiated a randomized trial by the Lung Cancer Study Group where 210 stage II-III NSCLC patients received complete (R0) surgical resection with or without adjuvant RT to 50 Gy. There was no statistically significant benefit in OS. However, there was a significant benefit to local recurrence for those who received PORT, defined as first recurrence in the ipsilateral lung or mediastinum. Twenty-one

patients (43%) experienced local recurrence with surgery alone versus only a single patient (3%) with adjuvant radiation. On multivariate analysis, patients with N2 disease seemed to benefit the most.[91] Similar randomized trials were conducted with varying results, leading to controversy surrounding PORT.[92,98-101]

The PORT metaanalysis attempted to address these inconsistencies by reviewing individual patient data from nine trials conducted between 1966 and 1988. A significant adverse effect was identified with a decrease in 2-year OS from 55% to 48% with PORT (HR 1.21 SS). Subgroup analysis showed no benefit in patients with stage III(N2) disease and a detriment for stage I NSCLC.[102] These early data are generally not considered translatable to the modern era of radiotherapy as old techniques (e.g., Co-60, large 2-D fields, and high dose) were used, likely resulting in excessive cardiopulmonary morbidity and mortality, despite the drastic benefits seen in local control with adjuvant radiotherapy in patients with positive margins or N2 disease.[103,104]

In a separate metaanalysis of 11 phase III trials, authors compared treatment outcomes of patients with stage I-III NSCLC treated with cobalt machines versus modern linear accelerators. Survival benefit for PORT was only significant in patients treated with LINACs (HR 0.76, $P = .02$), as well as a notable improvement on local control.[105] Unplanned nonrandomized analysis of patients treated with or without PORT (45−60 Gy) in the Adjuvant Navelbine International Trialist Association (ANITA) trial suggested a survival benefit with PORT in N2 patients, shown in Table 4.5 below.[106]

SEER and NCDB analyses of modern PORT in N2 patients suggest an OS benefit for incompletely resected stage III(N2) patients.[107-109] Therefore PORT should be considered in patients with evidence of N2 disease on surgical resection and in those with positive margins.

Postoperative Chemoradiation

Given the known survival advantage in patients treated with upfront chemoradiotherapy and questions surrounding appropriate adjuvant therapy in patients treated with upfront resection, the Eastern Cooperative Oncology Group (ECOG) conducted a randomized trial to investigate the possible benefits of adjuvant chemoradiation. From 1991 to 1997, 488 patients with stage II-III NSCLC were randomized to receive four cycles of cisplatin 60 mg/m^2 and etoposide 120 mg/m^2 with concurrent radiotherapy to 50.4 Gy or radiation alone after surgical resection. Fifty-four percent of patients had pN2 disease. After a median follow-up of 44 months, there were no differences in

TABLE 4.5
Survival Analysis of Patients Treated in the ANITA trial

	PORT		NO RT	
	Median OS (m)	**5-year OS**	**Median OS (m)**	**5-year OS**
Observation (pN1)	50.2	42.6%	25.9	31.4%
Chemotherapy (pN1)	46.6	40%	93.6	56.3%
Observation (pN2)	22.7	47.4%	12.7	34%
Chemotherapy (pN2)	47.4	21.3%	23.8	16.6%

OS, overall survival; *PORT*, postoperative radiation therapy.

survival or local recurrence. Interestingly patients who received adjuvant systemic therapy did not have a significant reduction in distant relapse outside of the central nervous system (CNS). However, 30% of patients were unable to complete all four cycles because of toxicity.[110] Before publication of these results, the Radiation Therapy Oncology Group (RTOG) initiated a feasibility study, RTOG 9705, eventually enrolling 88 eligible stage II-IIIA NSCLC patients who received postoperative chemoradiotherapy with concurrent paclitaxel and carboplatin. Four cycles of chemotherapy were delivered in 3-week cycles; paclitaxel dose was 135 mg/m^2 during radiotherapy and increased to 225 mg/m^2 for cycles 3 and 4, while carboplatin AUC 5 was used during radiation and increased to AUC 6 for cycles 3 and 4. 1-, 2-, and 3-year OS was 86%, 70%, and 61%, respectively. Survival, local recurrence, and distant relapse were noted to be slightly improved as compared with ECOG 9705.[111]

Despite our postoperative strategies, the majority of patients with LA-NSCLC die of lung cancer. Unfortunately past trials are fraught with deficiencies (poor stratification, inclusion of early-stage patients, archaic radiation techniques, etc.), which has led to difficult interpretation and the controversy we see today. Hopefully results of the currently enrolling Lung ART trial, a phase III study comparing PORT with no PORT in patients with NSCLC with mediastinal nodal involvement, will elucidate the role of PORT.[112] Until these results are finally available, PORT should be strongly considered in patients with pN2 disease and positive margins. In terms of sequencing, PORT should be delivered after adjuvant chemotherapy in patients with R0 margins. In patients with positive margins, concurrent chemotherapy can be considered or sequential radiotherapy followed by chemotherapy as local recurrence is the greatest risk factor in this group.[113]

Adjuvant Chemotherapy

After publication of the PORT metaanalysis in the early 1990s leading to declining PORT, the role of adjuvant systemic therapy in NSCLC began to generate great interest. In 1995 the Non-Small Cell Lung Cancer Collaborative Group published a metaanalysis of 52 randomized trials, suggesting a 5% survival advantage at 5 years in patients who received cisplatin-based chemotherapy.[114] This led to an eruption of clinical trials investigating adjuvant platinum-based chemotherapy in NSCLC.

From 1995 to 1999 the International Adjuvant Lung Cancer Trial randomized 1867 patients with resectable stage IA-IIIB NSCLC after R0 surgery to adjuvant cisplatin-based chemotherapy for 3–4 cycles or observation. Approximately 40% of patients were stage III. Although slow accruement caused early closure, a 4%–5% OS and PFS advantage was identified at 5 years ($P < .03$).[117] However, after an increased follow-up of 7.5 years, the survival benefit became nonsignificant.[115] Simultaneously the ANITA began a large trial that randomized 840 stage IB-IIIA patients with R0 resection to adjuvant vinorelbine plus cisplatin or observation. PORT was not mandated but encouraged in patients with node-positive disease. Thirty-nine percent of patients enrolled had stage IIIA disease. OS benefit was 8.6% at 5 years with chemotherapy and found to be most pronounced in patients with nodal disease on subset analysis. In this study, survival advantage was maintained at 7 years.[116]

Owing to inconsistent results for adjuvant chemotherapy, pooled analysis of individual patient data from five randomized trials [116–120] conducted after 1995 with patients who received adjuvant cisplatin-based chemotherapy (with or without sequential radiotherapy) for completely resected NSCLC was used to create the Lung Adjuvant Cisplatin Evaluation (LACE) analysis. Authors confirmed a 5.4% absolute survival advantage at 5 years in patients receiving adjuvant cisplatin-based chemotherapy. Stage II and III patients were found to benefit the most (HR 0.83 for stage II and III). Additionally, a significant interaction between chemotherapy and PS was identified. Patients with PS of 0 seemed to benefit the most, whereas adjuvant chemotherapy was thought to be detrimental in patients with PS ≥ 2.[121]

Adjuvant chemotherapy is highly recommended in patients with positive nodal disease or positive margins—usually concurrent or sequential with radiotherapy.[113] Thus in the setting of LA-NSCLC, most patients will require adjuvant chemotherapy. For completion, adjuvant chemotherapy may be considered in patients with T2 tumors and high-risk features, such as visceral pleural invasion, poor differentiation, LVI, size >4 cm, and concerns for nodal involvement without sampling.[122–124]

UNRESECTABLE LA-NSCLC

Most patients with unresectable LA-NSCLC will succumb to their disease in a short period of time if left untreated. Radiotherapy, especially with concurrent chemotherapy, offers the only chance of cure in this group of patients and remains a pivotal component of the treatment paradigm as chemotherapy alone offers poor local control durability.[125]

Radiation Alone

In 1973 the RTOG performed a dose-escalation trial (RTOG 7301) in an attempt to optimize dose and fractionation schedule in definitive treatment of LA-NSCLC. Three hundred sixty-five patients with unresectable NSCLC were randomized to one of the four treatment regimens: 40 Gy with a 2-week split course, 40 Gy in 4 weeks, 50 Gy in 5 weeks, or 60 Gy in 6 weeks. Tumor volumes were identified and treated using kilovoltage radiographs (two-dimensional planning). Long-term survival was exceptionally poor in all arms, but the 60 Gy arm had the best performance and a local control of approximately 60%.[228] To further explore dose escalation and alternative fractionation, the RTOG conducted a phase I/II trial (RTOG 8311), ultimately enrolling 848 unresectable NSCLC patients who were treated with 60.2–79.2 Gy in 1.2-Gy twice-daily fractions. No significant differences in acute and late toxicity were noted between arms (60.0, 64.8, 69.6, 74.4, and 79.2 Gy). However, the percentage of patients who developed severe pneumonitis did increase from 2.6% in the low-dose arm to 8.1% in the high-dose arm. A dose response to 69.6 Gy was noted

in patients with good PS and <6% weight loss.[120] Thus 69.6 Gy became the standard definitive dose for altered fractionation.

Building on these results, the United Kingdom conducted a randomized trial comparing continuous, hyperfractionated, accelerated radiotherapy versus conventional radiotherapy (60 Gy in 30 fractions) in 563 patients with NSCLC. Patients treated with altered fractionation received 36 fractions of 1.5 Gy three times a day over 12 consecutive days. Most patients (81%) had squamous cell histology. The alternate fractionation regimen was well tolerated and had slightly increased rates of esophagitis. A 9% absolute improvement in 2-year survival was noted for patients treated with altered fractionation (20%–29%) and also a 27% reduction in the relative risk of local progression was noted. Interestingly there was a significant reduction in the risk of metastasis in patients with squamous histology.[126,127] Although obviously effective, the logistics of the consecutive TID treatment for patients and practitioners likely inhibited the acceptance of this regimen in the United States.

Once three-dimensional conformal radiotherapy (3DCRT) became available, the RTOG further explored dose escalation by initiating a phase I/II dose escalation trial, RTOG 9311. Patients with stage I-III NSCLC were placed into dose-escalated groups based on the volume of the lung receiving at least 20 Gy (V20). Depending on their V20 percentage, patients received between 64.5 and 90.3 Gy of radiation. Locoregional control was >50%, and toxicity was acceptable up to 83.8 Gy in patients with V20 < 25% and 77.4 Gy with V20 between 25% and 36%. There were two grade 5 toxicities in the 90.3 Gy arm.[128] As practitioners gained experience with 3DCRT and toxicity data became available, tumor size was found to be highly prognostic for survival and local tumor control and potentially obviated by further dose escalation to the primary.[129–131]

Hypofractionation allows for dose escalation in terms of biologic effective dose (BED), which may improve survival in patients who do not receive chemotherapy.[132] MD Anderson reported a small retrospective series comparing 55 patients treated with a durable thoracic palliative regimen 45 Gy in 15 fractions versus the standard definitive regimen of 60–66 Gy in 30–33 fractions. Interestingly despite worse prognostic factors, the 45 Gy regimen had similar response rates, LR control, and OS.[133] Several phase I studies have reported varying fractionation schedules with BEDs >80 Gy and acceptable toxicity.[134–136] A phase III study that is currently enrolling in Texas is comparing the standard 60 Gy in 30 fractions with accelerated hypofractionated image–guided radiation therapy with 60 Gy in 15 fractions for patients with stage II-III NSCLC unable to tolerate concurrent chemoradiation.

Sequential Chemoradiation

Although radiotherapy does offer a chance for cure in patients with LA-NSCLC, approximately >60% will fail distally. In an attempt to address metastatic dissemination, the Cancer and Leukemia Group B (CALGB) conducted a randomized trial (CALGB 8433) to compare outcomes in 155 stage III NSCLC patients treated with two cycles of induction chemotherapy versus immediate radiotherapy. Enrolled patients had a PS 0–1, ≤5% weight loss, and no scalene or supraclavicular lymphadenopathy. Chemotherapy consisted of cisplatin 100 mg/m^2 on days 1 and 29 and vinblastine 5 mg/m^2 on days 1, 8, 15, 22, and 29. Patients who received induction chemotherapy had greater rates of adverse effects, including neutropenic infections, vomiting, and severe weight loss. However, median survival was significantly increased from 9.6 to 13.7 months for patients who received induction chemotherapy ($P = .0066$) with 5-year survival advantage of 17% versus 6%.[137,138] To confirm these results the intergroup randomized 458 stage II-IIIB NSCLC patients with decent PS and minimal weight loss to standard radiotherapy, sequential chemoradiation, or hyperfractionated radiotherapy. Induction chemotherapy was the same as used in CALGB 8433 (aka. the Dillman regimen). Median survival was significantly improved with induction chemotherapy (13.8 months) as compared with standard radiotherapy (11.4 months) and hyperfractionated radiotherapy (12.3 months).[139] These trials, along with several others,[140–142] defined the role of sequential chemotherapy in LA-NSCLC.

Sequential and Concurrent Chemoradiotherapy

Despite dose escalation, local recurrence can occur in 40%–60% of patients treated with radiation alone.[143] In the 1980s cisplatin was noted to have radiosensitizing properties and profound tumoricidal effects in animal studies.[144] After witnessing the early success of concurrent chemoradiation in head and neck patients, the EORTC conducted a phase II/III trial to elucidate the effects of concurrent chemoradiation with cisplatin on NSCLC. From 1984 to 1989, 331 patients with unresectable stage I-III NSCLC were randomized to radiotherapy alone, radiotherapy with weekly cisplatin 30 mg/m^2, or radiotherapy with daily cisplatin 6 mg/m^2. All treatment arms received split-course radiotherapy: 30 Gy in 2 weeks, followed by a 3-week break, then 25 Gy in

2 weeks. Concurrent chemoradiation significantly improved OS and local control, as compared with radiotherapy alone. Three-year OS was 2% with radiation alone, 13% with weekly cisplatin, and 16% with daily cisplatin. The survival benefit was felt to be due to improved local control as there were no differences in time to distant metastasis between groups.[145] With the exception of a CALGB trial using induction carboplatin, other trials conducted around the same period corroborated this survival benefit. In terms of toxicity, increased rates of esophagitis were consistently noted.[146–152] Additionally, among trials using platinum-based regimens, considerable variability existed with chemotherapeutic agent selection, dosing, and schedules.

Eventually the RTOG initiated a large multiinstitutional randomized trial (RTOG 9410) to test novel regimens against the Dillman regimen. Beginning in 1994, patients with stage II–III (98% stage III) unresectable NSCLC were randomized to sequential chemoradiation (arm 1), concurrent chemoradiation with vinblastine and cisplatin (arm 2), or hyperfractionated radiotherapy with concurrent cisplatin and oral etoposide (arm 3). Patients were required to have a Karnofsky PS (KPS) of ≥70 and ≤5% weight loss over 3 months. Radiation therapy was 63 Gy over 7 weeks in both arms 1 and 2 and 69.6 Gy over 6 weeks in 1.2 Gy twice-daily fractionations (delivered at least 6 hours apart). Table 4.6 below shows the results between the treatment arms.

Rates of nonhematologic toxicity, especially esophagitis, were significantly higher with concurrent chemotherapy. However, late esophageal toxicity was similar among the arms. Standard fractionation with concurrent chemotherapy had the best survival outcomes and response rates.[153] Additionally, a metaanalysis of six randomized trials using platinum-based concomitant chemotherapy corroborated these findings, showing an absolute survival benefit of 4.5% at 5 years in favor of concomitant chemoradiation at the cost of increased acute esophageal toxicity.[154]

After SWOG 8805 demonstrated encouraging survival in bimodality arms, many questioned whether inclusion of surgery or rather, accrual of fit patients able to tolerate trimodality therapy influenced survival outcomes. SWOG 9019 attempted to address this question by conducting a small trial including 50 patients with T4N0/1 (36%), T4N2 (24%), or N3 (40%) stage IIIB NSCLC ("bulky" stage IIIB). Patients received identical therapy as given in SWOG 8805. Three-year OS was 17%.[155] Although somewhat less than observed in SWOG 8805 due to inclusion of solely bulky disease, survival was considerably clinically improved over

TABLE 4.6
Results of RTOG 9410

	Median OS (m)	5-year OS	Response Rate	Clinical CR	Esophagitis
Arm 1	14.6	10%	61%	30%	4%
Arm 2	17	16%	70%	42%	22%
Arm 3	15.6	13%	65%	33%	45%

OS, overall survival; RTOG, Radiation Therapy Oncology Group.

historical comparisons with radiation alone and virtually identical to stage IIIB subset of SWOG 8805. Based on clinical and preclinical data, Choy et al. explored chemoradiotherapy with paclitaxel and carboplatin in 39 inoperable LA-NSCLC patients. Patients received radiation to 66 Gy over 7 weeks with concurrent paclitaxel 50 mg/m^2 and carboplatin AUC 2, followed by two cycles of consolidation paclitaxel 200 mg/m^2 and carboplatin AUC 6 starting 3 weeks after the last radiation session. This phase II study reported 2-year OS of 38%, comparing favorably to previous trials by the RTOG, EORTC, and West Japan Lung Cancer Group.[156] Interestingly 46% of patients developed grade 3/4 toxicity, whereas 20% of patients developed grade 3/4 esophagitis in SWOG 9019.

To compare novel chemotherapy regimens, the WJTOG conducted a phase III study including 456 patients with unresectable stage III NSCLC. Patients were randomized to 60 Gy over 7 weeks (with 1-week break) with concurrent mitomycin 8 mg/m^2, vindesine 3 mg/m^2, and cisplatin 80 mg/m^2; 60 Gy over 6 weeks with weekly irinotecan 20 mg/m^2 and carboplatin AUC 2 followed by two courses of irinotecan 50 mg/m^2 and carboplatin AUC 5; or 60 Gy over 6 weeks with weekly paclitaxel 40 mg/m^2 and carboplatin AUC 2, followed by two courses of paclitaxel 200 mg/m^2 and carboplatin AUC 5. There was no difference in OS at 5 years; however, toxicities were more favorable in patients receiving carboplatin and paclitaxel.[157] Moreover, the PROCLAIM trial randomized a similar group of patients (n = 598) to chemoradiotherapy with pemetrexed-cisplatin followed by consolidation with pemetrexed or chemoradiotherapy with etoposide-cisplatin followed by nonpemetrexed doublet consolidation. The study was closed early due to futility, with no significant difference in survival between arms. However, patients in the study arm did have significantly lower incidence of grade 3/4 events, 64% versus 79%.[158] Based on these results, concurrent carboplatin and paclitaxel or cisplatin and etoposide continue to be standard regimens for concurrent chemoradiation.

The accepted radiation dose (60–63 Gy in 1.8–2.0 Gy fractions) used for patients with stage III NSCLC was established in the 1970s by RTOG 7301. As discussed previously, RTOG 9311 further explored dose escalation in the 3-D conformal era, reaching doses of >80 Gy with radiation alone. At the time the maximum tolerated dose for concurrent chemoradiation was thought to be approximately 74 Gy based on several dose escalation trials using modern radiotherapy techniques with concurrent chemoradiotherapy.[159–164] In a groundbreaking trial the RTOG randomized 464 unresectable stage III NSCLC patients to 60, 74, 60 Gy plus cetuximab, or 74 Gy plus cetuximab. Radiation was given in 2 Gy fractions, and all patients received concurrent chemotherapy with paclitaxel 45 mg/m^2 and carboplatin AUC 2 once a week. This was followed by two cycles of consolidation paclitaxel 200 mg/m^2 and carboplatin AUC 6 2 weeks after completion of chemoradiation. Patients were staged with PET, and ineligible if contralateral hilar or supraclavicular lymph nodes were detected. To the surprise of the oncologic community, there was an 11% improvement in 2-year OS in the low-dose arm. This outcome is thought to be secondary to toxicity as patients who received high-dose chemoradiotherapy were significantly more likely to have severe esophagitis (21%) compared with patients in the low-dose arm (7%).[165] RTOG 0617 has established 60 Gy in 30 fractions as the standard dose in patients who receive chemoradiotherapy.

One should note that these trials included a highly select group of patients with good PS and minimal weight loss. Therefore selecting for tolerability is vital as treatment delays do seem to effect survival.[166] In patients thought to not tolerate concurrent chemoradiation, sequential chemoradiation or radiation alone should be used.

Consolidation Chemotherapy

Although strategies to improve locoregional control continue to evolve, distant relapse remains a major issue in NSCLC. Several trials have attempted to address potential eradication of distant micrometastatic disease using adjuvant systemic therapy with varying results. In the era of novel cytotoxic therapies, the SWOG designed a phase II trial (SWOG 9504) to attempt maximum cytoreduction with full-dose cisplatin and etoposide during thoracic radiotherapy, followed by consolidation docetaxel. Consolidation docetaxel was dosed at 75 mg/m^2 and began 4–6 weeks after definitive chemoradiotherapy. From 1996 to 1998, 83 eligible stage IIIB patients were enrolled. Median survival was 26 months, and 1-, 2-, and 3-year survival rates were 76%, 54%, and 37%, respectively. Results compared favorably to a predecessor trial, S9019, that used cisplatin and etoposide for consolidation with 1-, 2-, and 3-year survival rates of 58%, 34%, and 17%, respectively.[167]

To evaluate whether improvement in survival was due to consolidation docetaxel in SWOG 9504, the Hoosier Oncology Group and US Oncology conducted a randomized trial comparing consolidation docetaxel versus observation. Patients received cisplatin 50 mg/m^2 and etoposide 50 mg/m^2 concurrently with radiation therapy to 59.40 Gy. If no progression, patients were randomly assigned to docetaxel 75 mg/m^2 for three cycles versus observation. After enrolling 203 stage III patients, the trial was terminated early due to futility and showed no difference in OS between arms. Consolidation docetaxel substantially increased the risk of febrile neutropenia, grade 3/4 pneumonitis, hospitalization (29% vs. 8%), and premature death.[168] Therefore consolidation docetaxel was not recommended.

Another interesting multiinstitutional trial randomized 257 stage IIIA and IIIB NSCLC patients to induction chemotherapy followed by radiotherapy alone, induction chemotherapy followed by chemoradiotherapy, or chemoradiotherapy followed by consolidation chemotherapy. Induction and consolidation chemotherapy consisted of two cycles of paclitaxel 200 mg/m^2 and carboplatin AUC 6. Chemotherapy delivered during radiotherapy was weekly paclitaxel 45 mg/m^2 and carboplatin AUC 2. Median OS was seemingly improved for those treated with concurrent chemoradiation followed by consolidation chemotherapy but associated with increased acute toxicity. In patients who received induction chemotherapy followed by concurrent chemoradiation, only 46% of patients were able to complete planned 7 weekly cycles of chemotherapy and one-third did not complete planned radiotherapy.[169] Consequently chemotherapy should be delivered adjuvantly in most cases as to not delay or prevent patients from completing definitive treatment.

More recently, results of the KCSG-LU05-04 trial have been published. From 2005 to 2011, 437 patients with stage III NSCLC were randomly assigned to concurrent chemoradiotherapy with or without consolidation chemotherapy. Patients were given docetaxel 20 mg/m^2 and cisplatin 20 mg/m^2 every week for 6 weeks during radiation treatments (66 Gy in 33 fractions). Three cycles of docetaxel and cisplatin were given for consolidation. Most (92%) patients were staged with PET. The trial was negative, with no statistical difference between PFS and OS between arms.[170] These results were in line with a semirecent Japanese metaanalysis that was unable to identify a significant survival benefit with consolidation chemotherapy.[171]

Although adjuvant chemotherapy is typically prescribed after definitive chemoradiation, up to half of the patients are unable to receive consolidation chemotherapy due to progression or toxicity. The previously described large prospective trials fail to show significant benefit with the addition of adjuvant chemotherapy and possibly favor omission. At the least, inclusion should be decided on a case-by-case basis. The minimal benefits of adjuvant chemotherapy have led to much interest in pursuing targeted and immunotherapeutic options.

TARGETED THERAPIES

In patients with metastatic NSCLC, targeted antibodies have revolutionized systemic treatment options and are now considered primary treatment options in patients with targetable mutations.

Epidermal Growth Factor Receptor

The epidermal growth factor receptor (EGFR) gene is located in chromosome 7 at position 12,[172] encoding a transmembrane tyrosine kinase located on the surface of epithelial cells. About 90% of mutations occur on exon 19 (L858R), resulting in increased kinase activity and hyperactivation of downstream pathways.[37] Mutations involving the ATP-binding pocket of the EGFR occurs infrequently and correlates with improved clinical response to TKIs.[173] Mutations are found more frequently in nonsmokers, Asian women, and adenocarcinoma histology.[38] Resistance to TKIs is associated with KRAS mutations, acquired T790 M mutation in kinase domain, and amplification of alternative kinases.[39]

Cetuximab

The RTOG conducted a phase II study to investigate the feasibility of concurrent chemoradiotherapy with cetuximab in stage III NSCLC patients. Patients received weekly paclitaxel, carboplatin, and cetuximab (225 mg/m^2) for six cycles with daily radiotherapy to a total dose of 63 Gy in 35 fractions. All patients received two cycles of consolidation therapy with paclitaxel, carboplatin, and cetuximab. Therapy was tolerated fairly well and 2-year OS was 49%, which was considerably improved from historical controls.[174] Owing to these promising results, cetuximab was incorporated into RTOG 0617. Unfortunately RTOG 0617 failed to demonstrate a survival benefit with the addition of cetuximab to concurrent chemoradiation in unselected patients. However, in a planned subset analysis there was a significant survival benefit in high EGFR-expressing patients (42 vs. 21 months) with the addition of cetuximab.[165] Although theoretically beneficial in high EGFR expression patients, no clear advantage has been established in a randomized fashion, so its use is not recommended for definitive chemoradiotherapy in NSCLC.

Gefitinib

Gefitinib was the first anti-EGFR agent approved by the US Food and Drug Administration (FDA) for use as a single agent in chemorefractory patients.[175] The SWOG performed a phase III trial where unselected stage III NSCLC patients were treated with chemoradiation, consolidation with docetaxel, and then randomized to maintenance therapy with gefitinib 250 mg per day or placebo. At unplanned interim analysis there was no benefit to maintenance gefitinib, so the study was closed. Patients on the gefitinib maintenance arm actually demonstrated worse OS but this seemed to be related to disease progression rather than drug toxicity.[176] Additionally, the CALGB conducted a phase II study to evaluate the effects of adding gefitinib to sequential or concurrent chemoradiotherapy in patients with unresectable stage III NSCLC. Patients were categorized as poor risk ($\geq$5% weight loss and/or PS 2) or good risk (PS 0–1 and weight loss <5%). All patients received two cycles of induction chemotherapy with carboplatin AUC 6, paclitaxel 200 mg/m^2, and gefitinib 250 mg. The poor-risk group received gefitinib 250 mg per day with concurrent radiation to a total dose of 66 Gy in 33 fractions. Good-risk patients received the same therapy but also received weekly carboplatin AUC 2 and paclitaxel 50 mg/m^2. Interestingly survival was best in the poor-risk group with median OS of 19 versus 13.4 months in the good risk, suggesting the addition of gefitinib to chemoradiation may not be advantageous.[177] Regardless, further studies are needed to elucidate possible benefits of radiotherapy with gefitinib in poor-risk patients.

Erlotinib

Another EGFR inhibitor, erlotinib, has been heavily studied in NSCLC. The Tarceva Lung Cancer Investigation and Tarceva Responses in Conjunction with Paclitaxel and Carboplatin are two large phase III trials with >1000 patients that did not show a significant survival benefit with the addition of erlotinib to chemotherapy in unselected patients. Not surprisingly, outcomes were improved in never smokers (more likely to be EGFR positive).[178,179] In a phase I study Choong et al.[180] attempted to determine the maximum tolerated dose of erlotinib with chemoradiotherapy in patients with unresectable stage III NSCLC. Using standard chemoradiation regimens, erlotinib dose was escalated from 50 to 150 mg and given only during chemoradiation. Median survival was unimpressive in this unselected population. However, patients who developed a rash had 3-year OS of 53% versus 10% in those who did not. In a phase II study the CALGB randomized patients who were never or light smokers to erlotinib alone or erlotinib with carboplatin and paclitaxel. At a median follow-up of 30 months, there was no difference in PFS between the groups. When the groups were stratified by EGFR mutation status, PFS and OS were significantly improved as compared with patients without EGFR mutation. Interestingly median OS in patients with EGFR mutations was similar between the groups.[181] As we enter the era of targeted therapy, identifying patient characteristics (nonsmokers, women, and/or Asian) or simply testing for EGFR mutation status will likely help select for patients who benefit the most.

Bevacizumab and Thalidomide

One hallmark of cancer is the ability to induce angiogenesis as rapidly dividing cells need an adequate source of nutrients/oxygen and the ability to eliminate waste products.[182] Although many angiogenic factors have been identified, inhibition of vascular endothelial growth factor (VEGF)/vascular permeability factor has had some success in the clinic. Through interaction with tyrosine kinase receptors, VEGF expression induces endothelial cell proliferation and promotes angiogenesis.[183] Aberrant expression of similar growth factors in tumors leads to the rapid abnormal neovascularization seen in tumors.

Bevacizumab, a recombinant humanized monoclonal antibody, interacts with VEGF, inhibiting interaction with the VEGF receptor. Bevacizumab has been successfully used in colorectal cancer, glioblastoma, renal cell carcinoma, and ovarian cancer.[184] Unfortunately the use of bevacizumab concurrently with radiotherapy in NSCLC has been associated with significant toxicity, such as tracheoesophageal fistula formation.[185] Another agent, thalidomide, has also been somewhat unsuccessful in the clinic. Although exact mechanisms of antitumoral activity have yet to be elucidated, it is thought that thalidomide stimulates maturation and normalization of tumor vasculature.[186] The efficacy of thalidomide in patients with NSCLC was tested in ECOG 3598 that randomized patients with stage III NSCLC to definitive chemoradiation with or without thalidomide. There was no difference in survival between the arms, and greater rates of thrombosis/embolism were noted in patients who received thalidomide.[187]

Needless to say the use of antiangiogenic agents in patients with LA-NSCLC has not flourished clinically. Currently the traditional model of antiangiogenic agents limiting neovascularization and nutrient delivery is under question as evidence supporting the alternative promotion of tumoral vascular normalization is emerging.[183] Although contradictory to historic mechanisms, restoration of tumor vasculature may aid in adequate delivery of cytotoxic agents and maximize immune infiltration.[188]

Anaplastic Lymphoma Kinase

The anaplastic lymphoma kinase (ALK) gene is located on chromosome 2, mutated/rearranged in 3%–7% of lung cancers, and more common in young patients who have never smoked.[45,189,190] Although there are multiple mutational variants, the most common is the N-terminal fusion of echinoderm microtubule–associated protein–like 4 with the intracellular kinase domain of ALK, producing a cytoplasmic protein with constitutive kinase activity.[191–193]

Several inhibitors have been developed (e.g., crizotinib, ceritinib, and alectinib) and approved by the FDA.[190,194] Although initially designed as an MET inhibitor, crizotinib is effective in ALK-positive NSCLC.[44,46,190,195] In a randomized trial of 342 patients with mostly metastatic (98%) treatment-naïve ALK-positive NSCLC treated with crizotinib or platinum-based chemotherapy with pemetrexed, PFS was significantly improved by 4 months with crizotinib. There was no survival benefit; however, crossover was permitted. Unfortunately effects are not durable and

resistance eventually develops. Second-generation ALK inhibitors ceritinib,[196–198] alectinib,[199–201] and the recently approved brigatinib are often active in patients who progress or are intolerant of crizotinib. Interestingly alectinib appears to have CNS activity and may be an appealing upfront option in patients presenting with brain metastasis.[202] To date, there are no published trials assessing the effects of ALK inhibitors on definitive treatment of LA-NSCLC. We patiently await the results of the NRG phase II study with sequential crizotinib and chemoradiotherapy in stage III NSCLC.

IMMUNOTHERAPY

Historically NSCLC was thought to be nonimmunogenic. However, this does not seem to be the case given the results of recent trials,[203] creating significant excitement in the rapidly evolving landscape of immunotherapy in NSCLC.

Programmed Death Ligand 1

Programmed death ligand 1 (PD-L1; and its partner PD-L2) is a transmembrane protein expressed in normal tissues to inhibit the activity of T-cells and prevent autoimmunity. PD-L1 is commonly upregulated on the surface of tumor cells, binding to the programmed death 1 (PD-1) expressed on tumor-infiltrating lymphocytes, eventually causing a T-cell tolerance.[204,205] This represents one of the various mechanisms of immune evasion.

Assessing PD-L1 positivity in assays can be difficult as PD-L1 is commonly expressed on tumor-infiltrating inflammatory cells.[206] Regardless, several PD-1 inhibitors, nivolumab and pembrolizumab, have been developed to exploit this mechanism of immune escape and are now FDA approved for use in lung cancer. In a randomized trial of 582 patients with NSCLC who progressed on platinum-based chemotherapy, patients were treated with salvage nivolumab 3 mg/kg every 2 weeks or docetaxel 75 mg/m^2 every 3 weeks. Median OS was longer with nivolumab, 12.2 versus 9.4 months. Most patients had quantifiable expression, and patients with at least 1% expression derived benefit from nivolumab over docetaxel.[207] However, in the upfront setting, Checkmate 026 found no significant difference between PFS or OS in patients treated with nivolumab versus platinum doublet chemotherapy.[208,209] Similarly, benefits of pembrolizumab in patients with NSCLC were explored in two large trials KEYNOTE-010[210] and KEYNOTE 024.[211] Both trials were able to establish a significant survival benefit for those with high levels of PD-L1 expression in the second-line setting.

Monoclonal antibodies targeting PD-L1 have been developed and investigated in patients with NSCLC. In a large phase III trial patients with stage IIIB or IV NSCLC who had previously received 1–2 cytotoxic systemic regimens were randomized to either atezolizumab or docetaxel. OS was improved from 9.6 to 13.8 months with atezolizumab regardless of PD-L1 expression and was tolerated reasonably well with 15% related grade 3 or 4 events.[212] These exciting results have led to rapid incorporation of immunotherapy in the treatment paradigm of NSCLC, with the desire to identify immunogenic costimulators for synergistic effects.

Combining Immunotherapy and Radiotherapy

Enhancing responses to immunotherapy with radiation has shown to be feasible in preclinical and early clinical data and is now the subject of multiple clinical trials. Cell death by immunogenicity is one of the many postulated mechanisms of radiation injury. As previously discussed, tumor cells are thought to evade the immune system in part by expression of specific cell surface molecules. In vivo, doses up to 20 Gy have been shown to alter the expression of cell surface immune molecules, making tumor cells more amenable to immune system recognition and attack.[213] Unfortunately standard fraction radiotherapy (doses 1.8–3 Gy) does not seem to elicit the same response and likely repeatedly sterilizes immune infiltration, given the high radiosensitivity of lymphocytes.[214] Thus dose, fractionation schedule, volume of treated disease, and systemic therapy likely have varying immune-suppressive effects.

Immune response with varying dose and fractionation schedules in mice has mixed results.[215–219] However, preclinical data do suggest a dose threshold for immune stimulation. In one study, mice bearing murine melanoma tumors were treated with up to 15 Gy and followed up for treatment response and immune effects. Doses above 5 Gy per fraction were needed to produce immunostimulatory response, suggesting a potential threshold.[220] Although reports of abscopal effect after stereotactic body radiation therapy (SBRT) do exist,[221,222] radiation alone is probably not enough to illicit a clinically significant response in humans.[223,224] However, with the introduction of immune checkpoint inhibitors, immune priming may be the future as secondary analysis of KEYNOTE 001 suggested patients with advanced NSCLC treated with pembrolizumab and radiotherapy versus pembrolizumab alone have longer PFS and OS.[225,226] Publication of the PACIFIC trial corroborates these findings. The PACIFIC trial randomized 709 patients with locally advanced, unresectable, NSCLC at a 2:1 ratio to consolidation durvalumab or placebo. Median PFS, the primary endpoint, was an astounding 16.8 months in patients who received durvalumab versus 5.6 months with placebo. Benefits were noted across all prespecified subgroups and durvolumab was tolerated exceptionally well with clinically insignificant side effects as compared with placebo.[227] Although exciting and likely paradigm shifting, we await data on OS and long-term follow-up. Further understanding of immune effects, synergy with radiotherapy, and optimizing consolidative treatment options will be of pivotal importance moving forward.

RADIOTHERAPY
Dose

For more than 3 decades, RTOG 7301 defined the standard dose for patients receiving thoracic radiation. In this study, survival rates for all arms were very poor, but escalation to 60 Gy arm had superior survival and local control.[228] In 1983, RTOG 8311 published their results of dose escalation to 79.2 Gy and alternative fractionation, with a dose response to 69.6 Gy, establishing a new standard.[120] Once 3DCRT became available, the RTOG further explored dose escalation to 83.8 Gy in RTOG 9311, without excessive toxicity.[128] Eventually survival advantage of radiosensitization with concurrent chemotherapy was realized. However, appropriate dose with this new regimen had not been established. Multiple trials were able to show safety to a dose of approximately 74 Gy with chemotherapy using modern techniques.[159–164] In a landmark trial, RTOG 0617 showed a survival advantage in patients who received thoracic radiation to 60 versus 74 Gy with concurrent carboplatin and paclitaxel,[165] establishing the current standard dose of 60 Gy for chemoradiation in LA-NSCLC.

Despite these results, groups continue to explore dose escalation. An interesting study from the University of Kentucky evaluated the feasibility of conventional chemoradiotherapy followed by SBRT boost to residual primary disease on PET.[229–231] In combination with results from the PACIFIC trial, an SBRT boost at the end of treatment may modestly improve local control rates and promote antigen expression before consolidation with immunotherapy.

VOLUMES

Gross Tumor Volume

The gross tumor volume is typically defined as macroscopic disease seen on the planning CT scan, usually identified using lung windowing on planning CT. In patients with significant surrounding consolidation secondary to obstruction or lung collapse, a PET scan can help identify regions of gross disease. IV contrast is of particular importance when outlining gross nodal disease. Historically, comprehensive elective nodal coverage with 2-D techniques was used to cover all potentially draining nodal stations, producing large volumes with significant morbidity. Practice eventually transitioned to involved nodal coverage, which has been shown to decrease morbidity without increasing rates of nodal failure.[232] Lymph nodes with a short axis of $\geq$1 cm are considered involved[233] and included in nodal volumes, unless negative on EBUS or PET. As previously discussed, PET has a negative predictive value of 87%[21] and is particularly useful in ruling out suspicious nodes.

Clinical Target Volume

Microscopic extension of visualized gross disease is encompassed by volumetric expansion to create the clinical target volume (CTV). Based on pathologic examination, expansions of 5–9 mm are generally recommended to encompass 80%–90% of microscopic tumor extension.[234,235] Similarly gross nodal disease is usually expanded by 3- to 5-mm margin to encompass extranodal extension.[236] CTV volumes are typically trimmed to respect usual anatomic boundaries.

Planned Target Volume

To account for setup variations, CTV is expanded 3–5 mm to create the planned target volume (PTV). If setup is confirmed with port imaging, a PTV of 5 mm is typically used. However, PTV can be limited to 3 mm or less if dose reduction to nearby critical structures is needed, with daily cone-beam CT scans.

MODALITIES

Photons: 2-D, 3-D, and Intensity-Modulated Radiotherapy Planning

Before the adoption of CT-based planning, primary tumor volume and draining nodal stations were planned on plain films (aka. two-dimensional planning). Large fields were often used to ensure disease was encompassed in an attempt to prevent marginal failures. Once available, CT was quickly incorporated in treatment planning as accurate dose to tumor and critical structures could be calculated, termed 3DCRT. Although a significant upgrade from 2-D planning, limited field arrangements and constant beam dose prevented significant dose escalation and critical structure avoidance. In the early 2000s, intensity-modulated radiotherapy (IMRT) was developed. In IMRT the intensity of each beam is modified using dose rate and multileaf collimator alterations, leading to optimal tumor coverage. Using this technique highly conformal plans can be created, which considerably spare adjacent normal tissue (e.g., lungs, esophagus, heart, and spinal cord) without sacrificing tumor coverage. As opposed to static IMRT, volumetric-modulated arc therapy is dynamic and constantly modulates the beam as the gantry rotates around the patient.

Although the dose distribution advantages with IMRT have been shown across multiple disease sites,[237−242] secondary analysis of patients treated on RTOG 0617 has provided prospective acute and late toxicity comparisons for 3D versus IMRT in NSCLC. In this analysis, patients treated with IMRT were found to have significantly less $\geq$grade 3 pneumonitis, despite having larger treatment volumes. The heart was better spared with IMRT, which was associated with an OS benefit on adjusted analysis.[243] Furthermore, on a separate quality of life analysis, fewer patients who received IMRT had clinically meaningful decline in FACT-LCS as compared with 3DCRT.[244] In summary, advent of IMRT has provided a novel avenue for normal tissue sparing and dose escalation. As plans become increasingly conformal, knowledge surrounding anatomic boundaries, appropriate margins, and motion management are vital to prevent marginal failures.

Protons

Proton therapy has existed since the early 1950s and first used clinically at Lawrence Berkeley Laboratory.[245] A high voltage is applied to hydrogen gas, which strips the electrons from the hydrogen atoms, leaving positively charged protons. These protons are then injected into a particle accelerator and accelerated to an energy of approximately 250 MeV in a cyclotron or synchrotron before entering a patient. Although expensive and technically more challenging, proton therapy does have some dosimetric advantages over photon therapy. As protons are known to stop at a specific depth, termed the Bragg peak, they essentially have no exit dose, sparing tissues deep to the target. Disadvantages include increased neutron production and range uncertainties.

There are two main methodologies to deliver protons: passive scattering and scanning. In passive scattering the proton beam is modulated by a rotating range modulator that spreads out the Bragg peak and by a scatterer that widens the beam laterally before collimation by an aperture before entering the patient. Scanning technique magnetically steers the pencil beam, allowing for 2-D scanning of the target. The target is covered by layering dose via energy modulation of the beam, also known as intensity-modulated proton therapy.

Dosimetric benefits to proton therapy versus photon therapy have been described in multiple analyses.[239,246–248] However, the translational advantage in the clinic has been negligible. In a phase II study from MDACC, 44 patients with stage III NSCLC were treated to 74 Gy with protons (passive scatter) and concurrent carboplatin and paclitaxel. At a median follow-up of 19.7 months, no patients experienced grade 4 or 5 adverse events, and PFS was 63% at 1 year.[249] The Bayesian trial attempted to compare 3-D proton therapy (3DPT) versus IMRT in 150 patients with LA-NSCLC. IMRT and 3DPT plans were compared for each patient. Patients were eligible for randomization if both plans satisfied normal tissue constraints. Otherwise patients were treated with the more dosimetrically appealing plan or plan covered by insurance provider. Although only published in abstract form, there were no differences between rates of radiation pneumonitis or local recurrence between arms.[250] To date, no study has shown significant benefit with protons in terms of normal tissue toxicity or recurrence rates in locally advanced lung cancer. Owing to the limited number of facilities, expense, reimbursement, and lack of clinically proven benefit to date, IMRT with photons is considered the standard of care.

Carbon Ions

Carbon ions can be used for heavy ion therapy, offering highly conformal dose distribution due to an even sharper Brag peak and potentially greater biologic effectiveness as compared with photons and protons. The high-linear energy transfer of carbon ions makes this modality intriguing for use in malignancies radioresistant to photon therapy. This type of particle therapy is not currently available in the United States. But centers do exist in Japan, Germany, China, Italy, and Austria.[251] Installation costs are quite expensive at approximately 140 million USD—about twice as much as a proton facility. Outcomes for patients with early-stage lung cancer treated with carbon ions are comparable to those seen with SBRT.[252] Takahashi et al. conducted a phase I/II trial to determine the efficacy and toxicity in patients with inoperable stage IIA to IIIA NSCLC treated with carbon ions. Although relatively short follow-up, results were encouraging with local control rate of 93% at 2 years.[253] As this modality continues to evolve and cost decreases, carbon ions could potentially be another option in patients who cannot tolerate concurrent chemoradiotherapy.

REFERENCES

1. Siegel RL, Miller KD, Jemal A. Cancer statistics, 2017. *CA Cancer J Clin.* 2017;67(1):7–30. https://doi.org/10.3322/caac.21387.
2. *Browse the SEER Cancer Statistics Review 1975-2014.* https://seer.cancer.gov/csr/1975_2014/browse_csr.php?sectionSEL=15&pageSEL=sect_15_table.12.html.
3. Alberg AJ, Brock MV, Ford JG, Samet JM, Spivack SD. Epidemiology of lung cancer. *Chest.* 2013;143(5):e1S–e29S. https://doi.org/10.1378/chest.12-2345.
4. Pierce JP, Messer K, White MM, Cowling DW, Thomas DP. Prevalence of heavy smoking in California and the United States, 1965-2007. *JAMA.* 2011;305(11):1106–1112. https://doi.org/10.1001/jama.2011.334.
5. Team TNLSTR. Reduced lung-cancer mortality with low-dose computed tomographic screening. *N Engl J Med.* 2011;365(5):395–409. https://doi.org/10.1056/NEJMoa1102873.
6. Wagner H, Langer CJ. Non–small cell lung cancer. In: *Clinical Radiation Oncology.* 4th ed. Philadelphia, PA: Elsevier; 2016:809–842.e8. https://www.clinicalkey.com/#!/content/book/3-s2.0-B9780323240987000447.
7. Rami-Porta R, Asamura H, Travis WD, Rusch VW. Lung cancer - major changes in the American Joint Committee on Cancer eighth edition cancer staging manual. *CA Cancer J Clin.* 2017;67(2):138–155. https://doi.org/10.3322/caac.21390.
8. Chen VW, Ruiz BA, Hsieh M-C, Wu X-C, Ries LAG, Lewis DR. Analysis of stage and clinical/prognostic factors for lung cancer from SEER registries: AJCC staging and collaborative stage data collection system. *Cancer.* 2014;120(suppl 23):3781–3792. https://doi.org/10.1002/cncr.29045.
9. Berlin NI, Buncher CR, Fontana RS, Frost JK, Melamed MR. The National Cancer Institute cooperative early lung cancer detection program. Results of the initial screen (prevalence). Early lung cancer detection: introduction. *Am Rev Respir Dis.* 1984;130(4):545–549. https://doi.org/10.1164/arrd.1984.130.4.545.
10. Melamed MR, Flehinger BJ, Zaman MB, Heelan RT, Perchick WA, Martini N. Screening for early lung cancer. Results of the Memorial Sloan-Kettering study in New York. *Chest.* 1984;86(1):44–53.
11. Humphrey LL, Deffebach M, Pappas M, et al. Screening for lung cancer with low-dose computed tomography: a systematic review to update the US preventive services task force recommendation. *Ann Intern Med.* 2013;159(6):411–420. https://doi.org/10.7326/0003-4819-159-6-201309170-00690.

12. Horeweg N, Scholten ET, de Jong PA, et al. Detection of lung cancer through low-dose CT screening (NELSON): a prespecified analysis of screening test performance and interval cancers. *Lancet Oncol.* 2014;15(12): 1342−1350. https://doi.org/10.1016/S1470-2045(14) 70387-0.

13. Scholten ET, Horeweg N, de Koning HJ, et al. Computed tomographic characteristics of interval and post screen carcinomas in lung cancer screening. *Eur Radiol.* 2015; 25(1):81−88. https://doi.org/10.1007/s00330-014-3394-4.

14. Diaz LA, Bardelli A. Liquid biopsies: genotyping circulating tumor DNA. *J Clin Oncol.* 2014;32(6):579−586. https://doi.org/10.1200/JCO.2012.45.2011.

15. Party BTSS of CS of GBIW. Guidelines on the selection of patients with lung cancer for surgery. *Thorax.* 2001;56(2): 89−108. https://doi.org/10.1136/thorax.56.2.89.

16. Brunelli A, Kim AW, Berger KI, Addrizzo-Harris DJ. Physiologic evaluation of the patient with lung cancer being considered for resectional surgery: diagnosis and management of lung cancer, 3rd ed: American College of Chest Physicians evidence-based clinical practice guidelines. *Chest.* 2013;143(suppl 5):e166S−e190S. https://doi.org/10.1378/chest.12-2395.

17. Dwamena BA, Sonnad SS, Angobaldo JO, Wahl RL. Metastases from non-small cell lung cancer: mediastinal staging in the 1990s—meta-analytic comparison of PET and CT. *Radiology.* 1999;213(2):530−536. https://doi.org/10.1148/radiology.213.2.r99nv46530.

18. Toloza EM, Harpole L, McCrory DC. Noninvasive staging of non-small cell lung cancer: a review of the current evidence. *Chest.* 2003;123(1 suppl):137S−146S.

19. Marom EM, McAdams HP, Erasmus JJ, et al. Staging non-small cell lung cancer with whole-body PET. *Radiology.* 1999;212(3):803−809. https://doi.org/10.1148/radiology.212.3.r99se21803.

20. Bury T, Barreto A, Daenen F, Barthelemy N, Ghaye B, Rigo P. Fluorine-18 deoxyglucose positron emission tomography for the detection of bone metastases in patients with non-small cell lung cancer. *Eur J Nucl Med.* 1998;25(9):1244−1247.

21. Reed CE, Harpole DH, Posther KE, et al. Results of the American College of Surgeons Oncology Group Z0050 trial: the utility of positron emission tomography in staging potentially operable non-small cell lung cancer. *J Thoracic Cardiovasc Surg.* 2003;126(6):1943−1951. https://doi.org/10.1016/j.jtcvs.2003.07.030.

22. Rankin S. PET/CT for staging and monitoring non small cell lung cancer. *Cancer Imaging.* 2008; 8(Spec Iss A):S27−S31. https://doi.org/10.1102/1470-7330.2008.9006.

23. Nomori H, Watanabe K, Ohtsuka T, Naruke T, Suemasu K, Uno K. Evaluation of F-18 fluorodeoxyglucose (FDG) PET scanning for pulmonary nodules less than 3 cm in diameter, with special reference to the CT images. *Lung Cancer Amst Neth.* 2004;45(1):19−27. https://doi.org/10.1016/j.lungcan.2004.01.009.

24. Gould MK, Maclean CC, Kuschner WG, Rydzak CE, Owens DK. Accuracy of positron emission tomography for diagnosis of pulmonary nodules and mass lesions: a meta-analysis. *JAMA.* 2001;285(7):914−924. https://doi.org/10.1001/jama.285.7.914.

25. Rivera MP, Mehta AC, Wahidi MM. Establishing the diagnosis of lung cancer: diagnosis and management of lung cancer, 3rd ed: American College of Chest Physicians evidence-based clinical practice guidelines. *Chest.* 2013; 143(suppl 5):e142S−e165S. https://doi.org/10.1378/chest.12-2353.

26. Lemaire A, Nikolic I, Petersen T, et al. Nine-year single center experience with cervical mediastinoscopy: complications and false negative rate. *Ann Thorac Surg.* 2006; 82(4):1185−1190. https://doi.org/10.1016/j.athoracsur.2006.05.023.

27. Defranchi SA, Edell ES, Daniels CE, et al. Mediastinoscopy in patients with lung cancer and negative endobronchial ultrasound guided needle aspiration. *Ann Thorac Surg.* 2010;90(6):1753−1757. https://doi.org/10.1016/j.athoracsur.2010.06.052.

28. Annema JT, van Meerbeeck JP, Rintoul RC, et al. Mediastinoscopy vs endosonography for mediastinal nodal staging of lung cancer: a randomized trial. *JAMA.* 2010;304(20):2245−2252. https://doi.org/10.1001/jama.2010.1705.

29. Dela Cruz CS, Tanoue LT, Matthay RA. Lung cancer: epidemiology, etiology, and prevention. *Clin Chest Med.* 2011;32(4):605−644. https://doi.org/10.1016/j.ccm.2011.09.001.

30. Travis WD, Brambilla E, Noguchi M, et al. Diagnosis of lung adenocarcinoma in resected specimens: implications of the 2011 International Association for the Study of Lung Cancer/American Thoracic Society/ European Respiratory Society Classification. *Arch Pathol Lab Med.* 2012;137(5):685−705. https://doi.org/10.5858/arpa.2012-0264-RA.

31. Travis WD, Brambilla E, Nicholson AG, et al. The 2015 World health Organization classification of lung tumors. *J Thorac Oncol.* 2015;10(9):1243−1260. https://doi.org/10.1097/JTO.0000000000000630.

32. Anagnostou VK, Syrigos KN, Bepler G, Homer RJ, Rimm DL. Thyroid transcription factor 1 is an independent prognostic factor for patients with stage I lung adenocarcinoma. *J Clin Oncol.* 2009;27(2):271−278. https://doi.org/10.1200/JCO.2008.17.0043.

33. Rekhtman N, Ang DC, Sima CS, Travis WD, Moreira AL. Immunohistochemical algorithm for differentiation of lung adenocarcinoma and squamous cell carcinoma based on large series of whole-tissue sections with validation in small specimens. *Mod Pathol.* 2011;24(10):1348−1359. https://doi.org/10.1038/modpathol.2011.92.

34. Tam IYS, Chung LP, Suen WS, et al. Distinct epidermal growth factor receptor and KRAS mutation patterns in non−small cell lung cancer patients with different tobacco exposure and clinicopathologic features. *Clin Cancer Res.* 2006;12(5):1647−1653. https://doi.org/10.1158/1078-0432.CCR-05-1981.

35. Soung YH, Lee JW, Kim SY, et al. Mutational analysis of EGFR and K-RAS genes in lung adenocarcinomas. *Virchows Arch.* 2005;446(5):483–488. https://doi.org/10.1007/s00428-005-1254-y.
36. Shigematsu H, Gazdar AF. Somatic mutations of epidermal growth factor receptor signaling pathway in lung cancers. *Int J Cancer.* 2006;118(2):257–262. https://doi.org/10.1002/ijc.21496.
37. Ladanyi M, Pao W. Lung adenocarcinoma: guiding EGFR-targeted therapy and beyond. *Mod Pathol.* 2008;21(S2):S16–S22. https://doi.org/10.1038/modpathol.3801018.
38. Pao W, Miller V, Zakowski M, et al. EGF receptor gene mutations are common in lung cancers from "never smokers" and are associated with sensitivity of tumors to gefitinib and erlotinib. *Proc Natl Acad Sci U S A.* 2004;101(36):13306–13311. https://doi.org/10.1073/pnas.0405220101.
39. Fujimoto J, Wistuba II. Current concepts on the molecular pathology of non-small cell lung carcinoma. *Semin Diagn Pathol.* 2014;31(4):306–313. https://doi.org/10.1053/j.semdp.2014.06.008.
40. Ferguson KM, Berger MB, Mendrola JM, Cho H-S, Leahy DJ, Lemmon MA. EGF activates its receptor by removing interactions that autoinhibit ectodomain dimerization. *Mol Cell.* 2003;11(2):507–517. https://doi.org/10.1016/S1097-2765(03)00047-9.
41. Buttitta F, Barassi F, Fresu G, et al. Mutational analysis of the HER2 gene in lung tumors from Caucasian patients: mutations are mainly present in adenocarcinomas with bronchioloalveolar features. *Int J Cancer.* 2006;119(11):2586–2591. https://doi.org/10.1002/ijc.22143.
42. Langer CJ, Stephenson P, Thor A, Vangel M, Johnson DH, Eastern Cooperative Oncology Group Study 2598. Trastuzumab in the treatment of advanced non-small-cell lung cancer: is there a role? Focus on Eastern Cooperative Oncology Group study 2598. *J Clin Oncol.* 2004;22(7):1180–1187. https://doi.org/10.1200/JCO.2004.04.105.
43. Bergethon K, Shaw AT, Ignatius Ou S-H, et al. ROS1 rearrangements define a unique molecular class of lung cancers. *J Clin Oncol.* 2012;30(8):863–870. https://doi.org/10.1200/JCO.2011.35.6345.
44. Shaw AT, Ou S-HI, Bang Y-J, et al. Crizotinib in ROS1-rearranged non-small-cell lung cancer. *N Engl J Med.* 2014;371(21):1963–1971. https://doi.org/10.1056/NEJMoa1406766.
45. Wong DW-S, Leung EL-H, So KK-T, et al. The EML4-ALK fusion gene is involved in various histologic types of lung cancers from nonsmokers with wild-type EGFR and KRAS. *Cancer.* 2009;115(8):1723–1733. https://doi.org/10.1002/cncr.24181.
46. Sasaki T, Jänne PA. New strategies for treatment of ALK rearranged non-small cell lung cancers. *Clin Cancer Res.* 2011;17(23):7213–7218. https://doi.org/10.1158/1078-0432.CCR-11-1404.
47. Camidge DR, Ou S-HI, Shapiro G, et al. Efficacy and safety of crizotinib in patients with advanced c-MET-amplified non-small cell lung cancer (NSCLC). *J Clin Oncol.* 2014;32(suppl 15):8001. https://doi.org/10.1200/jco.2014.32.15_suppl.8001.
48. Awad MM, Oxnard GR, Jackman DM, et al. MET exon 14 mutations in non-small-cell lung cancer are associated with advanced age and stage-dependent MET genomic amplification and c-MET overexpression. *J Clin Oncol.* 2016;34(7):721–730. https://doi.org/10.1200/JCO.2015.63.4600.
49. Beau-Faller M, Ruppert A-M, Voegeli A-C, et al. MET gene copy number in non-small cell lung cancer: molecular analysis in a targeted tyrosine kinase inhibitor naïve cohort. *J Thorac Oncol.* 2008;3(4):331–339. https://doi.org/10.1097/JTO.0b013e318168d9d4.
50. Onitsuka T, Uramoto H, Ono K, et al. Comprehensive molecular analyses of lung adenocarcinoma with regard to the epidermal growth factor receptor, K-ras, MET, and hepatocyte growth factor status. *J Thorac Oncol.* 2010;5(5):591–596. https://doi.org/10.1097/JTO.0b013e3181d0a4db.
51. Wang R, Hu H, Pan Y, et al. RET fusions define a unique molecular and clinicopathologic subtype of non-small-cell lung cancer. *J Clin Oncol.* 2012;30(35):4352–4359. https://doi.org/10.1200/JCO.2012.44.1477.
52. Wan PTC, Garnett MJ, Roe SM, et al. Mechanism of activation of the RAF-ERK signaling pathway by oncogenic mutations of B-RAF. *Cell.* 2004;116(6):855–867. https://doi.org/10.1016/S0092-8674(04)00215-6.
53. Paik PK, Arcila ME, Fara M, et al. Clinical characteristics of patients with lung adenocarcinomas harboring BRAF mutations. *J Clin Oncol.* 2011;29(15):2046–2051. https://doi.org/10.1200/JCO.2010.33.1280.
54. Riely GJ, Politi KA, Miller VA, Pao W. Update on epidermal growth factor receptor mutations in non-small cell lung cancer. *Clin Cancer Res.* 2006;12(24):7232–7241. https://doi.org/10.1158/1078-0432.CCR-06-0658.
55. Warren GW, Alberg AJ, Kraft AS, Cummings KM. The 2014 Surgeon General's report: "The health consequences of smoking–50 years of progress": a paradigm shift in cancer care. *Cancer.* 2014;120(13):1914–1916. https://doi.org/10.1002/cncr.28695.
56. Parsons A, Daley A, Begh R, Aveyard P. Influence of smoking cessation after diagnosis of early stage lung cancer on prognosis: systematic review of observational studies with meta-analysis. *BMJ.* 2010;340:b5569. https://doi.org/10.1136/bmj.b5569.
57. Videtic GMM, Stitt LW, Dar AR, et al. Continued cigarette smoking by patients receiving concurrent chemoradiotherapy for limited-stage small-cell lung cancer is associated with decreased survival. *J Clin Oncol.* 2003;21(8):1544–1549. https://doi.org/10.1200/JCO.2003.10.089.

58. Roach MC, Rehman S, DeWees TA, Abraham CD, Bradley JD, Robinson CG. It's never too late: smoking cessation after stereotactic body radiation therapy for non-small cell lung carcinoma improves overall survival. *Pract Radiat Oncol.* 2016;6(1):12–18. https://doi.org/10.1016/j.prro.2015.09.005.

59. Berthiller J, Straif K, Boniol M, et al. Cannabis smoking and risk of lung cancer in men: a pooled analysis of three studies in Maghreb. *J Thorac Oncol.* 2008;3(12):1398–1403. https://doi.org/10.1097/JTO.0b013e31818ddcde.

60. Zhang LR, Morgenstern H, Greenland S, et al. Cannabis smoking and lung cancer risk: pooled analysis in the International Lung Cancer Consortium. *Int J Cancer.* 2015; 136(4):894–903. https://doi.org/10.1002/ijc.29036.

61. Callaghan RC, Allebeck P, Sidorchuk A. Marijuana use and risk of lung cancer: a 40-year cohort study. *Cancer Causes Control.* 2013;24(10):1811–1820. https://doi.org/10.1007/s10552-013-0259-0.

62. Moir D, Rickert WS, Levasseur G, et al. A comparison of mainstream and sidestream marijuana and tobacco cigarette smoke produced under two machine smoking conditions. *Chem Res Toxicol.* 2008;21(2):494–502. https://doi.org/10.1021/tx700275p.

63. Lane M, Smith FE, Sullivan RA, Plasse TF. Dronabinol and prochlorperazine alone and in combination as antiemetic agents for cancer chemotherapy. *Am J Clin Oncol.* 1990;13(6):480–484.

64. Nelson K, Walsh D, Deeter P, Sheehan F. A phase II study of delta-9-tetrahydrocannabinol for appetite stimulation in cancer-associated anorexia. *J Palliat Care.* 1994;10(1): 14–18.

65. Martini N, Flehinger BJ, Zaman MB, Beattie EJ. Results of resection in non-oat cell carcinoma of the lung with mediastinal lymph node metastases. *Ann Surg.* 1983; 198(3):386–397.

66. Pass HI, Pogrebniak HW, Steinberg SM, Mulshine J, Minna J. Randomized trial of neoadjuvant therapy for lung cancer: interim analysis. *Ann Thorac Surg.* 1992; 53(6):992–998.

67. Depierre A, Milleron B, Moro-Sibilot D, et al. Preoperative chemotherapy followed by surgery compared with primary surgery in resectable stage I (except T1N0), II, and IIIa non-small-cell lung cancer. *J Clin Oncol.* 2002;20(1): 247–253. https://doi.org/10.1200/JCO.2002.20.1.247.

68. Martini N, Kris MG, Gralla RJ, et al. The effects of preoperative chemotherapy on the resectability of non-small cell lung carcinoma with mediastinal lymph node metastases (N2 M0). *Ann Thorac Surg.* 1988;45(4):370–379.

69. Roth JA, Fossella F, Komaki R, et al. A randomized trial comparing perioperative chemotherapy and surgery with surgery alone in resectable stage IIIA non-small-cell lung cancer. *J Natl Cancer Inst.* 1994;86(9):673–680.

70. Rosell R, Gomez-Codina J, Camps C, et al. A randomized trial comparing preoperative chemotherapy plus surgery with surgery alone in patients with non-small-cell lung cancer. *N Engl J Med.* 1994;330(3):153–158. https://doi.org/10.1056/NEJM199401203300301.

71. Ichinose Y, Yosimori K, Yoneda S, Kuba M, Kudoh S, Niitani H. UFT plus cisplatin combination chemotherapy in the treatment of patients with advanced nonsmall cell lung carcinoma: a multiinstitutional phase II trial. For the Japan UFT Lung Cancer Study Group. *Cancer.* 2000; 88(2):318–323.

72. van Meerbeeck JP, Kramer GWPM, Van Schil PEY, et al. Randomized controlled trial of resection versus radiotherapy after induction chemotherapy in stage IIIA-N2 non-small-cell lung cancer. *J Natl Cancer Inst.* 2007; 99(6):442–450. https://doi.org/10.1093/jnci/djk093.

73. Betticher DC, Hsu Schmitz S-F, Tötsch M, et al. Mediastinal lymph node clearance after docetaxel-cisplatin neoadjuvant chemotherapy is prognostic of survival in patients with stage IIIA pN2 non-small-cell lung cancer: a multicenter phase II trial. *J Clin Oncol.* 2003;21(9): 1752–1759. https://doi.org/10.1200/JCO.2003.11.040.

74. Andre F, Grunenwald D, Pignon JP, et al. Survival of patients with resected N2 non-small-cell lung cancer: evidence for a subclassification and implications. *J Clin Oncol.* 2000;18(16):2981–2989. https://doi.org/10.1200/JCO.2000.18.16.2981.

75. Asamura H, Chansky K, Crowley J, et al. The International association for the study of lung cancer lung cancer staging project. *J Thorac Oncol.* 2015;10(12):1675–1684. https://doi.org/10.1097/JTO.0000000000000678.

76. Albain KS, Rusch VW, Crowley JJ, et al. Concurrent cisplatin/etoposide plus chest radiotherapy followed by surgery for stages IIIA (N2) and IIIB non-small-cell lung cancer: mature results of Southwest Oncology Group phase II study 8805. *J Clin Oncol Off.* 1995;13(8):1880–1892. https://doi.org/10.1200/JCO.1995.13.8.1880.

77. Faber LP, Kittle CF, Warren WH, et al. Preoperative chemotherapy and irradiation for stage III non-small cell lung cancer. *Ann Thorac Surg.* 1989;47(5):669–675; discussion 676–677.

78. Albain KS, Swann RS, Rusch VR, et al. Phase III study of concurrent chemotherapy and radiotherapy (CT/RT) vs CT/RT followed by surgical resection for stage IIIA(pN2) non-small cell lung cancer (NSCLC): outcomes update of North American Intergroup 0139 (RTOG 9309). *J Clin Oncol.* 2005;23(suppl 16):7014. https://doi.org/10.1200/jco.2005.23.16_suppl.7014.

79. Albain KS, Swann RS, Rusch VW, et al. Radiotherapy plus chemotherapy with or without surgical resection for stage III non-small-cell lung cancer: a phase III randomised controlled trial. *Lancet Lond Engl.* 2009;374(9687): 379–386. https://doi.org/10.1016/S0140-6736(09)60737-6.

80. Allen AM, Mentzer SJ, Yeap BY, et al. Pneumonectomy after chemoradiation. *Cancer.* 2008;112(5):1106–1113. https://doi.org/10.1002/cncr.23283.

81. Gudbjartsson T, Gyllstedt E, Pikwer A, Jönsson P. Early surgical results after pneumonectomy for non-small cell lung cancer are not affected by preoperative radiotherapy and chemotherapy. *Ann Thorac Surg.* 2008;86(2):376–382. https://doi.org/10.1016/j.athoracsur.2008.04.013.

82. Doddoli C, Barlesi F, Trousse D, et al. One hundred consecutive pneumonectomies after induction therapy for non-small cell lung cancer: an uncertain balance between risks and benefits. *J Thorac Cardiovasc Surg*. 2005;130(2):416–425. https://doi.org/10.1016/j.jtcvs.2004.11.022.

83. d'Amato TA, Ashrafi AS, Schuchert MJ, et al. Risk of pneumonectomy after induction therapy for locally advanced non-small cell lung cancer. *Ann Thorac Surg*. 2009;88(4):1079–1085. https://doi.org/10.1016/j.athoracsur.2009.06.025.

84. Martin J, Ginsberg RJ, Abolhoda A, et al. Morbidity and mortality after neoadjuvant therapy for lung cancer: the risks of right pneumonectomy. *Ann Thorac Surg*. 2001;72(4):1149–1154. https://doi.org/10.1016/S0003-4975(01)02995-2.

85. Pless M, Stupp R, Ris H-B, et al. Induction chemoradiation in stage IIIA/N2 non-small-cell lung cancer: a phase 3 randomised trial. *Lancet*. 2015;386(9998):1049–1056. https://doi.org/10.1016/S0140-6736(15)60294-X.

86. *NCCN Clinical Practice Guidelines in Oncology*. https://www.nccn.org/professionals/physician_gls/f_guidelines.asp#site.

87. Rusch VW, Giroux DJ, Kraut MJ, et al. Induction chemoradiation and surgical resection for superior sulcus non-small-cell lung carcinomas: long-term results of Southwest Oncology group trial 9416 (Intergroup trial 0160). *J Clin Oncol*. 2007;25(3):313–318. https://doi.org/10.1200/JCO.2006.08.2826.

88. Kunitoh H, Kato H, Tsuboi M, et al. Phase II trial of preoperative chemoradiotherapy followed by surgical resection in patients with superior sulcus non-small-cell lung cancers: report of Japan Clinical Oncology Group trial 9806. *J Clin Oncol Off*. 2008;26(4):644–649. https://doi.org/10.1200/JCO.2007.14.1911.

89. Pourel N, Santelmo N, Naafa N, et al. Concurrent cisplatin/etoposide plus 3D-conformal radiotherapy followed by surgery for stage IIB (superior sulcus T3N0)/III non-small cell lung cancer yields a high rate of pathological complete response. *Eur J Cardiothorac Surg*. 2008;33(5):829–836. https://doi.org/10.1016/j.ejcts.2008.01.063.

90. Gomez DR, Cox JD, Roth JA, et al. A prospective phase 2 study of surgery followed by chemotherapy and radiation for superior sulcus tumors. *Cancer*. 2012;118(2):444–451. https://doi.org/10.1002/cncr.26277.

91. Group TLCS. Effects of postoperative mediastinal radiation on completely resected stage II and stage III epidermoid cancer of the lung. *N Engl J Med*. 1986;315(22):1377–1381. https://doi.org/10.1056/NEJM198611273152202.

92. Stephens RJ, Girling DJ, Bleehen NM, Moghissi K, Yosef HM, Machin D. The role of post-operative radiotherapy in non-small-cell lung cancer: a multicentre randomised trial in patients with pathologically staged T1-2, N1-2, M0 disease. Medical Research Council Lung Cancer Working Party. *Br J Cancer*. 1996;74(4):632–639.

93. Kelsey CR, Light KL, Marks LB. Patterns of failure after resection of non–small-cell lung cancer: implications for postoperative radiation therapy volumes. *Int J Radiat Oncol*. 2006;65(4):1097–1105. https://doi.org/10.1016/j.ijrobp.2006.02.007.

94. Kirsh MM, Rotman H, Argenta L, et al. Carcinoma of the lung: results of treatment over ten years. *Ann Thorac Surg*. 1976;21(5):371–377.

95. Green N, Kurohara SS, George FW, Crews QE. Postresection irradiation for primary lung cancer. *Radiology*. 1975;116(02):405–407. https://doi.org/10.1148/116.2.405.

96. Choi NCH, Grillo HC, Gardiello M, Scannell JG, Wilkins EW. Basis for new strategies in postoperative radiotherapy of bronchogenic carcinoma. *Int J Radiat Oncol Biol Phys*. 1980;6(1):31–35. https://doi.org/10.1016/0360-3016(80)90199-6.

97. Newman SB, DeMeester TR, Golomb HM, Hoffman PC, Little AG, Raghavan V. Treatment of modified Stage II (T1 N1 M0, T2 N1 M0) non-small cell bronchogenic carcinoma. A combined modality approach. *J Thorac Cardiovasc Surg*. 1983;86(2):180–185.

98. Van Houtte P, Rocmans P, Smets P, et al. Postoperative radiation therapy in lung caner: a controlled trial after resection of curative design. *Int J Radiat Oncol Biol Phys*. 1980;6(8):983–986.

99. Lafitte JJ, Ribet ME, Prévost BM, Gosselin BH, Copin MC, Brichet AH. Postresection irradiation for T2 N0 M0 non-small cell carcinoma: a prospective, randomized study. *Ann Thorac Surg*. 1996;62(3):830–834.

100. Debevec M, Bitenc M, Vidmar S, et al. Postoperative radiotherapy for radically resected N2 non-small-cell lung cancer (NSCLC): randomised clinical study 1988–1992. *Lung Cancer*. 1996;14(1):99–107. https://doi.org/10.1016/0169-5002(95)00515-3.

101. Mayer R, Smolle-Juettner F-M, Szolar D, et al. Postoperative radiotherapy in radically resected non-small cell lung cancer. *Chest*. 1997;112(4):954–959. https://doi.org/10.1378/chest.112.4.954.

102. Postoperative radiotherapy in non-small-cell lung cancer: systematic review and meta-analysis of individual patient data from nine randomised controlled trials. *Lancet*. 1998;352(9124):257–263. https://doi.org/10.1016/S0140-6736(98)06341-7.

103. Bogart JA, Aronowitz JN. Localized non-small cell lung cancer: adjuvant radiotherapy in the era of effective systemic therapy. *Clin Cancer Res*. 2005;11(13 pt 2):5004s–5010s. https://doi.org/10.1158/1078-0432.CCR-05-9010.

104. Munro AJ. What now for postoperative radiotherapy for lung cancer? *Lancet*. 1998;352(9124):250–251. https://doi.org/10.1016/S0140-6736(98)22030-7.

105. Billiet C, Decaluwé H, Peeters S, et al. Modern postoperative radiotherapy for stage III non-small cell lung cancer may improve local control and survival: a meta-analysis. *Radiother Oncol*. 2014;110(1):3–8. https://doi.org/10.1016/j.radonc.2013.08.011.

106. Douillard J-Y, Rosell R, Lena MD, Riggi M, Hurteloup P, Mahe M-A. Impact of postoperative radiation therapy on survival in patients with complete resection and stage I, II, or IIIA non–small-cell lung cancer treated with adjuvant chemotherapy: the adjuvant Navelbine International Trialist Association (ANITA) Randomized Trial. *Int J Radiat Oncol Biol Phys.* 2008;72(3):695–701. https://doi.org/10.1016/j.ijrobp.2008.01.044.

107. Lally BE, Zelterman D, Colasanto JM, Haffty BG, Detterbeck FC, Wilson LD. Postoperative radiotherapy for stage II or III non–small-cell lung cancer using the surveillance, epidemiology, and end results database. *J Clin Oncol.* 2006;24(19):2998–3006. https://doi.org/10.1200/JCO.2005.04.6110.

108. Robinson CG, Patel AP, Bradley JD, et al. Postoperative radiotherapy for pathologic N2 non–small-cell lung cancer treated with adjuvant chemotherapy: a review of the National Cancer Data Base. *J Clin Oncol.* 2015;33(8):870–876. https://doi.org/10.1200/JCO.2014.58.5380.

109. Wang EH, Corso CD, Rutter CE, et al. Postoperative radiation therapy is associated with improved overall survival in incompletely resected stage II and III non–small-cell lung cancer. *J Clin Oncol.* 2015;33(25):2727–2734. https://doi.org/10.1200/JCO.2015.61.1517.

110. Keller SM, Adak S, Wagner H, et al. A randomized trial of postoperative adjuvant therapy in patients with completely resected stage II or IIIa non–small-cell lung cancer. *N Engl J Med.* 2000;343(17):1217–1222. https://doi.org/10.1056/NEJM200010263431703.

111. Bradley JD, Paulus R, Graham MV, et al. Phase II trial of postoperative adjuvant paclitaxel/carboplatin and thoracic radiotherapy in resected stage II and IIIA non–small-cell lung cancer: promising long-term results of the radiation therapy oncology group–RTOG 9705. *J Clin Oncol.* 2005;23(15):3480–3487. https://doi.org/10.1200/JCO.2005.12.120.

112. *Radiation Therapy in Treating Patients With Non Small Cell Lung Cancer That Has Been Completely Removed by Surgery - Full Text View - ClinicalTrials.gov.* https://clinicaltrials.gov/ct2/show/NCT00410683.

113. Bezjak A, Temin S, Franklin G, et al. Definitive and adjuvant radiotherapy in locally advanced non–small-cell lung cancer: American Society of Clinical Oncology Clinical Practice Guideline Endorsement of the American Society for Radiation Oncology Evidence-Based Clinical Practice Guideline. *J Clin Oncol.* 2015;33(18):2100–2105. https://doi.org/10.1200/JCO.2014.59.2360.

114. Chemotherapy in non-small cell lung cancer. A meta-analysis using updated data on individual patients from 52 randomised clinical trials. Non-small Cell Lung Cancer Collaborative Group. *BMJ.* 1995;311(7010):899–909.

115. Arriagada R, Dunant A, Pignon J-P, et al. Long-term results of the international adjuvant lung cancer trial evaluating adjuvant cisplatin-based chemotherapy in resected lung cancer. *J Clin Oncol.* 2010;28(1):35–42. https://doi.org/10.1200/JCO.2009.23.2272.

116. Douillard J-Y, Rosell R, Lena MD, et al. Adjuvant vinorelbine plus cisplatin versus observation in patients with completely resected stage IB–IIIA non-small-cell lung cancer (Adjuvant Navelbine International Trialist Association [ANITA]): a randomised controlled trial. *Lancet Oncol.* 2006;7(9):719–727. https://doi.org/10.1016/S1470-2045(06)70804-X.

117. Group TIALCTC. Cisplatin-based adjuvant chemotherapy in patients with completely resected non–small-cell lung cancer. *N Engl J Med.* 2004;350(4):351–360. https://doi.org/10.1056/NEJMoa031644.

118. Winton T, Livingston R, Johnson D, et al. Vinorelbine plus cisplatin vs. observation in resected non–small-cell lung cancer. *N Engl J Med.* 2005;352(25):2589–2597. https://doi.org/10.1056/NEJMoa043623.

119. Scagliotti GV, Fossati R, Torri V, et al. Randomized study of adjuvant chemotherapy for completely resected stage I, II, or IIIA non-small-cell Lung cancer. *J Natl Cancer Inst.* 2003;95(19):1453–1461.

120. Waller D, Peake MD, Stephens RJ, et al. Chemotherapy for patients with non-small cell lung cancer: the surgical setting of the big lung trial. *Eur J Cardiothorac Surg.* 2004;26(1):173–182. https://doi.org/10.1016/j.ejcts.2004.03.041.

121. Pignon J-P, Tribodet H, Scagliotti GV, et al. Lung adjuvant cisplatin evaluation: a pooled analysis by the LACE collaborative group. *J Clin Oncol.* 2008;26(21):3552–3559. https://doi.org/10.1200/JCO.2007.13.9030.

122. Strauss GM, Herndon JE, Maddaus MA, et al. Adjuvant paclitaxel plus carboplatin compared with observation in stage IB non-small-cell lung cancer: CALGB 9633 with the Cancer and Leukemia Group B, Radiation Therapy Oncology Group, and North Central Cancer Treatment Group Study Groups. *J Clin Oncol.* 2008;26(31):5043–5051. https://doi.org/10.1200/JCO.2008.16.4855.

123. Park SY, Lee JG, Kim J, et al. Efficacy of platinum-based adjuvant chemotherapy in T2aN0 stage IB non-small cell lung cancer. *J Cardiothorac Surg.* 2013;8:151. https://doi.org/10.1186/1749-8090-8-151.

124. NSCLC Meta-analyses Collaborative Group, Arriagada R, Auperin A, et al. Adjuvant chemotherapy, with or without postoperative radiotherapy, in operable non-small-cell lung cancer: two meta-analyses of individual patient data. *Lancet Lond Engl.* 2010;375(9722):1267–1277. https://doi.org/10.1016/S0140-6736(10)60059-1.

125. Kubota K, Furuse K, Kawahara M, et al. Role of radiotherapy in combined modality treatment of locally advanced non-small-cell lung cancer. *J Clin Oncol.* 1994;12(8):1547–1552. https://doi.org/10.1200/JCO.1994.12.8.1547.

126. Saunders M, Dische S, Barrett A, Harvey A, Griffiths G, Parmar M. Continuous, hyperfractionated, accelerated radiotherapy (CHART) versus conventional radiotherapy in non-small cell lung cancer: mature data from the randomised multicentre trial. *Radiother Oncol.* 1999;52(2):137–148. https://doi.org/10.1016/S0167-8140(99)00087-0.

127. Saunders MI, Dische S. Continuous, hyperfractionated, accelerated radiotherapy (CHART) in non-small cell carcinoma of the bronchus. *Int J Radiat Oncol Biol Phys*. 1990; 19(5):1211–1215.

128. Bradley J, Graham MV, Winter K, et al. Toxicity and outcome results of RTOG 9311: a phase I–II dose-escalation study using three-dimensional conformal radiotherapy in patients with inoperable non–small-cell lung carcinoma. *Int J Radiat Oncol Biol Phys*. 2005;61(2): 318–328. https://doi.org/10.1016/j.ijrobp.2004.06.260.

129. Hayman JA, Martel MK, Ten Haken RK, et al. Dose escalation in non-small-cell lung cancer using three-dimensional conformal radiation therapy: update of a phase I trial. *J Clin Oncol*. 2001;19(1):127–136. https:// doi.org/10.1200/JCO.2001.19.1.127.

130. Bradley JD, Ieumwananonthachai N, Purdy JA, et al. Gross tumor volume, critical prognostic factor in patients treated with three-dimensional conformal radiation therapy for non-small-cell lung carcinoma. *Int J Radiat Oncol*. 2002;52(1):49–57. https://doi.org/10.1016/ S0360-3016(01)01772-2.

131. Rengan R, Rosenzweig KE, Venkatraman E, et al. Improved local control with higher doses of radiation in large-volume stage III non–small-cell lung cancer. *Int J Radiat Oncol*. 2004;60(3):741–747. https:// doi.org/10.1016/j.ijrobp.2004.04.013.

132. Ramroth J, Cutter DJ, Darby SC, et al. Dose and fractionation in radiation therapy of curative intent for non-small cell lung cancer: meta-analysis of randomized trials. *Int J Radiat Oncol*. 2016;96(4):736–747. https://doi.org/ 10.1016/j.ijrobp.2016.07.022.

133. Nguyen LN, Komaki R, Allen P, Schea RA, Milas L. Effectiveness of accelerated radiotherapy for patients with inoperable non-small cell lung cancer (NSCLC) and borderline prognostic factors without distant metastasis: a retrospective review. *Int J Radiat Oncol*. 1999;44(5):1053–1056. https://doi.org/10.1016/S0360-3016(99)00130-3.

134. Cannon DM, Mehta MP, Adkison JB, et al. Dose-limiting toxicity after hypofractionated dose-escalated radiotherapy in non–small-cell lung cancer. *J Clin Oncol*. 2013;31(34):4343–4348. https://doi.org/10.1200/ JCO.2013.51.5353.

135. Cheung P, Faria S, Ahmed S, et al. Phase II study of accelerated hypofractionated three-dimensional conformal radiotherapy for stage T1-3 N0 M0 non–small cell lung cancer: NCIC CTG BR.25. *J Natl Cancer Inst*. 2014;8: 106. https://doi.org/10.1093/jnci/dju164.

136. Westover KD, Loo BW, Gerber DE, et al. Precision hypofractionated radiation therapy in poor performing patients with non-small cell lung cancer: phase 1 dose escalation trial. *Int J Radiat Oncol Biol Phys*. 2015;93(1): 72–81. https://doi.org/10.1016/j.ijrobp.2015.05.004.

137. Dillman RO, Seagren SL, Propert KJ, et al. A randomized trial of induction chemotherapy plus high-dose radiation versus radiation alone in stage III non-small-cell lung cancer. *N Engl J Med*. 1990;323(14):940–945. https:// doi.org/10.1056/NEJM199010043231403.

138. Dillman RO, Herndon J, Seagren SL, Eaton WL, Green MR. Improved survival in stage III non-small-cell lung cancer: seven-year follow-up of cancer and leukemia group B (CALGB) 8433 trial. *J Natl Cancer Inst*. 1996; 88(17):1210–1215.

139. Sause W, Kolesar P, Taylor S, et al. Final results of phase III trial in regionally advanced unresectable non-small cell lung cancer. *Chest*. 2000;117(2):358–364. https:// doi.org/10.1378/chest.117.2.358.

140. Le Chevalier T, Arriagada R, Quoix E, et al. Radiotherapy alone versus combined chemotherapy and radiotherapy in nonresectable non-small-cell lung cancer: first analysis of a randomized trial in 353 patients. *J Natl Cancer Inst*. 1991;83(6):417–423.

141. Cullen MH, Billingham LJ, Woodroffe CM, et al. Mitomycin, ifosfamide, and cisplatin in unresectable non-small-cell lung cancer: effects on survival and quality of life. *J Clin Oncol*. 1999;17(10):3188–3194. https:// doi.org/10.1200/JCO.1999.17.10.3188.

142. Morton RF, Jett JR, McGinnis WL, et al. Thoracic radiation therapy alone compared with combined chemoradiotherapy for locally unresectable non-small cell lung cancer. A randomized, phase III trial. *Ann Intern Med*. 1991;115(9):681–686.

143. Perez CA, Pajak TF, Rubin P, et al. Long-term observations of the patterns of failure in patients with unresectable non-oat cell carcinoma of the lung treated with definitive radiotherapy. Report by the Radiation Therapy Oncology Group. *Cancer*. 1987;59(11):1874–1881.

144. von der Maase H, Overgaard J, Vaeth M. Effect of cancer chemotherapeutic drugs on radiation-induced lung damage in mice. *Radiother Oncol*. 1986;5(3):245–257.

145. Schaake-Koning C, van den Bogaert W, Dalesio O, et al. Effects of concomitant cisplatin and radiotherapy on inoperable non-small-cell lung cancer. *N Engl J Med*. 1992;326(8):524–530. https://doi.org/10.1056/ NEJM199202203260805.

146. Clamon G, Herndon J, Cooper R, Chang AY, Rosenman J, Green MR. Radiosensitization with carboplatin for patients with unresectable stage III non–small-cell lung cancer: a phase III trial of the Cancer and Leukemia Group B and the Eastern Cooperative Oncology Group. *J Clin Oncol*. 1999;17(1):4. https://doi.org/10.1200/ JCO.1999.17.1.4.

147. Vokes EE, Herndon JE, Kelley MJ, et al. Induction chemotherapy followed by chemoradiotherapy compared with chemoradiotherapy alone for regionally advanced unresectable stage III non–small-cell lung cancer: cancer and leukemia group B. *J Clin Oncol*. 2007;25(13):1698–1704. https://doi.org/10.1200/ JCO.2006.07.3569.

148. Furuse K, Fukuoka M, Kawahara M, et al. Phase III study of concurrent versus sequential thoracic radiotherapy in combination with mitomycin, vindesine, and cisplatin in unresectable stage III non–small-cell lung cancer. *J Clin Oncol*. 1999;17(9):2692–2699. https://doi.org/ 10.1200/JCO.1999.17.9.2692.

149. Fournel P, Robinet G, Thomas P, et al. Randomized Phase III Trial of Sequential Chemoradiotherapy Compared With Concurrent Chemoradiotherapy in Locally Advanced Non–Small-Cell Lung Cancer: Groupe Lyon-Saint-Etienne d'Oncologie Thoracique–Groupe Français de Pneumo-Cancérologie NPC 95-01 Study. *J Clin Oncol.* 2005;23(25):5910–5917. https://doi.org/10.1200/JCO.2005.03.070.

150. Jeremic B, Shibamoto Y, Acimovic L, Milisavljevic S. Hyperfractionated radiation therapy with or without concurrent low-dose daily carboplatin/etoposide for stage III non-small-cell lung cancer: a randomized study. *J Clin Oncol.* 1996;14(4):1065–1070. https://doi.org/10.1200/JCO.1996.14.4.1065.

151. Lee JS, Scott C, Komaki R, et al. Concurrent chemoradiation therapy with oral etoposide and cisplatin for locally advanced inoperable non-small-cell lung cancer: radiation therapy oncology group protocol 91-06. *J Clin Oncol.* 1996;14(4):1055–1064. https://doi.org/10.1200/JCO.1996.14.4.1055.

152. Byhardt RW, Scott CB, Ettinger DS, et al. Concurrent hyperfractionated irradiation and chemotherapy for unresectable nonsmall cell lung cancer. Results of Radiation Therapy Oncology Group 90-15. *Cancer.* 1995;75(9):2337–2344.

153. Curran WJ, Paulus R, Langer CJ, et al. Sequential vs concurrent chemoradiation for stage III non–small cell lung cancer: randomized phase III trial RTOG 9410. *J Natl Cancer Inst.* 2011;103(19):1452–1460. https://doi.org/10.1093/jnci/djr325.

154. Aupérin A, Le Péchoux C, Rolland E, et al. Meta-analysis of concomitant versus sequential radiochemotherapy in locally advanced non–small-cell lung cancer. *J Clin Oncol.* 2010;28(13):2181–2190. https://doi.org/10.1200/JCO.2009.26.2543.

155. Albain KS, Crowley JJ, Turrisi AT, et al. Concurrent cisplatin, etoposide, and chest radiotherapy in pathologic stage IIIB non–small-cell lung cancer: a Southwest Oncology group phase II study, SWOG 9019. *J Clin Oncol.* 2002;20(16):3454–3460. https://doi.org/10.1200/JCO.2002.03.055.

156. Choy H, Akerley W, Safran H, et al. Multiinstitutional phase II trial of paclitaxel, carboplatin, and concurrent radiation therapy for locally advanced non-small-cell lung cancer. *J Clin Oncol.* 1998;16(10):3316–3322. https://doi.org/10.1200/JCO.1998.16.10.3316.

157. Yamamoto N, Nakagawa K, Nishimura Y, et al. Phase III study comparing second- and third-generation regimens with concurrent thoracic radiotherapy in patients with unresectable stage III non–small-cell lung cancer: West Japan thoracic oncology group WJTOG0105. *J Clin Oncol.* 2010;28(23):3739–3745. https://doi.org/10.1200/JCO.2009.24.5050.

158. Senan S, Brade A, Wang L, et al. PROCLAIM: randomized phase III trial of pemetrexed-cisplatin or etoposide-cisplatin plus thoracic radiation therapy followed by consolidation chemotherapy in locally advanced nonsquamous non–small-cell lung cancer. *J Clin Oncol.* 2016;34(9):953–962. https://doi.org/10.1200/JCO.2015.64.8824.

159. Bradley JD, Moughan J, Graham MV, et al. A phase I/II radiation dose escalation study with concurrent chemotherapy for patients with inoperable stages I to III non-small-cell lung cancer: phase I results of RTOG 0117. *Int J Radiat Oncol Biol Phys.* 2010;77(2):367–372. https://doi.org/10.1016/j.ijrobp.2009.04.029.

160. Bradley JD, Bae K, Graham MV, et al. Primary analysis of the phase II component of a phase I/II dose intensification study using three-dimensional conformal radiation therapy and concurrent chemotherapy for patients with inoperable non-small-cell lung cancer: RTOG 0117. *J Clin Oncol.* 2010;28(14):2475–2480. https://doi.org/10.1200/JCO.2009.27.1205.

161. Schild SE, McGinnis WL, Graham D, et al. Results of a Phase I trial of concurrent chemotherapy and escalating doses of radiation for unresectable non-small-cell lung cancer. *Int J Radiat Oncol Biol Phys.* 2006;65(4):1106–1111. https://doi.org/10.1016/j.ijrobp.2006.02.046.

162. Socinski MA, Blackstock AW, Bogart JA, et al. Randomized phase II trial of induction chemotherapy followed by concurrent chemotherapy and dose-escalated thoracic conformal radiotherapy (74 Gy) in stage III non-small-cell lung cancer: CALGB 30105. *J Clin Oncol.* 2008;26(15):2457–2463. https://doi.org/10.1200/JCO.2007.14.7371.

163. Stinchcombe TE, Lee CB, Moore DT, et al. Long-term follow-up of a phase I/II trial of dose escalating three-dimensional conformal thoracic radiation therapy with induction and concurrent carboplatin and paclitaxel in unresectable stage IIIA/B non-small cell lung cancer. *J Thorac Oncol.* 2008;3(11):1279–1285. https://doi.org/10.1097/JTO.0b013e31818b1971.

164. Machtay M, Bae K, Movsas B, et al. Higher biologically effective dose of radiotherapy is associated with improved outcomes for locally advanced non-small cell lung carcinoma treated with chemoradiation: an analysis of the Radiation Therapy Oncology Group. *Int J Radiat Oncol Biol Phys.* 2012;82(1):425–434. https://doi.org/10.1016/j.ijrobp.2010.09.004.

165. Bradley JD, Paulus R, Komaki R, et al. Standard-dose versus high-dose conformal radiotherapy with concurrent and consolidation carboplatin plus paclitaxel with or without cetuximab for patients with stage IIIA or IIIB non-small-cell lung cancer (RTOG 0617): a randomised, two-by-two factorial phase 3 study. *Lancet Oncol.* 2015;16(2):187–199. https://doi.org/10.1016/S1470-2045(14)71207-0.

166. Cox JD, Pajak TF, Asbell S, et al. Interruptions of high-dose radiation therapy decrease longterm survival of favorable patients with unresectable nonsmall cell carcinoma of the lung: analysis of 1244 cases from 3 radiation therapy oncology group (RTOG) trials. *Int J Radiat Oncol.* 1993;27(3):493–498. https://doi.org/10.1016/0360-3016(93)90371-2.

167. Gandara DR, Chansky K, Albain KS, et al. Consolidation docetaxel after concurrent chemoradiotherapy in stage IIIB non–small-cell lung cancer: phase II Southwest Oncology group study S9504. *J Clin Oncol.* 2003;21(10):2004–2010. https://doi.org/10.1200/JCO.2003.04.197.

168. Hanna N, Neubauer M, Yiannoutsos C, et al. Phase III study of cisplatin, etoposide, and concurrent chest radiation with or without consolidation docetaxel in patients with inoperable stage III non–small-cell lung cancer: the Hoosier Oncology Group and U.S. Oncology. *J Clin Oncol.* 2008;26(35):5755–5760. https://doi.org/10.1200/JCO.2008.17.7840.

169. Belani CP, Choy H, Bonomi P, et al. Combined chemoradiotherapy regimens of paclitaxel and carboplatin for locally advanced non–small-cell lung cancer: a randomized phase II locally advanced multi-modality protocol. *J Clin Oncol.* 2005;23(25):5883–5891. https://doi.org/10.1200/JCO.2005.55.405.

170. Ahn JS, Ahn YC, Kim J-H, et al. Multinational randomized phase III trial with or without consolidation chemotherapy using docetaxel and cisplatin after concurrent chemoradiation in inoperable stage III non–small-cell lung cancer: KCSG-LU05-04. *J Clin Oncol.* 2015;33(24):2660–2666. https://doi.org/10.1200/JCO.2014.60.0130.

171. Tsujino K, Kurata T, Yamamoto S, et al. Is consolidation chemotherapy after concurrent chemo-radiotherapy beneficial for patients with locally advanced non-small-cell lung cancer? A pooled analysis of the literature. *J Thorac Oncol.* 2013;8(9):1181–1189. https://doi.org/10.1097/JTO.0b013e3182988348.

172. Voldborg BR, Damstrup L, Spang-Thomsen M, Poulsen HS. Epidermal growth factor receptor (EGFR) and EGFR mutations, function and possible role in clinical trials. *Ann Oncol.* 1997;8(12):1197–1206.

173. Lynch TJ, Bell DW, Sordella R, et al. Activating mutations in the epidermal growth factor receptor underlying responsiveness of non–small-cell lung cancer to gefitinib. *N Engl J Med.* 2004;350(21):2129–2139. https://doi.org/10.1056/NEJMoa040938.

174. Blumenschein GR, Paulus R, Curran WJ, et al. Phase II study of cetuximab in combination with chemoradiation in patients with stage IIIA/B non-small-cell lung cancer: RTOG 0324. *J Clin Oncol.* 2011;29(17):2312–2318. https://doi.org/10.1200/JCO.2010.31.7875.

175. Harari PM, Allen GW, Bonner JA. Biology of interactions: antiepidermal growth factor receptor agents. *J Clin Oncol.* 2007;25(26):4057–4065. https://doi.org/10.1200/JCO.2007.11.8984.

176. Kelly K, Chansky K, Gaspar LE, et al. Phase III trial of maintenance gefitinib or placebo after concurrent chemoradiotherapy and docetaxel consolidation in inoperable stage III non–small-cell lung cancer: SWOG S0023. *J Clin Oncol.* 2008;26(15):2450–2456. https://doi.org/10.1200/JCO.2007.14.4824.

177. Ready N, Jänne PA, Bogart J, et al. Chemoradiotherapy and gefitinib in stage III non-small cell lung cancer with epidermal growth factor receptor and KRAS mutation analysis: cancer and leukemia group B (CALEB) 30106, a CALGB-stratified phase II trial. *J Thorac Oncol.* 2010;5(9):1382–1390. https://doi.org/10.1097/JTO.0b013e3181eba657.

178. Gatzemeier U, Pluzanska A, Szczesna A, et al. Phase III study of erlotinib in combination with cisplatin and gemcitabine in advanced non–small-cell lung cancer: the Tarceva Lung Cancer Investigation Trial. *J Clin Oncol.* 2007;25(12):1545–1552. https://doi.org/10.1200/JCO.2005.1474.

179. Herbst RS, Prager D, Hermann R, et al. TRIBUTE: a phase III trial of erlotinib hydrochloride (OSI-774) combined with carboplatin and paclitaxel chemotherapy in advanced non–small-cell lung cancer. *J Clin Oncol.* 2005;23(25):5892–5899. https://doi.org/10.1200/JCO.2005.02.840.

180. Choong NW, Mauer AM, Haraf DJ, et al. Phase I trial of erlotinib-based multimodality therapy for inoperable stage III non-small cell lung cancer. *J Thorac Oncol.* 2008;3(9):1003–1011. https://doi.org/10.1097/JTO.0b013e31818396a4.

181. Jänne PA, Wang X, Socinski MA, et al. Randomized phase II trial of erlotinib alone or with carboplatin and paclitaxel in patients who were never or light former smokers with advanced lung adenocarcinoma: CALGB 30406 trial. *J Clin Oncol.* 2012;30(17):2063–2069. https://doi.org/10.1200/JCO.2011.40.1315.

182. Hanahan D, Weinberg RA. Hallmarks of cancer: the next generation. *Cell.* 2011;144(5):646–674. https://doi.org/10.1016/j.cell.2011.02.013.

183. Petrova TV, Makinen T, Alitalo K. Signaling via vascular endothelial growth factor receptors. *Exp Cell Res.* 1999;253(1):117–130. https://doi.org/10.1006/excr.1999.4707.

184. Ferrara N, Hillan KJ, Novotny W. Bevacizumab (Avastin), a humanized anti-VEGF monoclonal antibody for cancer therapy. *Biochem Biophys Res Commun.* 2005;333(2):328–335. https://doi.org/10.1016/j.bbrc.2005.05.132.

185. Spigel DR, Hainsworth JD, Yardley DA, et al. Tracheoesophageal fistula formation in patients with lung cancer treated with chemoradiation and bevacizumab. *J Clin Oncol.* 2010;28(1):43–48. https://doi.org/10.1200/JCO.2009.24.7353.

186. Lebrin F, Srun S, Raymond K, et al. Thalidomide stimulates vessel maturation and reduces epistaxis in individuals with hereditary hemorrhagic telangiectasia. *Nat Med.* 2010;16(4):420–428. https://doi.org/10.1038/nm.2131.

187. Schiller JH, Dahlberg SE, Mehta M, Johnson DH. A phase III trial of carboplatin, paclitaxel, and thoracic radiation therapy with or without thalidomide in patients with stage III non-small cell carcinoma of the lung (NSCLC): E3598. *J Clin Oncol.* 2009;27(15S):7503. https://doi.org/10.1200/jco.2009.27.15s.7503.

188. Jiang W, Huang Y, An Y, Kim BYS. Remodeling tumor vasculature to enhance delivery of intermediate-sized nanoparticles. *ACS Nano.* 2015;9(9):8689–8696. https://doi.org/10.1021/acsnano.5b02028.

189. Roskoski R. Anaplastic lymphoma kinase (ALK): structure, oncogenic activation, and pharmacological inhibition. *Pharmacol Res.* 2013;68(1):68–94. https://doi.org/10.1016/j.phrs.2012.11.007.

190. Kwak EL, Bang Y-J, Camidge DR, et al. Anaplastic lymphoma kinase inhibition in non–small-cell lung cancer. *N Engl J Med.* 2010;363(18):1693–1703. https://doi.org/10.1056/NEJMoa1006448.

191. Shaw AT, Yeap BY, Mino-Kenudson M, et al. Clinical features and outcome of patients with non-small-cell lung cancer who harbor EML4-ALK. *J Clin Oncol.* 2009;27(26):4247–4253. https://doi.org/10.1200/JCO.2009.22.6993.

192. Chiarle R, Voena C, Ambrogio C, Piva R, Inghirami G. The anaplastic lymphoma kinase in the pathogenesis of cancer. *Nat Rev Cancer.* 2008;8(1):11–23. https://doi.org/10.1038/nrc2291.

193. Cataldo KA, Jalal SM, Law ME, et al. Detection of t(2;5) in anaplastic large cell lymphoma: comparison of immunohistochemical studies, FISH, and RT-PCR in paraffin-embedded tissue. *Am J Surg Pathol.* 1999;23(11):1386–1392.

194. Shaw AT, Kim TM, Crinò L, et al. Ceritinib versus chemotherapy in patients with ALK-rearranged non-small-cell lung cancer previously given chemotherapy and crizotinib (ASCEND-5): a randomised, controlled, open-label, phase 3 trial. *Lancet Oncol.* 2017;18(7):874–886. https://doi.org/10.1016/S1470-2045(17)30339-X.

195. Solomon BJ, Mok T, Kim D-W, et al. First-line crizotinib versus chemotherapy in ALK-positive lung cancer. *N Engl J Med.* 2014;371(23):2167–2177. https://doi.org/10.1056/NEJMoa1408440.

196. Khozin S, Blumenthal GM, Zhang L, et al. FDA approval: ceritinib for the treatment of metastatic anaplastic lymphoma kinase–positive non–small cell lung cancer. *Clin Cancer Res.* 2015;21(11):2436–2439. https://doi.org/10.1158/1078-0432.CCR-14-3157.

197. Soria J-C, Tan DSW, Chiari R, et al. First-line ceritinib versus platinum-based chemotherapy in advanced ALK-rearranged non-small-cell lung cancer (ASCEND-4): a randomised, open-label, phase 3 study. *Lancet.* 2017;389(10072):917–929. https://doi.org/10.1016/S0140-6736(17)30123-X.

198. Scagliotti G, Kim TM, Crinò L, et al. Ceritinib vs chemotherapy (CT) in patients (pts) with advanced anaplastic lymphoma kinase (ALK)-rearranged (ALK+) non-small cell lung cancer (NSCLC) previously treated with CT and crizotinib (CRZ): results from the confirmatory phase 3 ASCEND-5 study. *Ann Oncol.* 2016;27(suppl_6). https://doi.org/10.1093/annonc/mdw435.41.

199. Ou S-HI, Ahn JS, De Petris L, et al. Alectinib in crizotinib-refractory ALK-rearranged non-small-cell lung cancer: a phase II global study. *J Clin Oncol.* 2016;34(7):661–668. https://doi.org/10.1200/jco.2016.34.4_suppl.661.

200. Shaw AT, Gandhi L, Gadgeel S, et al. Alectinib in ALK-positive, crizotinib-resistant, non-small-cell lung cancer: a single-group, multicentre, phase 2 trial. *Lancet Oncol.* 2016;17(2):234–242. https://doi.org/10.1016/S1470-2045(15)00488-X.

201. Avrillon V, Pérol M. Alectinib for treatment of ALK-positive non-small-cell lung cancer. *Future Oncol Lond Engl.* 2017;13(4):321–335. https://doi.org/10.2217/fon-2016-0386.

202. Wardak Z, Choy H. Improving treatment options for brain metastases from ALK-positive non–small-cell lung cancer. *J Clin Oncol.* 2016;34(34):4064–4065. https://doi.org/10.1200/JCO.2016.69.9587.

203. Melosky B, Chu Q, Juergens R, Leighl N, McLeod D, Hirsh V. Pointed progress in second-line advanced non-small-cell lung cancer: the rapidly evolving field of checkpoint inhibition. *J Clin Oncol.* 2016;34(14):1676–1688. https://doi.org/10.1200/JCO.2015.63.8049.

204. Pardoll DM. The blockade of immune checkpoints in cancer immunotherapy. *Nat Rev Cancer.* 2012;12(4):252–264. https://doi.org/10.1038/nrc3239.

205. Robainas M, Otano R, Bueno S, Ait-Oudhia S. Understanding the role of PD-L1/PD1 pathway blockade and autophagy in cancer therapy. *OncoTargets Ther.* 2017;10:1803–1807. https://doi.org/10.2147/OTT.S132508.

206. Herbst RS, Soria J-C, Kowanetz M, et al. Predictive correlates of response to the anti-PD-L1 antibody MPDL3280A in cancer patients. *Nature.* 2014;515(7528):563–567. https://doi.org/10.1038/nature14011.

207. Borghaei H, Paz-Ares L, Horn L, et al. Nivolumab versus docetaxel in advanced nonsquamous non–small-cell lung cancer. *N Engl J Med.* 2015;373(17):1627–1639. https://doi.org/10.1056/NEJMoa1507643.

208. Socinski M, Creelan B, Horn L, et al. NSCLC, metastatic-CheckMate 026: a phase 3 trial of nivolumab vs investigator's choice (IC) of platinum-based doublet chemotherapy (PT-DC) as first-line therapy for stage iv/recurrent programmed death ligand 1 (PD-L1)–positive NSCLC. *Ann Oncol.* 2016;27(suppl 6). https://doi.org/10.1093/annonc/mdw435.39.

209. Carbone DP, Reck M, Paz-Ares L, et al. First-line nivolumab in stage IV or recurrent non–small-cell lung cancer. *N Engl J Med.* 2017;376(25):2415–2426. https://doi.org/10.1056/NEJMoa1613493.

210. Herbst RS, Baas P, Kim D-W, et al. Pembrolizumab versus docetaxel for previously treated, PD-L1-positive, advanced non-small-cell lung cancer (KEYNOTE-010): a randomised controlled trial. *Lancet.* 2016;387(10027):1540–1550. https://doi.org/10.1016/S0140-6736(15)01281-7.

211. Reck M, Rodríguez-Abreu D, Robinson AG, et al. Pembrolizumab versus chemotherapy for PD-L1–positive non–small-cell lung cancer. *N Engl J Med.* 2016;375(19):1823–1833. https://doi.org/10.1056/NEJMoa1606774.

212. Rittmeyer A, Barlesi F, Waterkamp D, et al. Atezolizumab versus docetaxel in patients with previously treated non-small-cell lung cancer (OAK): a phase 3, open-label, multicentre randomised controlled trial. *Lancet*. 2017; 389(10066):255–265. https://doi.org/10.1016/S0140-6736(16)32517-X.

213. Garnett CT, Palena C, Chakarborty M, Tsang K-Y, Schlom J, Hodge JW. Sublethal irradiation of human tumor cells modulates phenotype resulting in enhanced killing by cytotoxic T lymphocytes. *Cancer Res*. 2004; 64(21):7985–7994. https://doi.org/10.1158/0008-5472.CAN-04-1525.

214. Lee Y, Auh SL, Wang Y, et al. Therapeutic effects of ablative radiation on local tumor require CD8+ T cells: changing strategies for cancer treatment. *Blood*. 2009; 114(3):589–595. https://doi.org/10.1182/blood-2009-02-206870.

215. Reits EA, Hodge JW, Herberts CA, et al. Radiation modulates the peptide repertoire, enhances MHC class I expression, and induces successful antitumor immunotherapy. *J Exp Med*. 2006;203(5):1259–1271. https://doi.org/10.1084/jem.20052494.

216. Dewan MZ, Galloway AE, Kawashima N, et al. Fractionated but not single-dose radiotherapy induces an immune-mediated abscopal effect when combined with anti-CTLA-4 antibody. *Clin Cancer Res*. 2009;15(17): 5379–5388. https://doi.org/10.1158/1078-0432.CCR-09-0265.

217. Abuodeh Y, Venkat P, Kim S. Systematic review of case reports on the abscopal effect. *Curr Probl Cancer*. 2016;40(1):25–37. https://doi.org/10.1016/j.currproblcancer.2015.10.001.

218. Chajon E, Castelli J, Marsiglia H, Crevoisier RD. The synergistic effect of radiotherapy and immunotherapy: a promising but not simple partnership. *Crit Rev Oncol Hematol*. 2017;111:124–132. https://doi.org/10.1016/j.critrevonc.2017.01.017.

219. Habets THPM, Oth T, Houben AW, et al. Fractionated radiotherapy with 3 x 8 Gy induces systemic anti-tumour responses and abscopal tumour inhibition without modulating the humoral anti-tumour response. *PLoS One*. 2016;11(7):e0159515. https://doi.org/10.1371/journal.pone.0159515.

220. Schaue D, Ratikan JA, Iwamoto KS, McBride WH. Maximizing tumor immunity with fractionated radiation. *Int J Radiat Oncol*. 2012;83(4):1306–1310. https://doi.org/10.1016/j.ijrobp.2011.09.049.

221. Wersäll PJ, Blomgren H, Pisa P, Lax I, Kälkner K-M, Svedman C. Regression of non-irradiated metastases after extracranial stereotactic radiotherapy in metastatic renal cell carcinoma. *Acta Oncol*. 2006;45(4):493–497. https://doi.org/10.1080/02841860600604611.

222. Postow MA, Callahan MK, Barker CA, et al. Immunologic correlates of the abscopal effect in a patient with melanoma. *N Engl J Med*. 2012;366(10):925–931. https://doi.org/10.1056/NEJMoa1112824.

223. Demaria S, Formenti SC. Radiation as an immunological adjuvant: current evidence on dose and fractionation. *Front Oncol*. 2012;2. https://doi.org/10.3389/fonc.2012.00153.

224. Baird JR, Monjazeb AM, Shah O, et al. Stimulating innate immunity to enhance radiation therapy–induced tumor control. *Int J Radiat Oncol Biol Phys*. 2017;99(2):362–373. https://doi.org/10.1016/j.ijrobp.2017.04.014.

225. Garon EB, Rizvi NA, Hui R, et al. Pembrolizumab for the treatment of non–small-cell lung cancer. *N Engl J Med*. 2015;372(21):2018–2028. https://doi.org/10.1056/NEJMoa1501824.

226. Shaverdian N, Lisberg AE, Bornazyan K, et al. Previous radiotherapy and the clinical activity and toxicity of pembrolizumab in the treatment of non-small-cell lung cancer: a secondary analysis of the KEYNOTE-001 phase 1 trial. *Lancet Oncol*. 2017;18(7):895–903. https://doi.org/10.1016/S1470-2045(17)30380-7.

227. Antonia SJ, Villegas A, Daniel D, et al. Durvalumab after chemoradiotherapy in stage III non–small-cell lung cancer. *N Engl J Med*. 2017. https://doi.org/10.1056/NEJMoa1709937.

228. Perez CA, Stanley K, Rubin P, et al. A prospective randomized study of various irradiation doses and fractionation schedules in the treatment of inoperable non-oat-cell carcinoma of the lung. Preliminary report by the radiation therapy oncology group. *Cancer*. 1980; 45(11):2744–2753. https://doi.org/10.1002/1097-0142 (19800601)45:11<2744::AID-CNCR2820451108>3.0. CO;2-U.

229. Kumar S, Feddock J, Li X, et al. Update of a prospective study of stereotactic body radiation therapy for post-chemoradiation residual disease in stage II/III non-small cell lung cancer. *Int J Radiat Oncol Biol Phys*. 2017;99(3):652–659. https://doi.org/10.1016/j.ijrobp. 2017.07.036.

230. Higgins KA, Pillai RN, Chen Z, et al. Concomitant chemotherapy and radiotherapy with SBRT boost for unresectable, stage III non-small cell lung cancer: a phase I Study. *J Thorac Oncol*. September 2017. https://doi.org/10.1016/j.jtho.2017.07.036.

231. Hepel JT, Leonard KL, Safran H, et al. Stereotactic body radiation therapy boost after concurrent chemoradiation for locally advanced non-small cell lung cancer: a phase 1 dose escalation study. *Int J Radiat Oncol*. 2016;96(5):1021–1027. https://doi.org/10.1016/j.ijrobp.2016.08.032.

232. Rosenzweig KE, Sura S, Jackson A, Yorke E. Involved-field radiation therapy for inoperable non–small-cell lung cancer. *J Clin Oncol*. 2007;25(35):5557–5561. https://doi.org/10.1200/JCO.2007.13.2191.

233. Glazer GM, Gross BH, Quint LE, Francis IR, Bookstein FL, Orringer MB. Normal mediastinal lymph nodes: number and size according to American Thoracic Society mapping. *Am J Roentgenol*. 1985;144(2):261–265. https://doi.org/10.2214/ajr.144.2.261.

234. Giraud P, Antoine M, Larrouy A, et al. Evaluation of microscopic tumor extension in non-small-cell lung cancer for three-dimensional conformal radiotherapy planning. *Int J Radiat Oncol Biol Phys.* 2000;48(4): 1015–1024.

235. Grills IS, Fitch DL, Goldstein NS, et al. Clinicopathologic analysis of microscopic extension in lung adenocarcinoma: defining clinical target volume for radiotherapy. *Int J Radiat Oncol Biol Phys.* 2007;69(2):334–341. https://doi.org/10.1016/j.ijrobp.2007.03.023.

236. Yuan S, Meng X, Yu J, et al. Determining optimal clinical target volume margins on the basis of microscopic extracapsular extension of metastatic nodes in patients with non-small-cell lung cancer. *Int J Radiat Oncol Biol Phys.* 2007;67(3):727–734. https://doi.org/10.1016/j.ijrobp.2006.08.057.

237. Jiang Z-Q, Yang K, Komaki R, et al. Long-term clinical outcome of intensity-modulated radiotherapy for inoperable non-small cell lung cancer: the MD Anderson experience. *Int J Radiat Oncol Biol Phys.* 2012;83(1): 332–339. https://doi.org/10.1016/j.ijrobp.2011.06.1963.

238. McCloskey P, Balduyck B, Van Schil PE, Faivre-Finn C, O'Brien M. Radical treatment of non-small cell lung cancer during the last 5 years. *Eur J Cancer Oxf Engl.* 2013;49(7):1555–1564. https://doi.org/10.1016/j.ejca.2012.12.023.

239. Wu VWC, Kwong DLW, Sham JST. Target dose conformity in 3-dimensional conformal radiotherapy and intensity modulated radiotherapy. *Radiother Oncol.* 2004;71(2):201–206. https://doi.org/10.1016/j.radonc.2004.03.004.

240. Grills IS, Yan D, Martinez AA, Vicini FA, Wong JW, Kestin LL. Potential for reduced toxicity and dose escalation in the treatment of inoperable non-small-cell lung cancer: a comparison of intensity-modulated radiation therapy (IMRT), 3D conformal radiation, and elective nodal irradiation. *Int J Radiat Oncol Biol Phys.* 2003; 57(3):875–890.

241. Liu HH, Wang X, Dong L, et al. Feasibility of sparing lung and other thoracic structures with intensity-modulated radiotherapy for non-small-cell lung cancer. *Int J Radiat Oncol Biol Phys.* 2004;58(4):1268–1279. https://doi.org/10.1016/j.ijrobp.2003.09.085.

242. Liao ZX, Komaki RR, Thames HD, et al. Influence of technologic advances on outcomes in patients with unresectable, locally advanced non-small-cell lung cancer receiving concomitant chemoradiotherapy. *Int J Radiat Oncol Biol Phys.* 2010;76(3):775–781. https://doi.org/10.1016/j.ijrobp.2009.02.032.

243. Chun SG, Hu C, Choy H, et al. Impact of intensity-modulated radiation therapy technique for locally advanced non–small-cell lung cancer: a secondary analysis of the NRG oncology RTOG 0617 randomized clinical trial. *J Clin Oncol.* 2016;35(1):56–62. https://doi.org/10.1200/JCO.2016.69.1378.

244. Movsas B, Hu C, Sloan J, et al. Quality of life analysis of a radiation dose-escalation study of patients with non-small-cell lung cancer: a secondary analysis of the radiation therapy oncology group 0617 randomized clinical trial. *JAMA Oncol.* 2016;2(3):359–367. https://doi.org/10.1001/jamaoncol.2015.3969.

245. Tobias CA, Lawrence JH, Born JL, et al. Pituitary irradiation with high-energy proton beams a preliminary report. *Cancer Res.* 1958;18(2):121–134.

246. Nichols RC, Huh SH, Hoppe BS, et al. Protons safely allow coverage of high-risk nodes for patients with regionally advanced non-small-cell lung cancer. *Technol Cancer Res Treat.* 2011;10(4):317–322. https://doi.org/10.7785/tcrt.2012.500208.

247. Kesarwala AH, Ko CJ, Ning H, et al. Intensity-modulated proton therapy for elective nodal irradiation and involved-field radiation in the definitive treatment of locally advanced non-small-cell lung cancer: a dosimetric study. *Clin Lung Cancer.* 2015;16(3):237–244. https://doi.org/10.1016/j.cllc.2014.12.001.

248. Chang JY, Zhang X, Wang X, et al. Significant reduction of normal tissue dose by proton radiotherapy compared with three-dimensional conformal or intensity-modulated radiation therapy in stage I or stage III non–small-cell lung cancer. *Int J Radiat Oncol Biol Phys.* 2006; 65(4):1087–1096. https://doi.org/10.1016/j.ijrobp.2006.01.052.

249. Chang JY, Komaki R, Lu C, et al. Phase II study of high-dose proton therapy with concurrent chemotherapy for unresectable stage III non-small cell lung cancer. *Cancer.* 2011;117(20):4707–4713. https://doi.org/10.1002/cncr.26080.

250. Liao ZX, Lee JJ, Komaki R, et al. Bayesian randomized trial comparing intensity modulated radiation therapy versus passively scattered proton therapy for locally advanced non-small cell lung cancer. *J Clin Oncol.* 2016;34(suppl 15):8500. https://doi.org/10.1200/JCO.2016.34.15_suppl.8500.

251. PTCOG - Facilities in Operation. https://www.ptcog.ch/index.php/facilities-in-operation.

252. Demizu Y, Fujii O, Iwata H, Fuwa N. Carbon ion therapy for early-stage non-small-cell lung cancer. *Biomed Res Int.* 2014;2014. https://doi.org/10.1155/2014/727962.

253. Takahashi W, Nakajima M, Yamamoto N, et al. A prospective nonrandomized phase I/II study of carbon ion radiotherapy in a favorable subset of locally advanced non-small cell lung cancer (NSCLC). *Cancer.* 2015;121(8):1321–1327. https://doi.org/10.1002/cncr.29195.

CHAPTER 5

First-Line Therapy for Wild-Type Patients

MICHAEL J. JELINEK, MD • JYOTI D. PATEL, MD

Lung cancer remains the leading cause of cancer-related deaths in the United States and the world. Adenocarcinoma histology contributes approximately 40% of all lung cancer cases and is now the most prevalent type of non–small-cell lung cancer (NSCLC) with an increasing incidence.[1] Systemic therapy is the mainstay of treatment as most patients present with either advanced-stage disease or relapse after definitive therapy for early-stage disease. For some advanced-stage adenocarcinoma patients, somatic driver mutations in the epidermal growth factor receptor (EGFR) or chromosomal translocations resulting in activated alkaline lymphoma kinase (ALK) fusion or ROS1 fusion allow for highly effective small molecule tyrosine kinase inhibitors that result in dramatic and durable responses. However, only a fraction of patients with advanced lung adenocarcinoma have these oncogenic driver mutations (EGFR, ALK, and ROS1 incidence is approximately 17%, 8%, and 1%–2%, respectively).[2] For the large number of patients without these driver mutations, the so-called wild-type patients, chemotherapy, antiangiogenic agents, and immunotherapy are the mainstay of initial treatment.

CHEMOTHERAPY

For patients with wild-type lung adenocarcinoma, chemotherapy has historically been the backbone of first-line treatment. In 1969, Green et al. published one of the pioneering studies demonstrating improvement in survival with alkylating agents in lung cancer.[3] Over the next 30 years, many chemotherapeutic agents were tested with only a few showing consistent activity in NSCLC—cisplatin, mitomycin C, vinblastine, ifosfamide, and etoposide.[4] In 1995, the NSCLC Collaborative Group published the first meta-analysis demonstrating a survival benefit of treating NSCLC with chemotherapy.[5] Eleven trials conducted from 1970 to 1988 with a total of 1190 patients demonstrated a 10% reduction in the risk of death for those who received chemotherapy compared with those who received supportive care alone. Alkylating agents were found to be detrimental, and thus cisplatin-based regimens emerged as the primary treatment modality. These trials took place before the introduction of effective antinausea drugs, and cisplatin therapy was associated with high emetogenic potential. Unfortunately, none of these studies effectively measured the quality of life. Nevertheless, significant debate arose over the relatively small benefit of chemotherapy compared with the toxic side effects.

Because of the overall survival advantage, cisplatin-based therapy became the standard of care for fit patients. The NSCLC Collaborative Group updated the original meta-analysis to include trials containing more modern chemotherapy regimens. This meta-analysis included 16 randomized trials from 1982 to 2001 demonstrating an absolute 1-year overall survival benefit of 9% when chemotherapy was added to best supportive care. The 1-year overall survival was increased from 20% to 29%, and the median overall survival was increased from 4.5 to 6 months.[6] Again a 10% benefit in overall survival was demonstrated despite the inclusion of more modern agents. However, in the later trials, antiemetics were available to provide a more tolerable cisplatin-based regimen. For the trials measuring quality of life, there was either unchanged or improved quality of life in patients receiving chemotherapy. This helped quell some of the debate, but the fact remained that multiple analyses only demonstrated a small clinical benefit (on the matter of weeks) to using chemotherapy.

Because of the small clinical benefit and the possible risks associated with chemotherapy, the number of chemotherapy agents used in combination came into question. As more chemotherapy agents emerged,

Pulmonary Adenocarcinoma: Approaches to Treatment. https://doi.org/10.1016/B978-0-323-55433-6.00005-5

a 2004 meta-analysis analyzed the role of a doublet regimen compared with a single-agent regimen and to a triplet regimen.[7] Compared with the single-agent regimen, doublet chemotherapy provided an improved objective tumor response rate (26% vs. 13%, odds ratio [OR] 0.42, $P < .001$) and 1-year survival (35% vs. 30%, OR 0.80, $P < .001$) although causing more grade 3 and 4 toxicities. The triplet regimen was associated with a significantly increased objective response rate (ORR) (31% vs. 23%, OR 0.66, $P < .001$) but did not provide a 1-year survival benefit (OR 1.01, $P = .88$) when compared with the doublet regimen. As expected, the triplet regimens generally caused more grade 3 and 4 toxicities including neutropenia, thrombocytopenia, anemia, infection, and mucositis. From these data, doublet therapy became the standard of care as it provided equally effective survival while lessening the side effect profile compared with triplet therapy.

Previous trials had not directly investigated the optimal agent to pair with cisplatin, and no overwhelming data were available to support one agent over another. The Eastern Cooperative Oncology Group (ECOG) 1594 hoped to answer this question by comparing four regimens - cisplatin in combination with paclitaxel, gemcitabine, or docetaxel or carboplatin in combination with paclitaxel. None of these regimens provided a significant survival advantage over the others.[8] As a result of this trial, ECOG recommended that further trials use carboplatin and paclitaxel as the standard regimen in the metastatic setting due to similar efficacy and an improved toxicity profile. However, the trial was designed as a superiority trial rather than a noninferiority trial, making it difficult to determine the level of equivalence between the two platinum regimens. This necessitated further analysis of whether cisplatin or carboplatin was more beneficial in NSCLC.

Many randomized controlled trials were conducted hoping to determine the superiority of cisplatin or carboplatin. Three meta-analyses have analyzed this question, and all three have shown similar results. The first demonstrated a higher response rate among cisplatin-based regimens, but this did not lead to a survival advantage.[9] The second meta-analysis included 2968 individual patient data derived from trials occurring in 1990–2004. These data demonstrated that carboplatin had a significantly lower response rate when substituted for cisplatin (24% vs. 30%, OR 1.37, $P < .001$). There was a trend towards better overall survival in the cisplatin group (9.1 vs. 8.4 months, hazard ratio [HR] 1.07, $P = .10$) although nonsignificant. However, in a subset analysis of nonsquamous

histology, carboplatin was associated with a significantly worse mortality (HR 1.12). Despite the small survival benefit, cisplatin was associated with more toxicity, including nausea, vomiting, and nephrotoxicity. Carboplatin was more frequently associated with severe thrombocytopenia.[10] The most recent meta-analysis analyzed twice the number of trials and over double the patients compared with the largest of the aforementioned meta-analyses. Again cisplatin provided an overall better response rate, but there was no survival advantage when compared with carboplatin.[11]

Cisplatin consistently demonstrates improvement in response rate compared with carboplatin, but there was no survival advantage in the metastatic setting. The side effect profile of each drug was similar between the included trials. Cisplatin was commonly associated with nephrotoxicity, nausea, and vomiting, whereas carboplatin had significantly more thrombocytopenia. In practice, patients who are being treated with curative intent are treated with a cisplatin-based regimen if there are no contraindications. In the metastatic, palliative setting, a carboplatin-based regimen is used, particularly in the United States. One could argue that with improved antiemetics, cisplatin-based therapy could become a reasonable option to use. However, the consistent occurrence of grade 3 and 4 nephrotoxicity with cisplatin does not outweigh the response benefit compared with carboplatin. In the palliative setting, carboplatin is much better tolerated and is not limited by a survival disadvantage.

While newer third-generation chemotherapies were being combined with platinum agents, investigators were questioning whether these newer agents could be combined to provide a better toxicity and response profile than platinum-based therapy. Multiple randomized clinical trials were performed comparing the combination of a platinum-agent and a third-generation chemotherapy (gemcitabine, paclitaxel, docetaxel, or vinorelbine) with two third-generation agents. These were formally analyzed in a meta-analysis showing that platinum-based doublets provided a slightly higher 1-year survival (RR 1.08, 95% CI 1.01–1.16, $P = .03$) than nonplatinum doublets.[12] If patients are ineligible for platinum-based therapy, combinations of gemcitabine with docetaxel, paclitaxel, or vinorelbine are reasonable options based on these studies.

Until this point, doublet combinations of platinum compounds with gemcitabine, vinorelbine, or taxanes were the preferred regimens for all NSCLCs. After gaining approval for second-line treatment of advanced NSCLC,[13] pemetrexed was tested in a phase III, noninferiority trial comparing cisplatin and gemcitabine versus cisplatin and pemetrexed in the front-line treatment of advanced NSCLC.[14] Survival was similar between the two arms, and the pemetrexed group experienced less adverse events. In a prespecified subset analysis, cisplatin and pemetrexed had a significantly better overall survival in adenocarcinoma patients than cisplatin and gemcitabine (12.6 vs. 10.9 months, HR 0.84, $P = .03$). A second study analyzing the efficacy of pemetrexed versus docetaxel in the second-line setting also demonstrated the benefit of pemetrexed in the nonsquamous subgroup.[15] Based on these data, ease of administration, and favorable toxicity profile, pemetrexed has become a preferred partner to combine with platinum in the front-line setting for adenocarcinoma.

Despite the data that have led to the widespread use of pemetrexed in nonsquamous histologies, many questions remain about the data itself. The results were based on one of 19 subgroup analyses. Additionally, in an era of financial toxicity, oncologists must weigh perceived and actual benefit with cost. However, owing to the tolerability and ease of administration, it is unlikely that the use of pemetrexed for lung adenocarcinoma will change substantially in the near future. Table 5.1 lists the approved first-line doublet chemotherapy options for adenocarcinoma patients with good performance status according to the National Comprehensive Cancer Network (NCCN) guidelines.

TABLE 5.1
Approved First-Line Doublet Chemotherapy Options for Good Performance Status Patients

Cisplatin	Docetaxel
	Etoposide
	Gemcitabine
	Paclitaxel
	Pemetrexed
Carboplatin	Nab-paclitaxel
	Docetaxel
	Etoposide
	Gemcitabine
	Paclitaxel
	Pemetrexed
Gemcitabine	Docetaxel
	Vinorelbine

DURATION OF CHEMOTHERAPY

As combination chemotherapy became an accepted and rationale strategy to increase response and tolerability and decrease resistance, investigators focused on delivering additional therapy to provide survival benefit. One of the earliest trials with modern chemotherapy regimens randomized patients to receive carboplatin and paclitaxel for four cycles or continuously until disease progression. Both the arms received a median number of four treatment cycles. Of the patients assigned to receive four cycles of chemotherapy, only 57% received the full treatment course. Of the 116 patients in the continuous arm, 42% tolerated five or more cycles, and 18% received eight or more cycles. The overall ORR was similar between the two arms, and all responses occurred within the first four cycles. There was no survival or quality of life benefit between the two arms.[16] From this trial, there appeared to be no benefit of extending treatment beyond the standard four cycles.

As more trials began to investigate the length of treatment, multiple meta-analyses attempted to determine the optimal treatment duration. A meta-analysis of 3027 patients demonstrated a significantly improved progression-free survival (HR 0.75, $P < .00001$) and overall survival (HR 0.92, $P = .03$) when chemotherapy was extended beyond the standard number of four cycles.[17] This analysis included a heterogeneous group of trials that generally included four versus six cycles of chemotherapy. This led to a subsequent meta-analysis evaluating the differences between six or fewer cycles of planned first-line chemotherapy.[18] There was no statistical overall survival benefit to patients assigned to six cycles of chemotherapy. A small progression-free survival benefit was shown in those who were assigned to six cycles (6.09 vs. 5.33 months, HR 0.79, $P = .0007$). However, it is important to note that the analysis was based on intention-to-treat, and only 53% of the patients in the six-cycle cohort actually received the intended six cycles. Thus it is difficult to interpret the accuracy of the results. Regardless, with the addition of immunotherapy to the front-line setting discussed later, four cycles of platinum-based therapy with a third generation chemotherapy or pemetrexed followed by maintenance therapy is a general standard of care.

BEVACIZUMAB

Although front-line chemotherapy has been shown to have a survival benefit as well as improve the quality of life, the median survival of NSCLC patients remains poor. The strategy of adding other biologic agents is best exemplified by the addition of bevacizumab. Bevacizumab is a recombinant humanized monoclonal antibody that targets the vascular endothelial growth factor (VEGF). As a mediator of angiogenesis and microvascular permeability, VEGF is essential for tumor growth and metastasis. Because VEGF overexpression in lung cancer portends a poor prognosis, targeting VEGF became a therapeutic strategy.[19]

One of the initial bevacizumab trials enrolled all NSCLC patients to carboplatin and paclitaxel alone or with the addition of 7.5 mg/kg or 15 mg/kg of bevacizumab. The high-dose cohort experienced a higher response rate (31.5% vs. 18.8%) and significantly longer time to progression (7.4 vs. 4.2 months, $P = .023$) than the control group. The high-dose cohort experienced a 3-month survival advantage although this was not significant ($P = .63$). An exploratory analysis demonstrated a survival advantage in nonsquamous histology. From this study arose the concern of administering bevacizumab to patients with squamous cell histology. There were six life-threating episodes of pulmonary hemorrhage which may have been associated with squamous cell tumors (4 of 13 squamous, and 2 of 54 nonsquamous). Other associations were centrally located tumors, proximity to major blood vessels, and tumor cavitation.[20] After this trial, only nonsquamous patients were able to participate in efficacy trials for bevacizumab.

The ECOG 4599 trial randomized 878 patients with recurrent or advanced nonsquamous NSCLC to paclitaxel and carboplatin with or without 15 mg/kg of bevacizumab.[21] After six cycles, bevacizumab continued every 3 weeks until disease progression. The bevacizumab cohort had a 2-month overall survival advantage compared with the standard group (12.3 vs. 10.3 months, HR 0.79, $P = .003$). Similarly, patients receiving bevacizumab had a significantly improved progression-free survival (6.2 vs. 4.5 months, $P < .001$) and ORR (35% vs. 15%, $P < .001$). The bevacizumab arm experienced more major bleeding episodes than the control group (4.4% vs. 0.7%). There were 15 treatment-related deaths in the bevacizumab group and two deaths in the standard group. Attributable causes of death in the bevacizumab cohort included pulmonary hemorrhage, febrile neutropenia, cerebrovascular accident, gastrointestinal hemorrhage, and pulmonary embolism.

The ECOG 4599 trial was followed shortly by the AVAiL trial that assigned 1043 patients with advanced nonsquamous NSCLC to cisplatin and gemcitabine in addition to 7.5 mg/kg of bevacizumab, 15 mg/kg of bevacizumab, or placebo.[22,23] After completing a maximum of six cycles, patients were continued on bevacizumab or placebo maintenance therapy. Of note, the trial was designed to compare each bevacizumab arm to placebo and not to each other. Progression-free survival was significantly greater in patients receiving low- or high-dose bevacizumab although the absolute difference was modest (6.7 vs. 6.5 vs. 6.1 months for low dose, high dose, and placebo, respectively). Overall survival was not different between the three arms. Patients receiving bevacizumab were more likely to experience hypertension, bleeding, and proteinuria than those in the control group.

Despite both of these large phase III studies showing a progression-free survival benefit, the AVAiL trial did not demonstrate a prolonged overall survival. The authors of the AVAiL trial suggest a few reasons for this discrepancy. The population in the AVAiL trial had more favorable prognostic features that may have led to the better overall survival in the standard chemotherapy group than in the historical controls. Additionally, during the AVAiL trial, more efficacious second-line therapies were available on disease progression and may have contributed to the increased survival among both arms. Eventually a meta-analysis including ECOG 4599, AVAiL, and two phase II trials demonstrated a significantly increased overall survival (HR 0.90, $P = .03$) and progression-free survival (HR 0.72, $P < .001$) with the addition of bevacizumab to standard front-line chemotherapy.[24]

Further data were collected regarding the safety of bevacizumab in the SAiL and ARIES cohort trials.[25,26] SAiL was a phase IV trial of more than 2200 patients investigating the role of bevacizumab in the front-line setting in combination with chemotherapy. Adverse events included venous thromboembolism (8%), hypertension (6%), bleeding (4%), proteinuria (3%), and pulmonary hemorrhage (1%). The ARIES trial of more than 1500 patients demonstrated similar rates of adverse events to the SAiL trial. Based on a significant amount of safety data, a panel of experts concluded that the major exclusion criteria for receiving bevacizumab are predominantly squamous histology and/or a history of grade 2 or more pulmonary hemorrhage. These groups were excluded from the aforementioned trials, and thus no formal conclusion could be drawn. Central tumors, proximity to blood vessels, cavitation, age, performance status, and anticoagulation status were not associated with increased adverse events and should not affect eligibility for bevacizumab.[27]

There is an obvious safety concern using bevacizumab in the setting of brain metastases. However, multiple trials have demonstrated the safety of using bevacizumab in patients with asymptomatic brain metastases. A retrospective analysis of 17 studies, 13 of which were randomized controlled trials, including various cancer types, demonstrated similar rates of cerebral hemorrhage regardless of whether patients received bevacizumab. Of the 8443 patients in randomized clinical trials, 187 patients had CNS metastases. Three of 91 patients (3.3%) receiving bevacizumab experienced grade 4 cerebral hemorrhage compared with one of 96 patients (1.0%) not receiving bevacizumab.[28] The same investigator group performed the phase II BRAIN trial evaluating the safety of bevacizumab in chemotherapy-naïve or pretreated NSCLC patients with asymptomatic untreated brain metastases. Of the 91 patients enrolled, only one developed a nonfatal intracranial bleed.[29] Thus patients with asymptomatic brain metastases should be eligible for bevacizumab.

MAINTENANCE THERAPY

As discussed earlier, extending initial platinum-based chemotherapy beyond the traditional four to six cycles has provided little clinical benefit. Maintenance therapy was designed as an extension of platinum-based chemotherapy to provide continued response. Maintenance therapy is generally used for an undetermined amount of time until disease progression or significant toxicity. There are two general types of maintenance therapy—continuous and switch—which are initiated immediately after four to six cycles of platinum-based therapy. Continuous therapy uses agent(s) effective during induction chemotherapy to prolong time to progression. Switch therapy uses an agent not used during induction chemotherapy to prevent resistance and progression. As the platinum component of chemotherapy provides most of the side effects, multiple third-generation chemotherapy agents and targeted agents have been evaluated in this setting. Trials have examined the role of continuation and switch maintenance strategies as well as combination therapy in the maintenance setting. Most of these strategies have demonstrated some progression-free survival advantages.

Pemetrexed is the most widely used and preferred chemotherapeutic agent in the maintenance setting of adenocarcinoma. Two large prospective trials have investigated the role of maintenance single-agent pemetrexed. First, the JMEN study evaluated pemetrexed versus best supportive care as switch maintenance therapy after four to six cycles of nonpemetrexed platinum-doublet therapy. All histological subtypes were included because data about the ineffectiveness of pemetrexed in squamous cancers were not available. In the total population, pemetrexed improved the progression-free survival and overall survival. A subgroup analysis demonstrated a progression-free (4.6 vs. 2.7 months, HR 0.51, $P < .0001$) and overall (16.8 vs. 11.5 months, HR 0.73, $P = .026$) survival advantage in adenocarcinoma patients.[30] Of note, about one-third of the patients on the discontinuation arm did not receive any therapy after discontinuation potentially leading to the significant difference in the overall survival.

The second large trial demonstrating the role of pemetrexed in the continuous maintenance setting was the PARAMOUNT trial. Nine hundred thirty-nine nonsquamous NSCLC patients received a four-cycle induction phase of cisplatin and pemetrexed. Nonprogressing patients (n = 539) were randomized in a 2:1 fashion to receive maintenance pemetrexed or best supportive care. Progression-free survival (3.9 vs. 2.6 months, HR 0.64, $P = .0002$) and overall survival (13.9 vs. 11.0 months, HR 0.76, $P = .0195$) were significantly better in the pemetrexed group than in the placebo group.[31–33] Because of these trials, pemetrexed is often used in the maintenance setting, generally as continuous therapy.

In light of the survival advantages of pemetrexed[14] and bevacizumab[21] in adenocarcinoma, the PointBreak trial enrolled 939 treatment-naïve patients who were randomly assigned to carboplatin, pemetrexed, and bevacizumab or to carboplatin, paclitaxel, and bevacizumab. Those who did not progress after four cycles of treatment continued on bevacizumab. In addition, patients randomized to the pemetrexed group received maintenance pemetrexed. Progression-free survival was slightly prolonged in the pemetrexed group compared with that in the paclitaxel cohort (6.0 vs. 5.6 months, HR 0.83, $P = .012$). The primary endpoint of overall survival was not met. Additionally, overall survival was shorter than in other recent trials containing pemetrexed-based therapies. However, patients on PointBreak were randomized before induction, whereas the other large trials randomized patients after induction therapy, thereby selecting out good responders.[34]

After demonstrating the role of bevacizumab and pemetrexed in the maintenance setting, the AVAPERL trial became the first to directly compare these agents in the maintenance setting. Patients received cisplatin, pemetrexed, and bevacizumab as primary therapy. Nonprogressing patients were randomized to maintenance pemetrexed and bevacizumab or bevacizumab alone. The trial met its primary endpoint of progression-free survival with a median of 7.4 months in the combination group compared with 3.7 months in the bevacizumab-alone cohort (HR 0.57, $P < .001$).[35] Although not statistically significant, the overall survival was prolonged in the combination group (17.1 vs. 13.2 months, HR 0.87, $P = .29$).[36]

Other chemotherapeutic agents have been tested in the maintenance setting, mainly gemcitabine and docetaxel. In the IFT trial, after receiving four cycles of induction cisplatin and gemcitabine, 464 NSCLC patients randomly received maintenance gemcitabine, erlotinib, or observation. The trial design only allowed for each of the agents to be compared to observation rather than to each other. Although there was a significantly improved progression-free survival and a trend toward better overall survival in the gemcitabine maintenance group, subgroup analysis demonstrated little benefit in patients with adenocarcinoma.[37] In the study by Fidias et al., the strategy of switch maintenance effectively tested early or late second-line treatment. Five hundred sixty-six NSCLC patients received four cycles of gemcitabine plus carboplatin. The 309 patients who did not progress were assigned to immediate maintenance therapy with docetaxel or observation with docetaxel treatment on disease progression. Progression-free survival was significantly improved with the immediate administration of docetaxel compared with the delayed group (5.7 vs. 2.7 months, $P = .001$). However, overall survival only trended toward a benefit to immediate docetaxel (12.3 vs. 9.7 months, $P = .0853$). Notably the study was underpowered to detect an overall survival advantage of less than 4 months. Thus the benefit of docetaxel in this setting appears to be the additional therapy rather than the timing.[38]

Of brief mention, erlotinib has also been studied as a single-agent maintenance therapy in patients without a driver mutation after it was shown to have a survival benefit in patients with previously treated NSCLC.[39] Initially two large phase III trials were conducted to evaluate erlotinib's role in this setting. The SATURN trial enrolled patients, regardless of the EGFR status, who did not progress after standard platinum induction therapy to erlotinib maintenance or placebo. Among the entire population, there was a statistically significant but clinically insignificant 1-week progression-free survival benefit (HR 0.71, $P < .0001$).[40] The ATLAS trial investigated the strategy of combination bevacizumab and erlotinib in the maintenance setting. After receiving four cycles of platinum-based chemotherapy and bevacizumab, patients who had not progressed received bevacizumab maintenance with or without erlotinib regardless of EGFR status. A statistically significant difference in the progression-free survival was seen between

patients receiving erlotinib compared with bevacizumab alone (4.8 vs. 3.7 months, $P < .001$).[41] Finally the IUNO trial enrolled only patients with wild-type EGFR to maintenance erlotinib or placebo after completing four cycles of platinum-based chemotherapy without progression. There was no progression-free or overall survival benefit.[42] After the result of these trials and gains in our understanding of the biology of EGFR, erlotinib has little role as maintenance therapy in the first-line setting of wild-type disease.

There remains some debate about the appropriate maintenance strategy as multiple approaches have been studied—single versus combination, continuous versus switch, and bevacizumab versus pemetrexed. The trials involving bevacizumab maintenance also included bevacizumab in the induction phase. Thus it is difficult to determine whether the survival advantage occurred because of adding bevacizumab to the induction or maintenance aspect of therapy. An exploratory retrospective analysis of ECOG 4599 attempted to evaluate the role of bevacizumab alone in the maintenance setting. Patients eligible for maintenance therapy after receiving either induction regimen were evaluated. Postinduction progression-free and overall survivals were improved in the bevacizumab arm.[43] In addition, the strategy of maintenance bevacizumab and pemetrexed compared with pemetrexed alone has never been directly compared. The lack of comparative data leads to continued debate about the appropriate maintenance regimen. The ongoing ECOG 5508 trial will likely shed more light on the matter. This trial will treat nonsquamous patients with carboplatin, paclitaxel, and bevacizumab induction therapy followed by randomization to one of three maintenance strategies: pemetrexed alone, bevacizumab alone, or pemetrexed and bevacizumab. This trial will help adjudicate the differences between single versus combination, continuous versus switch, and pemetrexed versus bevacizumab maintenance therapy. However, the results will unlikely change clinical practice with the addition of immunotherapy to the front-line and maintenance setting.

Despite the statistical survival benefit of maintenance therapy, the quality of life and financial implications become important considerations as the survival benefit is at best 3 months. The quality of life was analyzed in the aforementioned studies with various measures. Unlike chemotherapy for lung cancer, maintenance therapy has generally not provided an improvement in the quality of life based on various measures. In the JMEN study, patients receiving pemetrexed maintenance experienced pain at a later point compared with those on best supportive care.[44] However, there are no overwhelming data to demonstrate a quality of life benefit from maintenance therapy. Another factor is the financial toxicity of maintenance strategy especially with specialized drugs such as pemetrexed bevacizumab, and now, immunotherapy. A cost-effectiveness model comparing multiple induction-maintenance sequences in nonsquamous NSCLC hoped to compare these various strategies based on cost and efficacy. Gemcitabine and cisplatin followed by best supportive care was the baseline induction treatment to which other regimens were compared. From this analysis, the strategy of cisplatin and pemetrexed with or without maintenance pemetrexed had similar cost-effectiveness to the reference regimen of gemcitabine and cisplatin. Adding bevacizumab to carboplatin and paclitaxel with maintenance bevacizumab was not cost-effective, and the reference regimen had lower costs and better or equivalent outcomes.[45] Thus it is important to participate in shared decision-making with patients to determine the best treatment strategy.

IMMUNOTHERAPY

With the advent of checkpoint inhibitors, the landscape of treating NSCLC dramatically changed. Nivolumab, a programmed death-1 (PD-1) inhibitor, was the first immunotherapy to gain approval in the second-line setting due to an overall survival benefit when compared with docetaxel.[46] Despite a low response rate and an overall survival not dramatically improved, nivolumab provided long, durable responses and remissions that were relatively unprecedented. With further understanding and development of these agents, immunotherapy has moved to the front-line setting of treating lung adenocarcinoma.

Pembrolizumab, another PD-1 antibody, was the first immunotherapy agent to gain FDA approval as first-line therapy for a subset of NSCLC patients. The KEYNOTE-024 trial enrolled treatment-naïve advanced NSCLC patients with tumor cell programmed death ligand 1 (PD-L1) staining of at least 50% to either pembrolizumab monotherapy or standard platinum-doublet chemotherapy. More than 1700 patients were screened for the trial, and approximately 30% of patients had PD-L1 staining greater than 50%. Of those 500 patients, 305 entered randomization. The overall response rate and duration of response to pembrolizumab were 45% and 12.1 months compared with 28% and 5.7 months for standard therapy, respectively. The primary endpoint, progression-free survival, was significantly prolonged in patients receiving pembrolizumab

(10.3 vs. 6.0 months, HR 0.50, $P < .001$). Similarly, pembrolizumab provided an overall survival benefit of 30.0 months compared to 14.2 months in the chemotherapy arm (HR 0.63, p = 0.002).[47] Not only did pembrolizumab result in improvements in survival, it was also more tolerable. More than half of the standard chemotherapy patients experienced a severe treatment-related adverse event. Conversely, one-quarter of patients suffered severe adverse events in the experimental group.[48] Now, regardless of tumor histology, patients with PD-L1 status 50% or greater are eligible for front-line pembrolizumab.

With the success of front-line pembrolizumab in PD-L1–high patients, nivolumab was tested in a similar but slightly different fashion. The CheckMate 026 trial enrolled 541 treatment-naïve patients with advanced NSCLC. Patients were randomized to nivolumab or standard first-line platinum-doublet chemotherapy. However, unlike KEYNOTE-024, this trial included all PD-L1–positive patients defined as PD-L1 staining of at least 1% on tumor cells. The analysis, though, only included the 423 patients who had PD-L1 staining 5% or greater. Among these patients, ORR (26% vs. 34%), progression-free survival (4.2 vs. 5.9 months), and overall survival (14.4 vs. 13.2 months) were not improved with nivolumab compared with standard chemotherapy, respectively.[49] Perhaps as a result of a less stringent PD-L1 cutoff, the front-line nivolumab trial was negative.

After the establishment of PD-1/-L1 antibodies as single-agent treatment of advanced NSCLC, the next trials questioned whether immunotherapy could be combined with chemotherapy in the front-line setting. One of the first published studies of combination therapy paired ipilimumab, a cytotoxic T-lymphocyte antigen-4 (CTLA-4) inhibitor, with standard front-line chemotherapy in patients with nonsquamous cell carcinoma. Patients were randomized to carboplatin, paclitaxel, and one of three arms—placebo, concurrent ipilimumab (four doses of concurrent followed by two doses of placebo plus carboplatin and paclitaxel), and phased ipilimumab (two cycles of placebo plus carboplatin and paclitaxel followed by four doses of all the three agents). Phased ipilimumab improved immune-related progression-free survival (HR 0.72, $P = .05$) and progression-free survival (HR 0.69, $P = .02$) compared with the control. However, there was no overall survival benefit among either arm when compared with the control. The rate of grade 3 and 4 adverse events was similar in all the arms.[50] At this point, ipilimumab has no approval as a single or combination agent in NSCLC.

With the success of single agent PD-1 inhibitors, numerous combination trials have completed or are ongoing. The KEYNOTE-189 trial was the first phase III trial to demonstrate survival advantages adding immunotherapy to front-line chemotherapy in unselected patients. This trial randomized 616 treatment-naïve, metastatic, non-squamous NSCLC patients to chemotherapy (cisplatin or carboplatin and peme-trexed) plus or minus pembrolizumab. The PFS was 8.8 months in the chemoimmunotherapy arm compared to 4.9 months in the chemotherapy cohort (HR 0.52, p < 0.0001). Overall survival was 69% at 12 months in the combination group versus 49% in the chemotherapy group (HR 0.49, p < 0.001). No significant additional toxicity was seen in the combination group. The overall survival benefit was strongly influenced by PD-L1 expression. For patients with PD-L1 ≥ 50%, 12 month OS was 73% vs 48% with and without immunotherapy, respectively. For those with no PD-L1 expression, 12 month OS was 62% and 52% with and without immunotherapy. Approximately 33% of patients on the placebo arm crossed over to receive pembrolizumab monotherapy at disease progression.[51]

Additionally, the IMPower 150 trial, - a multi-arm, multi-endpoint trial randomized 1202 patients to 1) atezolizumab, carboplatin, paclitaxel (ACP), 2) bevacizumab, carboplatin, paclitaxel (BCP), or 3) atezolizumab, bevacizumab, carboplatin, paclitaxel (ABCP). ABCP was compared to BCP prior to ACP being compared to BCP. The available published data analyzed the PFS between ABCP and BCP. The median PFS in the ABCP group was 8.3 months compared to 6.8 months in the BCP group (HR 0.62, p < 0.001). Interim analysis of overall survival for the ABCP and BCP groups was 19.2 vs 14.7 months (HR 0.78, p = 0.02). No additional unexpected toxicities were seen. Of note, patients with EGFR or ALK genomic alterations were included if they had progressed on one tyrosine kinase inhibitor. Amongst the 13% of patients with EGFR/ALK alterations, the PFS was 9.7 months in those who received ABCP and 6.1 months in the BCP cohort (HR 0.59, p=0.025).[52] CheckMate 227 was a multi-part, multi-arm phase III clinical trial comparing nivolumab, nivolumab plus ipilimumab, and nivolumab plus chemotherapy vs chemotherapy alone. Part 1 of the trial investigated survival benefits of nivolumab plus ipilimumab vs chemotherapy based off tumor mutational burden. An elevated tumor mutational burden was defined as 10 or more mutations per megabase. PFS was analyzed with respect to tumor mutational burden. Amongst all patients with available tumor mutational burden analysis, 44.2% had 10 or more mutations per megabase. The 1-year PFS rate and PFS was 42.6% and 7.2 months amongst the

TABLE 5.2
Selected Ongoing/Partially Reported First-Line Phase III Immunotherapy Trials in Advanced Non-Small Cell Lung Adenocarcinoma

Name/Identifier	Treatment	Histology	PD-L1 Status
CheckMate 227 NCT02477826	PD-L1 ≥ 1%: Nivolumab versus nivolumab + ipilimumab versus chemotherapy PD-L1 ≤ 1%: Nivolumab + ipilimumab versus nivolumab + chemotherapy versus chemotherapy	All	All
CheckMate 9LA NCT03215706	Nivolumab + ipilimumab + chemotherapy versus chemotherapy	All	All
KEYNOTE 042 NCT02220894	Pembrolizumab versus chemotherapy	All	≥1%
KEYNOTE 189 NCT02578680	Chemotherapy + pembrolizumab versus chemotherapy	Nonsquamous	All
IMpower 150 NCT02366143	Atezolizumab + chemotherapy +/− bevacizumab versus chemotherapy + bevacizumab	Nonsquamous	All
IMpower 130 NCT02367781	Atezolizumab + chemotherapy versus chemotherapy	Nonsquamous	All
MYSTIC NCT02453282	Durvalumab + tremelimumab versus durvalumab versus chemotherapy	All	All
NEPTUNE NCT02542293	Durvalumab + tremelimumab versus chemotherapy	All	All

nivolumab plus ipilimumab group and 13.2% and 5.5 months in the chemotherapy alone arm (HR 0.58, p < 0.001). These results held true regardless of PD-L1 status or tumor histology.[53]

Table 5.2 includes selected ongoing phase III clinical trials that are ongoing or awaiting final data maturation. Understandably there is much excitement surrounding immunotherapy due to the potential for long durable responses. However, response rates occur in a minority of patients and durable responses in even less. As we progress further in our knowledge of immunotherapy, especially in combination regimens, it becomes our responsibility to have sound scientific rationale for these studies. Unfortunately only 3% of patients participate in clinical trials causing about one-fifth of all cancer-related trials to close early.[54] Obviously we can work at recruiting more patients for these trials, but at the same time we should be collectively offering the most rational science for patients.

We also need to develop a better understanding of those who will respond to immunotherapy. Overall, PD-L1 is a poor biomarker for response as it has various detection antibodies, different immunohistochemical cutoffs for positivity, heterogeneity of expression within tumors, and induction by sources other than the tumor. There are patients with no PD-L1 expression who have clinical responses as well as a large proportion of patients with high PD-L1 expression who receive no benefit. There is significant interest now in developing better predictors of response. Tumor mutational burden has demonstrated promise as a predictive biomarker for response to checkpoint inhibitors.[48] Other investigational markers to predict response include tumor burden,[55] inflammatory markers, and T-cell clonality.[56] With more sensitive and specific biomarkers, we can ideally choose who will benefit from these therapies from the beginning and avoid unnecessary toxicities of traditional chemotherapy. Additionally, with further advances, we will likely be able to manipulate the immune response to enhance the effects of checkpoint inhibitors.

ELDERLY PATIENTS

Lung cancer primarily affects older patients. The median age of diagnosis is 70 years, and nearly 70% of patients are 65 years or older at the time of diagnosis.[57] Thus there is a large proportion of patients who are at higher risk for treatment and have a general worse prognosis at the time of diagnosis. In addition, most clinical trials do not include this patient population making it difficult to determine the applicability in this particular group.

Because of the frailty of this population and the lack of inclusion in clinical trials, many investigations have attempted to determine whether alternative treatment regimens could provide an outcome benefit with a better toxicity profile.

The first strategy used was single-agent therapy with third-generation chemotherapy. The landmark ELVIS trial was one of the first to demonstrate the ability of single-agent chemotherapy to provide a survival benefit while maintaining quality of life. Advanced-stage patients who were older than 70 years and had an ECOG performance status of 0–2 were randomized to vinorelbine for a maximum of six cycles or best supportive care alone. Of note the primary outcome of the trial was quality of life and not survival. Patients receiving chemotherapy scored better on quality of life functioning scales, but they also reported more toxicity-related symptoms. Statistically, vinorelbine provided a modest improvement in median survival of 28 weeks compared with 21 weeks for best supportive care (HR 0.65, $P = .03$).[58] Unfortunately, accrual was cut short at 191 patients with a goal of 350. This early closure obviously brings the validity of the survival data into question. From these data, treatment strategies for this higher risk group of patients began to develop.

Although there are other single agents that have demonstrated activity in treatment-naïve patients, only docetaxel has been investigated specifically in the elderly. The WJTOG 9904 trial enrolled patients aged 70 years or above with a performance status between 0 and 2 and randomly assigned them to docetaxel or vinorelbine. Results demonstrated that docetaxel was as good as vinorelbine in treating elderly patients. Median overall survival was 14.3 months in the docetaxel group compared with 9.9 months in the vinorelbine cohort (HR 0.78, $P = .138$) although results were not significant. Progression-free survival (5.5 vs. 3.1 months, $P < .001$) and response rate (22.7% vs. 9.9%, $P = .019$) were significantly better for those receiving docetaxel. Docetaxel was associated with more grade 3 or 4 neutropenia, but side effects did not change quality of life compared with the side effects caused by vinorelbine.[59]

After demonstrating that single-agent chemotherapy could provide benefit to the elderly, the next logical step was to determine whether combination therapy could improve outcomes while maintaining quality of life. There have been multiple clinical trials conducted to answer this question; however, these have provided conflicting results. The MILES trial was the largest of the trials enrolling 698 patients aged 70 years and above to single-agent vinorelbine, single-agent gemcitabine, or combination vinorelbine and gemcitabine. Response rate, median survival, and quality of life were similar among all three groups. The combination regimen was slightly more toxic than either single agent.[60] In contrast, a French intergroup trial, IFCT-0501, enrolled 451 patients aged 70–89 years to combination carboplatin and paclitaxel or either single-agent gemcitabine or vinorelbine. Of note, patients of either group were treated with erlotinib at treatment failure regardless of mutational status. Overall survival was significantly improved in the combination chemotherapy arm compared with that in the single-agent chemotherapy arm (10.3 vs. 6.2 months, HR 0.64, $P < .0001$). Progression-free survival was also significantly prolonged in the combination arm (6.0 vs. 2.8 months, HR 0.51, $P < .0001$). Grade 3–4 cytopenia and peripheral neuropathy were significantly greater in the doublet chemotherapy arm. Quality-of-life measures were similar among doublet and single-agent chemotherapy.[61]

These two trials represent the difficulty of developing a specific regimen to encompass all elderly patients. The French trial, unlike the MILES trial, included a platinum agent which, in the general population, already has demonstrated a survival advantage.[11] A large meta-analysis specifically analyzed randomized control trials that were designed for patients aged 70 years or above or with prespecified subgroup analyses for the elderly. Platinum combination therapy appeared to improve overall survival (HR 0.76, 95% CI 0.69 to 0.85) and ORR (RR 1.57, 95% CI 1.32 to 1.85) when compared with nonplatinum therapy.[62] The inclusion of a platinum agent could play a role in the difference in outcomes demonstrated in the French trial and the MILES trial. The same meta-analysis[62] also showed, although with low-quality evidence, that nonplatinum single agents had similar effects on overall and progression-free survival as nonplatinum combination therapy. Thus the most ideal regimen includes doublet platinum therapy.

As with the general population, the use of bevacizumab in combination with systemic chemotherapy in the elderly has come into question. There have been no specific trials investigating its role only in the elderly population. However, many of the trials establishing the use of bevacizumab in the front-line setting also had subgroup analyses to investigate its role in the elderly. A subgroup analysis of ECOG 4599 demonstrated that elderly patients (as defined 70 years or older) had trends toward better response rate (29% vs. 17%, $P = .067$) and progression-free survival (5.9 vs. 4.9 months, $P = .063$), but no difference in overall

survival (11.3 vs. 12.1 months, $P = .40$). More importantly grade 3 to 5 toxicities were significantly higher in the elderly population (87% vs. 61%, $P < .001$).[63] Retrospective data from the AVAiL trial yielded a progression-free survival benefit to lower dose bevacizumab 7.5 mg/kg (HR 0.71, $P = .023$); however, there was no overall survival advantage when compared with chemotherapy alone. The toxicity profile among elderly and young patients was similar.[64] Observational data including 1500 Medicare patients aged 65 years or above showed no survival benefit by adding bevacizumab to carboplatin and paclitaxel.[65] Overall, from these data, bevacizumab has not been shown to provide a survival benefit in the elderly. There appears to be a greater tendency toward toxicity, even fatal complications. If used, bevacizumab must cautiously be prescribed for the elderly population.

The aforementioned trials have attempted to provide a better guide to treating elderly patients but, in essence, may have added further complexity to the situation. These trials included or analyzed only elderly patients, but a majority had a performance status 0–1. Many of these were fit elderly patients whom oncologists likely had little hesitancy enrolling on a clinical trial with doublet chemotherapy. As elderly patients are significantly underrepresented in clinical trials but make up a majority of the lung cancer population, we should be encouraging inclusion of healthy elderly patients onto investigational regimens. The heterogeneity that exists in younger patients still exists in the elderly. The choice of therapy should be made on similar grounds as for younger patients with the addition of further geriatric assessment. Now with immunotherapy in the clinical armamentarium, a well-tolerated, effective treatment exists for patients of all ages. For elderly patients who are not candidates for chemotherapy, the use of checkpoint inhibitors becomes a clear first-line option.

IMPAIRED PERFORMANCE STATUS

Many trials have lumped elderly patients and impaired performance status patients into the same category. However, as mentioned earlier, the elderly population is similarly heterogeneous as a younger population. Just as we differentiate between young and old patients, we also evaluate elderly patients based on their performance status. Thus it seems counterintuitive to include these populations in the same group. Unfortunately, because of this generalizability, poor performance status patients have been grossly understudied. On the other hand, a significant number of patients present with a poor performance status. Based on a study in 2008, the prevalence of poor performance status, defined as an ECOG status of 2–4, was 48% when reported by patients and 34% when judged by providers.[66] Many of the aforementioned studies performed in the elderly population included a small portion of patients with a performance status of 2. However, no conclusions can be made in this population because it would be severely underpowered. This is the case for most studies investigating the role of treatment in poor performance status patients as only a few trials have exclusively included this patient population.

Historically the standard of care for patients with a poor performance status was single-agent chemotherapy. More recently ASCO guidelines included combination therapy as an option for patients with a performance status of 2.[51] Two large phase III trials comparing single-agent versus combination therapy included a planned subgroup analysis for patients with an ECOG performance status of 2. The CALGB 9730 trial randomized patients to receive paclitaxel alone or in combination with carboplatin. Ninety-nine of the 561 patients had a performance status of 2. Among this small subset of patients, the 1-year survival was 18% versus 10% (HR 0.60, $P = .016$) in favor of combination therapy with similar toxicities between the two arms.[67] The IFCT-0501 trial discussed earlier included 27% of patients with a performance status of 2. Similarly this trial demonstrated a survival benefit (HR 0.63, CI 0.43–0.91) to combination therapy among poor performance status patients.[61]

Zukin et al. became the first to evaluate the question of single versus doublet therapy specifically in patients with an ECOG performance status of 2. More than 200 patients with a performance status of 2 were randomized to single-agent pemetrexed or combination carboplatin and pemetrexed in the front-line setting. Two independent investigators had to concur on performance status assignment. Of note, more than 60% of the patients were enrolled at one center raising the potential for selection bias. Response rates (23.8% vs. 10.3%, $P = .032$), progression-free survival (5.8 vs. 2.8 months, HR 0.46, $P < .001$), and overall survival (9.3 vs. 5.3 months, HR 0.62, $P = .001$) were all significantly improved in patients receiving combination chemotherapy. Anemia and neutropenia were significantly higher in the combination arm. There were four treatment-related deaths on the combination arm. The authors concluded that carboplatin and pemetrexed can be given safely to nonsquamous patients with a poor performance status.[68]

The multicenter randomized phase III CAPPA-2 trial looked at the benefit of cisplatin in performance status

2 patients. Treatment-naïve performance status 2 patients were randomly assigned to cisplatin and gemcitabine or gemcitabine alone. The study sample size was amended due to slow accrual, and the trial was stopped early based on preliminary results of the above trial by Zukin et al. Only 57 patients were accrued to this study, but based on the available data, overall survival (5.9 vs. 3.0 months, HR 0.52, $P = .039$) and progression-free survival (3.3 vs. 1.7 months, HR 0.49, $P = .017$) were significantly prolonged in the combination arm. Hematologic toxicity was more frequent in the combination arm. There were no treatment-related deaths. The authors concluded that cisplatin and gemcitabine could be an option for performance status 2 patients with the caveat of a significantly underpowered study.[69]

The aforementioned studies demonstrated the feasibility, safety, and benefit to combination therapy in patients with poor performance status. Subsequently a few trials have investigated whether certain regimens were superior in this setting. ECOG 1599 was a spin-off of the ECOG 1594 trial specific to poor performance status patients. The regimens used were based on the results of the ECOG 1594 trial. Carboplatin and paclitaxel was the least toxic regimen, and cisplatin and gemcitabine provided the best median overall survival among performance status 2 patients in ECOG 1594. ECOG 1599 enrolled 100 eligible treatment-naïve patients and randomly assigned them to either of the aforementioned regimens. Response rates, time to progression, overall survival, and 1-year survival were not significantly different between the two arms. As expected, carboplatin and paclitaxel were associated with more neuropathy and neutropenia, and cisplatin and gemcitabine caused more thrombocytopenia and creatinine elevation. Once again, doublet therapy provided benefit but remained relatively inferior to patients with performance status of 0–1.[70]

The phase III STELLAR-3 trial enrolled advanced NSCLC patients with an ECOG performance status of 2 and randomized them to either paclitaxel poliglumex and carboplatin or standard paclitaxel and carboplatin. Overall survival, response rate, and disease control rate were similar between both the arms. Notably, though, overall survival among both the arms was close to 8 months, which is higher than that of historical controls with a performance status of 2. The authors noted a difference in survival among geographical regions where patients from Eastern Europe had significantly better survivals. The authors remarked about the subjective nature of performance status which could have led to more fit patients ending up on the trial in this region.[71]

As with all patients, the entire clinical context must be taken into account to prescribe the safest therapy for their underlying disease. Because of the subjectivity and fluidity of performance status, it is important to continually reevaluate a patient's functional ability. Patients with a poor performance status require careful selection of the appropriate regimen as their outcomes are worse than healthier patients. Many of the aforementioned trials have demonstrated the benefit of chemotherapy in this setting. For patients with metastatic adenocarcinoma, carboplatin and pemetrexed is a reasonable option in patients with a poor performance status. Single-agent pemetrexed is an alternative option for patients who are at higher risk for toxicity. However, immunotherapy can be considered a front-line option in this particular patient population. As immunotherapy is generally better tolerated, it may provide an option for patients who would otherwise not be eligible for any other treatment modalities. Finally, patients with an ECOG performance status of 3–4 should not receive chemotherapy as it likely increases toxicity and possibly hastens death.

CONCLUSIONS

Over the past 20 years, treatment for lung adenocarcinoma has advanced beyond chemotherapy alone. For wild-type patients, we have discussed multiple regimens that are used in the front-line setting (Table 5.3). For patients with PD-L1 staining ≥ 50%, pembrolizumab is a clear choice for front-line treatment as it offers a higher response rate, increased survival and less toxicity. There is now further evidence that immunotherapy can effectively be brought to the front-line setting in combination with chemotherapy. For patients with low or intermediate PD-L1 staining, pembrolizumab plus carboplatin and pemetrexed is the new front-line option. Patients with negative PD-L1 status can be treated with chemoimmunotherapy as well; however, subgroup analyses demonstrate a much smaller benefit in this population. For patients with a contraindication to immunotherapy, a platinum-based doublet regimen with or without bevacizumab followed by maintenance therapy is an appropriate treatment regimen. We favor carboplatin and pemetrexed with or without bevacizumab followed by pemetrexed maintenance therapy due to favorable toxicity profile. Carboplatin, paclitaxel, and bevacizumab followed by bevacizumab maintenance is also an appropriate front-line regimen. For patients who have borderline performance status, it is appropriate to treat with chemoimmunotherapy although with greater caution. In the elderly, a comprehensive geriatric assessment should be performed before treatment. Based on these evaluations, treatment for this population should be stratified based on performance status similar to younger populations. For individuals with poor performance status at the time of diagnosis, palliative measures should be the focus of care (Fig. 5.1).

Regardless of the anticancer treatment a patient receives, palliative care has proven essential in lung cancer patients. A seminal article for palliative care randomized lung cancer patients to early palliative care or standard management. Early palliative care included a formal meeting with a palliative care physician and advanced practice nurses followed by at least monthly meetings at the discretion of the patient and the treating team. Unsurprisingly there were improvements in the

TABLE 5.3 Common First-Line Regimens for Lung Adenocarcinoma				
Trial	Regimen	ORR, %	PFS, mo.	OS, mo.
ECOG 1594[8]	Carboplatin + paclitaxel	17	3.1	8.1
Scagliotti et al.[14]	Cisplatin + pemetrexed	31	4.8	12.6[a]
ECOG 4599 (Ref. [21])	Carboplatin + paclitaxel + bevacizumab	35	6.2	12.3
PointBreak[34]	Carboplatin + pemetrexed + bevacizumab with pemetrexed/bevacizumab maintenance	34	6.0	12.6
	Carboplatin + paclitaxel + bevacizumab with bevacizumab maintenance	33	5.6	13.4
KEYNOTE-024[47,48]	Pembrolizumab[#]	45	10.3	NR
KEYNOTE 189[51]	Carboplatin + pemetrexed + pembrolizumab	48	8.8	NR

[a] Overall survival in adenocarcinoma subanalysis; #PD-L1 ≥ 50%.
mo = months; *ORR* = objective response rate; *OS* = overall survival; *PFS* = progression-free survival.

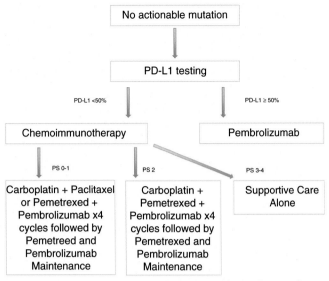

FIG. 5.1 General decision tree for patients with newly diagnosed lung adenocarcinoma with no actionable mutations. Patients are first stratified based on PD-L1 status followed by performance status. PD-L1, programmed death ligand 1.

quality of life and mood among the patients who received early palliative care. Additionally, patients who received palliative care had less aggressive end-of-life care defined as receiving chemotherapy within 14 days of death, no hospice care, or admission to hospice 3 days or less before death (33% vs. 54%, $P = .05$). Despite having less aggressive end-of-life care, palliative care patients had a longer median overall survival than those of the standard management cohort (11.6 vs. 8.9 months, $P = .02$).[72] With all lung cancer patients, the importance of incorporating palliative care is vital to completely treating the patient.

We have clearly made strides improving the survival of patients with metastatic disease. Despite this improvement, there is much work to be done to reach survivals comparable to other cancer types. There is much promise in the future with combination immunotherapies, incorporation of radiation therapy, antibody-drug conjugates, and nanoparticles. Treatment will continue to become more individualized as our therapies become more targeted. As we move forward with our understanding of the immune system, we will ideally be able to offer less toxic regimens than our standard chemotherapies. If the last 10 years of advancement has shown us anything, it is that we should expect bigger breakthroughs in the near future.

REFERENCES

1. Dela Cruz CS, Tanoue LT, Matthay RA. Lung cancer: epidemiology, etiology, and prevention. *Clin Chest Med.* 2011; 32(4):605–644.
2. Kris MG, Johnson BE, Berry LD, et al. Using multiplexed assays of oncogenic drivers in lung cancers to select targeted drugs. *JAMA.* 2014;311(19):1998–2006.
3. Green RA, Humphrey E, Close H, Patno ME. Alkylating agents in bronchogenic carcinoma. *Am J Med.* 1969; 46(4):516–525.
4. Johnson DH. Evolution of cisplatin-based chemotherapy in non-small cell lung cancer: a historical perspective and the eastern cooperative oncology group experience. *Chest.* 2000;117(4 suppl 1):133S–137S.
5. Group N-SCLCC. Chemotherapy in non-small cell lung cancer: a meta-analysis using updated data on individual patients from 52 randomized clinical trials. *BMJ.* 1995; 311(7010):899–909.
6. Group NM-AC. Chemotherapy in addition to supportive care improves survival in advanced non-small-cell lung cancer: a systematic review and meta-analysis of individual patient data from 16 randomized controlled trials. *J Clin Oncol.* 2008;26(28):4617–4625.
7. Delbaldo C, Michiels S, Syz N, Soria JC, Le Chevalier T, Pignon JP. Benefits of adding a drug to a single-agent or a 2-agent chemotherapy regimen in advanced non-small-cell lung cancer: a meta-analysis. *JAMA.* 2004;292(4):470–484.
8. Schiller JH, Harrington D, Belani CP, et al. Comparison of four chemotherapy regimens for advanced non-small-cell lung cancer. *N Engl J Med.* 2002;346(2):92–98.

9. Hotta K, Matsuo K, Ueoka H, Kiura K, Tabata M, Tanimoto M. Meta-analysis of randomized clinical trials comparing Cisplatin to Carboplatin in patients with advanced non-small-cell lung cancer. *J Clin Oncol.* 2004; 22(19):3852—3859.

10. Ardizzoni A, Boni L, Tiseo M, et al. Cisplatin- versus carboplatin-based chemotherapy in first-line treatment of advanced non-small-cell lung cancer: an individual patient data meta-analysis. *J Natl Cancer Inst.* 2007;99(11): 847—857.

11. Jiang J, Liang X, Zhou X, Huang R, Chu Z. A meta-analysis of randomized controlled trials comparing carboplatin-based to cisplatin-based chemotherapy in advanced non-small cell lung cancer. *Lung Cancer.* 2007;57(3):348—358.

12. Rajeswaran A, Trojan A, Burnand B, Giannelli M. Efficacy and side effects of cisplatin- and carboplatin-based doublet chemotherapeutic regimens versus non-platinum-based doublet chemotherapeutic regimens as first line treatment of metastatic non-small cell lung carcinoma: a systematic review of randomized controlled trials. *Lung Cancer.* 2008;59(1):1—11.

13. Hanna N, Shepherd FA, Fossella FV, et al. Randomized phase III trial of pemetrexed versus docetaxel in patients with non-small-cell lung cancer previously treated with chemotherapy. *J Clin Oncol.* 2004;22(9):1589—1597.

14. Scagliotti GV, Parikh P, von Pawel J, et al. Phase III study comparing cisplatin plus gemcitabine with cisplatin plus pemetrexed in chemotherapy-naive patients with advanced-stage non-small-cell lung cancer. *J Clin Oncol.* 2008;26(21):3543—3551.

15. Scagliotti G, Hanna N, Fossella F, et al. The differential efficacy of pemetrexed according to NSCLC histology: a review of two Phase III studies. *Oncologist.* 2009;14(3): 253—263.

16. Socinski MA, Schell MJ, Peterman A, et al. Phase III trial comparing a defined duration of therapy versus continuous therapy followed by second-line therapy in advanced-stage IIIB/IV non-small-cell lung cancer. *J Clin Oncol.* 2002;20(5):1335—1343.

17. Soon YY, Stockler MR, Askie LM, Boyer MJ. Duration of chemotherapy for advanced non-small-cell lung cancer: a systematic review and meta-analysis of randomized trials. *J Clin Oncol.* 2009;27(20):3277—3283.

18. Rossi A, Chiodini P, Sun JM, et al. Six versus fewer planned cycles of first-line platinum-based chemotherapy for non-small-cell lung cancer: a systematic review and meta-analysis of individual patient data. *Lancet Oncol.* 2014; 15(11):1254—1262.

19. Zhan P, Wang J, Lv XJ, et al. Prognostic value of vascular endothelial growth factor expression in patients with lung cancer: a systematic review with meta-analysis. *J Thorac Oncol.* 2009;4(9):1094—1103.

20. Johnson DH, Fehrenbacher L, Novotny WF, et al. Randomized phase II trial comparing bevacizumab plus carboplatin and paclitaxel with carboplatin and paclitaxel alone in previously untreated locally advanced or metastatic non-small-cell lung cancer. *J Clin Oncol.* 2004;22(11): 2184—2191.

21. Sandler A, Gray R, Perry MC, et al. Paclitaxel-carboplatin alone or with bevacizumab for non-small-cell lung cancer. *N Engl J Med.* 2006;355(24):2542—2550.

22. Reck M, von Pawel J, Zatloukal P, et al. Phase III trial of cisplatin plus gemcitabine with either placebo or bevacizumab as first-line therapy for nonsquamous non-small-cell lung cancer: AVAiL. *J Clin Oncol.* 2009;27(8):1227—1234.

23. Reck M, von Pawel J, Zatloukal P, et al. Overall survival with cisplatin-gemcitabine and bevacizumab or placebo as first-line therapy for nonsquamous non-small-cell lung cancer: results from a randomised phase III trial (AVAiL). *Ann Oncol.* 2010;21(9):1804—1809.

24. Soria JC, Mauguen A, Reck M, et al. Systematic review and meta-analysis of randomised, phase II/III trials adding bevacizumab to platinum-based chemotherapy as first-line treatment in patients with advanced non-small-cell lung cancer. *Ann Oncol.* 2013;24(1):20—30.

25. Crino L, Dansin E, Garrido P, et al. Safety and efficacy of first-line bevacizumab-based therapy in advanced non-squamous non-small-cell lung cancer (SAiL, MO19390): a phase 4 study. *Lancet Oncol.* 2010;11(8):733—740.

26. Fischbach N, Spigel DR, Brahmer J, et al. Preliminary safety and effectiveness of bevacizumab- (BV) based treatment in subpopulations of patients with non-small cell lung cancer (NSCLC) from the ARIES study: a BV treatment observational cohort study (OCS). *J Thorac Oncol.* 2009;4(9):S360.

27. Reck M, Barlesi F, Crino L, et al. Predicting and managing the risk of pulmonary haemorrhage in patients with NSCLC treated with bevacizumab: a consensus report from a panel of experts. *Ann Oncol.* 2012;23(5): 1111—1120.

28. Besse B, Lasserre SF, Compton P, Huang J, Augustus S, Rohr UP. Bevacizumab safety in patients with central nervous system metastases. *Clin Cancer Res.* 2010;16(1): 269—278.

29. Besse B, Le Moulec S, Mazieres J, et al. Bevacizumab in patients with nonsquamous non-small cell lung cancer and asymptomatic, untreated brain metastases (brain): a non-randomized, phase II study. *Clin Cancer Res.* 2015;21(8): 1896—1903.

30. Ciuleanu T, Brodowicz T, Zielinski C, et al. Maintenance pemetrexed plus best supportive care versus placebo plus best supportive care for non-small-cell lung cancer: a randomised, double-blind, phase 3 study. *Lancet.* 2009; 374(9699):1432—1440.

31. Paz-Ares L, de Marinis F, Dediu M, et al. Maintenance therapy with pemetrexed plus best supportive care versus placebo plus best supportive care after induction therapy with pemetrexed plus cisplatin for advanced non-squamous non-small-cell lung cancer (PARAMOUNT): a double-blind, phase 3, randomised controlled trial. *Lancet Oncol.* 2012;13(3):247—255.

32. Paz-Ares LG, de Marinis F, Dediu M, et al. PARAMOUNT: final overall survival results of the phase III study of maintenance pemetrexed versus placebo immediately after induction treatment with pemetrexed plus cisplatin for

advanced nonsquamous non-small-cell lung cancer. *J Clin Oncol.* 2013;31(23):2895–2902.

33. Reck M, Paz-Ares LG, de Marinis F, et al. PARAMOUNT: descriptive subgroup analyses of final overall survival for the phase III study of maintenance pemetrexed versus placebo following induction treatment with pemetrexed plus cisplatin for advanced nonsquamous non-small-cell lung cancer. *J Thorac Oncol.* 2014;9(2):205–213.

34. Patel JD, Socinski MA, Garon EB, et al. PointBreak: a randomized phase III study of pemetrexed plus carboplatin and bevacizumab followed by maintenance pemetrexed and bevacizumab versus paclitaxel plus carboplatin and bevacizumab followed by maintenance bevacizumab in patients with stage IIIB or IV nonsquamous non-small-cell lung cancer. *J Clin Oncol.* 2013;31(34):4349–4357.

35. Barlesi F, Scherpereel A, Rittmeyer A, et al. Randomized phase III trial of maintenance bevacizumab with or without pemetrexed after first-line induction with bevacizumab, cisplatin, and pemetrexed in advanced nonsquamous non-small-cell lung cancer: AVAPERL (MO22089). *J Clin Oncol.* 2013;31(24):3004–3011.

36. Barlesi F, Scherpereel A, Gorbunova V, et al. Maintenance bevacizumab-pemetrexed after first-line cisplatin-pemetrexed-bevacizumab for advanced nonsquamous nonsmall-cell lung cancer: updated survival analysis of the AVAPERL (MO22089) randomized phase III trial. *Ann Oncol.* 2014;25(5):1044–1052.

37. Perol M, Chouaid C, Perol D, et al. Randomized, phase III study of gemcitabine or erlotinib maintenance therapy versus observation, with predefined second-line treatment, after cisplatin-gemcitabine induction chemotherapy in advanced non-small-cell lung cancer. *J Clin Oncol.* 2012;30(28):3516–3524.

38. Fidias PM, Dakhil SR, Lyss AP, et al. Phase III study of immediate compared with delayed docetaxel after front-line therapy with gemcitabine plus carboplatin in advanced non-small-cell lung cancer. *J Clin Oncol.* 2009;27(4):591–598.

39. Shepherd FA, Rodrigues Pereira J, Ciuleanu T, et al. Erlotinib in previously treated non-small-cell lung cancer. *N Engl J Med.* 2005;353(2):123–132.

40. Cappuzzo F, Ciuleanu T, Stelmakh L, et al. Erlotinib as maintenance treatment in advanced non-small-cell lung cancer: a multicentre, randomised, placebo-controlled phase 3 study. *Lancet Oncol.* 2010;11(6):521–529.

41. Johnson BE, Kabbinavar F, Fehrenbacher L, et al. ATLAS: randomized, double-blind, placebo-controlled, phase IIIB trial comparing bevacizumab therapy with or without erlotinib, after completion of chemotherapy, with bevacizumab for first-line treatment of advanced non-small-cell lung cancer. *J Clin Oncol.* 2013;31(31):3926–3934.

42. Cicenas S, Geater SL, Petrov P, et al. Maintenance erlotinib versus erlotinib at disease progression in patients with advanced non-small-cell lung cancer who have not progressed following platinum-based chemotherapy (IUNO study). *Lung Cancer.* 2016;102:30–37.

43. Lopez-Chavez A, Young T, Fages S, et al. Bevacizumab maintenance in patients with advanced non-small-cell lung cancer, clinical patterns, and outcomes in the Eastern Cooperative Oncology Group 4599 Study: results of an exploratory analysis. *J Thorac Oncol.* 2012;7(11):1707–1712.

44. Belani CP, Brodowicz T, Ciuleanu TE, et al. Quality of life in patients with advanced non-small-cell lung cancer given maintenance treatment with pemetrexed versus placebo (H3E-MC-JMEN): results from a randomised, double-blind, phase 3 study. *Lancet Oncol.* 2012;13(3):292–299.

45. Kumar G, Woods B, Hess LM, et al. Cost-effectiveness of first-line induction and maintenance treatment sequences in non-squamous non-small cell lung cancer (NSCLC) in the U.S. *Lung Cancer.* 2015;89(3):294–300.

46. Borghaei H, Paz-Ares L, Horn L, et al. Nivolumab versus docetaxel in advanced nonsquamous non-small-cell lung cancer. *N Engl J Med.* 2015;373(17):1627–1639.

47. Brahmer J, Rodriguez-Abreu D, Robinson A, et al. OA 17.06 Updated analysis of KEYNOTE-024: pembrolizumab vs platinum-based chemotherapy for advanced NSCLC with PD-L1 TPS 50+%. *J Thorac Oncol.* 2017;12(11):S1793–S1794.

48. Reck M, Rodriguez-Abreu D, Robinson AG, et al. Pembrolizumab versus chemotherapy for PD-L1-Positive Non-Small-Cell Lung Cancer. *N Engl J Med.* 2016;375(19):1823–1833.

49. Carbone DP, Reck M, Paz-Ares L, et al. First-line nivolumab in stage IV or recurrent non-small-cell lung cancer. *N Engl J Med.* 2017;376(25):2415–2426.

50. Lynch TJ, Bondarenko I, Luft A, et al. Ipilimumab in combination with paclitaxel and carboplatin as first-line treatment in stage IIIB/IV non-small-cell lung cancer: results from a randomized, double-blind, multicenter phase II study. *J Clin Oncol.* 2012;30(17):2046–2054.

51. Gandhi L, Rodriguez-Abreu D, Gadgeel S, et al. Pembrolizumab plus Chemotherapy in Metastatic Non-Small-Cell Lung Cancer. *N Engl J Med.* 2018;378(22):2078–2092.

52. Socinski MA, Jotte RM, Capuzzo F, et al. Atezolizumab for First-Line Treatment of Metastatic Nonsquamous NSCLC. *N Engl J Med.* 2018;378(24):2288–2301.

53. Hellmann MD, Ciuleanu TE, Pluzanski A, et al. Nivolumab plus Ipilimumab in Lung Cancer with a High Tumor Mutational Burden. *N Engl J Med.* 2018;378(22):2093–2104.

54. Medicine Io. *Transforming Clinical Research in the United States: Challenges and Opportunities: Workshop Summary.* Washington, DC: The National Academies Press; 2010. https://doi.org/10.17226/12900.

55. Huang AC, Postow MA, Orlowski RJ, et al. T-cell invigoration to tumour burden ratio associated with anti-PD-1 response. *Nature.* 2017;545(7652):60–65.

56. Inoue H, Park JH, Kiyotani K, et al. Intratumoral expression levels of PD-L1, GZMA, and HLA-A along with oligoclonal T cell expansion associate with response to nivolumab in metastatic melanoma. *Oncoimmunology.* 2016;5(9):e1204507.

57. *Surveillance Epidemiology and End Results Database*; 2017. https://seer.cancer.gov/statfacts/html/lungb.html.

58. Effects of vinorelbine on quality of life and survival of elderly patients with advanced non-small-cell lung cancer. The Elderly Lung Cancer Vinorelbine Italian Study Group. *J Natl Cancer Inst*. 1999;91(1):66−72.

59. Kudoh S, Takeda K, Nakagawa K, et al. Phase III study of docetaxel compared with vinorelbine in elderly patients with advanced non-small-cell lung cancer: results of the West Japan Thoracic Oncology Group Trial (WJTOG 9904). *J Clin Oncol*. 2006;24(22):3657−3663.

60. Gridelli C, Perrone F, Gallo C, et al. Chemotherapy for elderly patients with advanced non-small-cell lung cancer: the Multicenter Italian Lung Cancer in the Elderly Study (MILES) phase III randomized trial. *J Natl Cancer Inst*. 2003;95(5):362−372.

61. Quoix E, Zalcman G, Oster JP, et al. Carboplatin and weekly paclitaxel doublet chemotherapy compared with monotherapy in elderly patients with advanced non-small-cell lung cancer: IFCT-0501 randomised, phase 3 trial. *Lancet*. 2011;378(9796):1079−1088.

62. Santos FN, Castria TB, Cruz MR, Riera R. Chemotherapy for advanced non-small cell lung cancer in the elderly population. *Sao Paulo Med J*. 2016;134(5):465−466.

63. Ramalingam SS, Dahlberg SE, Langer CJ, et al. Outcomes for elderly, advanced-stage non small-cell lung cancer patients treated with bevacizumab in combination with carboplatin and paclitaxel: analysis of Eastern Cooperative Oncology Group Trial 4599. *J Clin Oncol*. 2008;26(1):60−65.

64. Leighl NB, Zatloukal P, Mezger J, et al. Efficacy and safety of bevacizumab-based therapy in elderly patients with advanced or recurrent nonsquamous non-small cell lung cancer in the phase III BO17704 study (AVAiL). *J Thorac Oncol*. 2010;5(12):1970−1976.

65. Zhu J, Sharma DB, Gray SW, Chen AB, Weeks JC, Schrag D. Carboplatin and paclitaxel with vs without bevacizumab in older patients with advanced non-small cell lung cancer. *JAMA*. 2012;307(15):1593−1601.

66. Lilenbaum RC, Cashy J, Hensing TA, Young S, Cella D. Prevalence of poor performance status in lung cancer patients: implications for research. *J Thorac Oncol*. 2008;3(2):125−129.

67. Lilenbaum RC, Herndon 2nd JE, List MA, et al. Single-agent versus combination chemotherapy in advanced non-small-cell lung cancer: the cancer and leukemia group B (study 9730). *J Clin Oncol*. 2005;23(1):190−196.

68. Zukin M, Barrios CH, Pereira JR, et al. Randomized phase III trial of single-agent pemetrexed versus carboplatin and pemetrexed in patients with advanced non-small-cell lung cancer and Eastern Cooperative Oncology Group performance status of 2. *J Clin Oncol*. 2013;31(23):2849−2853.

69. Morabito A, Gebbia V, Di Maio M, et al. Randomized phase III trial of gemcitabine and cisplatin vs. gemcitabine alone in patients with advanced non-small cell lung cancer and a performance status of 2: the CAPPA-2 study. *Lung Cancer*. 2013;81(1):77−83.

70. Langer C, Li S, Schiller J, et al. Randomized phase II trial of paclitaxel plus carboplatin or gemcitabine plus cisplatin in Eastern Cooperative Oncology Group performance status 2 non-small-cell lung cancer patients: ECOG 1599. *J Clin Oncol*. 2007;25(4):418−423.

71. Langer CJ, O'Byrne KJ, Socinski MA, et al. Phase III trial comparing paclitaxel poliglumex (CT-2103, PPX) in combination with carboplatin versus standard paclitaxel and carboplatin in the treatment of PS 2 patients with chemotherapy-naive advanced non-small cell lung cancer. *J Thorac Oncol*. 2008;3(6):623−630.

72. Temel JS, Greer JA, Muzikansky A, et al. Early palliative care for patients with metastatic non-small-cell lung cancer. *N Engl J Med*. 2010;363(8):733−742.

CHAPTER 6

Lung Adenocarcinoma: Second-Line Treatment

BHAVISHA A. PATEL, MD • STEPHEN V. LIU, MD

INTRODUCTION

A discussion of second-line therapy for the treatment of adenocarcinoma of the lung has never been more relevant. In two short decades, the first agent approved in this setting, docetaxel, has been joined by multiple agents in various classes. Advances in the delivery of first-line therapy have come in the form of more effective agents, better patient selection, and improved supportive care. Coupled with earlier detection of lung cancer and rapid initiation of therapy, these advances have had the downstream effect of increasing the number of patients eligible for second-line systemic therapy. Fortunately, there is no longer a solitary approved treatment; selecting a second-line regimen from among the numerous options is influenced by many patient-specific factors. Treatment decisions are largely guided by the first-line therapy already given. Beyond that, the efficacy of each regimen is balanced by its unique safety profile in the context of individual comorbidities.

The genomic profile of the cancer is also critical in defining the treatment strategy. For patients whose tumors harbor an actionable molecular alteration, targeted therapy is the preferred initial and often subsequent therapy. It is critical that the genomic identity is established for every patient with advanced pulmonary adenocarcinoma. When molecular testing was not feasible or not performed at diagnosis, it must be pursued later in the treatment course, ideally before second-line therapy is initiated. If an actionable alteration is identified, it dramatically alters the treatment strategy, as well as the prognosis. These treatments are discussed elsewhere in this text. Here, we review second-line therapy for adenocarcinoma of the lung that does not harbor an actionable genomic aberration.

CYTOTOXIC CHEMOTHERAPY— MONOTHERAPY

Docetaxel

Docetaxel was the first agent approved in the second-line setting for the treatment of non–small cell lung cancer (NSCLC) after it was associated with improved survival when compared with best supportive care or with ifosfamide or vinorelbine monotherapy. In a randomized phase III study, patients with advanced NSCLC who had received prior platinum-containing chemotherapy were randomized to receive docetaxel or best supportive care.[1] Although docetaxel was initially administered at a dose of 100 mg/m^2 every 21 days, due to excess toxicity, the study was amended to implement a lower dose of docetaxel at 75 mg/m^2. The primary endpoint was overall survival and 204 patients were randomized: 100 to best supportive care, 49 to docetaxel at the 100 mg/m^2 dose, and 55 to the 75 mg/m^2 dose. Although the objective response rate was only 5.8%, docetaxel conferred an overall survival advantage with a median overall survival of 7.0 months as compared with 4.6 months with best supportive care ($P = .047$). The subset of patients treated with docetaxel 75 mg/m^2 fared better with a median survival of 7.5 months and a 1-year survival rate of 37% compared with 12% in the best supportive care arm. Notable toxicity with docetaxel at the 75 mg/m^2 dose included neutropenia (67% grade 3 or 4), febrile neutropenia (1.8%), nausea (36.4% any grade, 3.6% grade 3 or 4), and sensory neuropathy (20% any grade, 1.8% grade 3 or 4).

A second phase III trial, the TAX 320 study, included 373 patients with advanced NSCLC, 50% of whom had adenocarcinoma.[2] Patients were randomized to receive docetaxel 100 mg/m^2, docetaxel 75 mg/m^2, or to a control arm where patients could receive weekly either

Pulmonary Adenocarcinoma: Approaches to Treatment. https://doi.org/10.1016/B978-0-323-55433-6.00006-7

vinorelbine 30 mg/m^2 or ifosfamide 2 mg/m^2/day on days 1 through 3 in a 21-day cycle. For this study, the primary endpoint was also overall survival. Docetaxel achieved an overall response rate of 10.8% at the 100 mg/m^2 dose and 6.7% at the 75 mg/m^2 dose compared with 0.8% in the control arm. No difference was noted in median overall survival, although the 1-year survival rate favored docetaxel 75 mg/m^2: 32% versus 10% in the control arm. Of note, prior treatment with paclitaxel did not influence the survival rate. Docetaxel was associated with a greater risk of grade 4 neutropenia (77% at 100 mg/m^2 and 54% at 75 mg/m^2 compared with 31% in the control arm) and febrile neutropenia (12% at 100 mg/m^2, 8% at 75 mg/m^2, and 1% in the control arm); however, there was no statistically significant difference in the rate of discontinuation due to treatment-related adverse events.

Alternate dosing of docetaxel was explored to mediate toxicity. A weekly dose of 35 mg/m^2 was compared with a dose of 75 mg/m^2 given every 21 days. The two regimens had similar response rates (10.5% vs. 12.6%) with no significant difference in median overall survival (9.2 months vs. 6.3 months, $P = .07$).[3] Toxicity did favor the weekly approach with a lower incidence of grade 3 or 4 neutropenia (4.8% vs. 20.6%). However, a randomized trial comparing quality of life on the weekly versus the 3-weekly docetaxel regimen showed no significant difference between the two dosing regimens.[4] Docetaxel emerged as the standard second-line regimen for patients previously treated with platinum-based chemotherapy and remains a commonly used agent today.

Pemetrexed

The folate antimetabolite pemetrexed is one of the most commonly used cytotoxic agents used in the treatment of nonsquamous NSCLC. Pemetrexed has a prominent role in the first-line and maintenance treatment of pulmonary adenocarcinoma but its first indication was as second-line therapy.[5] A phase III trial compared pemetrexed 500 mg/m^2 with docetaxel 75 mg/m^2, both given in 21-day cycles until progression or unacceptable toxicity.[6] Patients randomized to pemetrexed received oral folic acid at a dose of 350−1000 mcg daily and a 1000 mcg injection of vitamin B12 1−2 weeks prior to starting therapy and every 9 weeks during treatment. Premedication for patients receiving pemetrexed included dexamethasone 4 mg by mouth for 3 days starting the day before pemetrexed, and in the docetaxel arm, premedication included dexamethasone 8 mg by mouth for 3 days starting the day before docetaxel. The primary

endpoint was to compare overall survival. This large study randomized 571 patients; patients were enrolled independent of histology, although approximately half of the patients had adenocarcinoma (54.4% in the pemetrexed arm, 49.3% in the docetaxel arm). There was no significant difference between pemetrexed and docetaxel in objective response rate (9.1% vs. 8.8%), median progression-free survival (PFS, 2.9 months in both arms), median overall survival (8.3 months vs. 7.9 months), or 1-year survival rate (29.7% in both arms). Docetaxel was associated with higher rates of grade 3 or 4 neutropenia (40.2% vs. 5.3%), febrile neutropenia (12.7 vs. 1.9%), sensory neuropathy (any grade, 15.9% vs. 4.9%), and diarrhea (any grade, 24.3% vs. 12.8%; grade 3 or 4, 2.5% vs. 0.4%), but lower rates of nausea (any grade, 16.7% vs. 30.9%), rash (any grade, 6.2% vs. 14.0%), and alanine aminotransferase (ALT) elevation (any grade, 1.4% vs. 7.9%; grade 3 or 4, 0% vs. 1.9%). Pemetrexed remains an appropriate second-line regimen for adenocarcinoma of the lung, although a significant subset of patients will have already received pemetrexed as part of first-line or maintenance therapy.

Other Cytotoxic Agents

While not approved in the second-line setting, multiple other cytotoxic agents are occasionally called upon clinically. The data supporting their use is sparse, primarily based on efficacy seen in smaller phase II studies. Use of these cytotoxic agents as second-line therapy for pulmonary adenocarcinoma will steadily decrease as more efficacious and better tolerated treatments continue to emerge, but unique clinical situations may arise where these agents have some relevance.

Gemcitabine is a pyrimidine antimetabolite that targets DNA polymerase and ribonucleotide reductase.[7] A phase II study of gemcitabine 1000 mg/m^2 given weekly for 3 out of 4 weeks included 83 patients, 45% of whom had adenocarcinoma. Gemcitabine demonstrated a response rate of 19%, equal across histologic subtypes.[8] Median survival was 34 weeks with a 1-year survival rate of 45%. The main adverse event was hematologic toxicity including grade 3 or 4 leukopenia (7%) and grade 3 thrombocytopenia (7%). A separate phase II study of gemcitabine using the same dose and schedule achieved similar results.[9] In a study of 32 patients (29 evaluable) with previously treated NSCLC, 63% of whom had adenocarcinoma, the response rate was 20.6% including 1 patient who achieved a complete response. The duration of response was 7 months. Median PFS was 3 months and median overall survival was 5.5 months.

Irinotecan was studied alone at a dose of 300 mg/m^2 or in combination with gemcitabine 1000 mg/m^2 on days 1 and 8 of a 21-day cycle as second-line treatment for patients with advanced NSCLC that progressed after cisplatin plus docetaxel.[10] The study randomized 147 patients and did not show a difference in survival between the two arms. In the irinotecan monotherapy arm, the objective response rate was 4.2% which included one complete response. Median time to progression was 5.0 months, and median survival was 7.0 months with a 1-year survival rate of 29%.

Paclitaxel in the second-line setting was explored in several different trials. Early in its development, the optimal dosing schedule of paclitaxel was not known, and many studies utilized a 24-h infusion. A randomized study compared two dosing schedules of paclitaxel in patients previously treated with chemotherapy.[11] Patients were randomized to receive paclitaxel 135 mg/m^2 or 200 mg/m^2 and were also randomized to receive treatment as a 1-h infusion on day 1 or split into three separate 1-h infusions given on days 1—3. The response rate was 25% overall, but responses were more common with the 200 mg/m^2 dose compared with the 135 mg/m^2 dose (31% vs. 12%). There was no notable difference in the 1-day versus 3-day comparison. In a phase II study of 38 patients with NSCLC, the majority of whom had adenocarcinoma,[12] patients received paclitaxel 100 mg/m^2 weekly for up to 21 weeks or until disease progression or unacceptable toxicity. The response rate was 16% with a median time to progression of 20 weeks and a median overall survival of 58 weeks.

The oral formulation of the topoisomerase-I inhibitor topotecan was compared with that of docetaxel in the second-line setting.[13] This noninferiority study included 829 patients who were randomized to receive oral topotecan 2.3 mg/m^2/day for five consecutive days or docetaxel 75 mg/m^2 in 21-day cycles. The response rate with topotecan was 5% with a median time to progression of 11.3 weeks and a median overall survival of 27.9 weeks. The primary toxicity encountered with topotecan was myelosuppression with notable rates of grade 3 or 4 neutropenia (50%), anemia (26%), and thrombocytopenia (26%).

Another oral agent that has been compared with docetaxel in this setting is S-1, an oral fluoropyrimidine. A phase II study of S-1 monotherapy as second-line therapy for NSCLC showed initial promise.[14] With a sample size of 50 patients, S-1 given orally twice daily (with dosage determined by a nomogram based on body surface area) for 28 days in 6-week cycles was associated with a response rate of 12.5%. The median PFS was 2.5 months with a median overall survival of 8.2 months and a 1-year survival rate of 29.6%. This prompted a large randomized study comparing oral S-1 with docetaxel.[15] This noninferiority study included 1154 patients randomized to S-1 or docetaxel (60 mg/m^2 in Japan and 75 mg/m^2 in all other countries). The study did demonstrate noninferiority. Median overall survival was 12.75 months with S-1 and 12.52 months with docetaxel (HR 0.945; 95% CI 0.833—1.073). The response rate was 8.3%, with S-1 and there was significant improvement in the EORTC QLQ-C30 global health status with therapy. While the results are encouraging, S-1 is not yet available in all parts of the world.

Prior to the development of modern era cytotoxic agents, vinorelbine was commonly used as part of initial therapy for pulmonary adenocarcinoma, and its use was extrapolated to the second-line setting if not given with initial therapy. The TAX 320 study, discussed above, included vinorelbine as one of the treatments in the control arm, where the response rate was 0.8%. In a phase II study of vinorelbine given 25 mg/m^2 weekly, no responses were seen in the first 15 patients included.[16] The study was stopped. With multiple other options available, vinorelbine is not typically considered part of standard second-line therapy.

COMBINATION CHEMOTHERAPY

In an effort to improve outcomes, cytotoxic combinations have been studied in the second-line setting. The addition of carboplatin to docetaxel was explored in a randomized phase III study of 132 patients who had received one prior line of platinum-free and docetaxel-free chemotherapy.[17] Patients received docetaxel 50 mg/m^2 every 2 weeks and were randomized to receive carboplatin AUC 4 with each infusion. The combination was associated with a modest improvement in PFS (3.33 months vs. 2.60 months, $P = .012$) but no difference in response rate (10.4% vs. 7.7%, $P = .764$) or median overall survival (10.27 months vs. 7.70 months, $P = .550$). Outcomes were not reported by histologic subtype, although adenocarcinoma was the most frequently reported histology.

Similar results were noted with pemetrexed combinations in two similar studies, NVALT7 and GOIRC 02—2006. The NVALT7 study randomized 240 patients with NSCLC (45% adenocarcinoma) who had progressed after platinum-based chemotherapy to receive pemetrexed 500 mg/m^2 monotherapy or in combination with carboplatin area under the curve (AUC) 5.[18] The combination did have a higher response rate

(16.8% vs. 5.8%, $P = .006$) and a longer time to progression (4.2 months vs. 2.8 months, $P = .004$), but no significant difference in overall survival was noted (8.0 vs. 7.6 months). The GOIRC 02−2006 study included patients with advanced NSCLC with progression during or after platinum-based chemotherapy.[19] Patients received pemetrexed 500 mg/m^2 with or without carboplatin AUC 5 for up to four cycles. The study did not meet its primary endpoint, with no difference noted in PFS with the combination (3.5 months vs. 3.6 months). There was also no difference in response rate (12.6% vs. 12.5%) or overall survival (9.2 months vs. 8.8 months). In the subgroup of patients with adenocarcinoma, there was no benefit to the addition of carboplatin, although there was an improvement in patients with squamous tumors. A planned pooled analysis of NVALT7 and GOIRC 02−2006 included 479 patients (81.4% with nonsquamous histology) and showed a higher response rate with combination therapy (15% vs. 9%) but no significant difference in median PFS (3.9 months vs. 3.0 months, $P = .07$) or in overall survival (8.7 months with the combination vs. 8.2 months with pemetrexed alone, $P = .316$).

Oxaliplatin is a platinum-agent that is not cross-tolerant with cisplatin or carboplatin and was explored as second-line therapy in NSCLC. A phase II study of 50 patients with NSCLC (38% with adenocarcinoma and 40% not otherwise specified) compared docetaxel 75 mg/m^2 alone or in combination with oxaliplatin 70 mg/m^2 given on day 2 in a 21-day cycle.[20] The combination was superior to monotherapy with a higher response rate (20% vs. 8%) and improved PFS (5.0 months vs. 1.7 months) and overall survival (11.0 months vs. 7.1 months), although the combination has not been developed further. Similarly, the addition of irinotecan (60 mg/m^2 days 1 and 8) to docetaxel 75 mg/m^2 in a 21-day cycle was explored in a randomized phase II study of 130 patients.[21] The combination prolonged time to tumor progression (6.4 months vs. 5.6 months, $P = .065$) with no significant change in response rate (20% vs. 14%), overall survival (6.5 months vs. 6.4 months) or 1-year survival rate (37% versus 34%), and an increase in grade 3 or 4 thrombocytopenia (17% vs. 6%, $P = .04$) and diarrhea (12% vs. 3%, $P = .05$). The combination of docetaxel and gemcitabine was the focus of JCOG0104 but was stopped due to high incidence of interstitial lung disease including several fatal cases.[22] Overall, 130 patients were randomized and there was no notable difference in survival (10.3 months with the combination vs. 10.1 months with monotherapy, $P = .36$).

While many other regimens have been explored with varying levels of success, combination chemotherapy is not standard second-line therapy for pulmonary adenocarcinoma following first-line platinum doublet chemotherapy. It would be appropriate, however, for patients who receive an alternate first-line therapy. For patients whose tumors harbor an actionable genomic alteration, such as an activating mutation in epidermal growth factor receptor (EGFR), the preferred first-line therapy is an EGFR tyrosine kinase inhibitor. At the time of progression, platinum doublet chemotherapy could be considered as second-line therapy for those patients if there are no preferred targeted options available. Likewise, for any patients initially treated with targeted therapy, application of the standard first-line treatment algorithm with doublet chemotherapy would be appropriate in later lines. This subset of patients is discussed elsewhere, although it is worth noting that with the transition to second-line chemotherapy, continuation of the original EGFR kinase inhibitor is not recommended. In the phase III IMPRESS trial, patients with an EGFR mutant NSCLC who progressed after a period of disease control with gefitinib were randomized to receive platinum doublet chemotherapy alone (cisplatin 75 mg/m^2 with pemetrexed 500 mg/m^2) or with continuation of their prior gefitinib.[23] Continuation of gefitinib did not improve PFS with a median PFS of 5.4 months in both arms. With longer follow-up, continuation of gefitinib had a negative impact on survival with a median overall survival of 13.4 months in the gefitinib plus chemotherapy arm and 19.5 months in the chemotherapy alone arm (HR 1.44; 95% CI 1.07−1.94).[24]

The integration of immunotherapy, specifically checkpoint inhibitors, in the initial treatment of pulmonary adenocarcinoma has created another group of patients where combination chemotherapy should be considered as second-line therapy. For patients whose tumors highly express programmed death receptor-1 ligand (PD-L1) by the Dako 22C3 immunohistochemistry (IHC) assay, the standard first-line therapy is pembrolizumab, a monoclonal antibody targeting programmed death receptor-1 (PD-1).[25] For patients who progress during pembrolizumab treatment, platinum doublet chemotherapy should be considered as second-line therapy. The increasingly complex landscape of lung cancer therapy will continue to alter the semantics when describing treatment options, but any patients who do not receive first-line platinum doublet therapy should be considered for such therapy in the second-line setting. We must acknowledge, however, that outcomes may not be the same in these settings and the sequence of therapy holds significance.

Treatment with checkpoint inhibitors can have durable effects on a host immune response and the tumor microenvironment. This could have a favorable impact on subsequent cytotoxic chemotherapy but may also influence toxicity. It is simply not yet clear what specific impact this will have on second-line cytotoxic therapy or how this should influence selection of second-line agents. More data are needed.

TARGETED AGENTS
Epidermal Growth Factor Receptor
Agents targeting EGFR have met with mixed success in the management of NSCLC. In tumors that harbor a sensitizing mutation in EGFR, use of EGFR tyrosine kinase inhibitors has been very effective and well tolerated, emerging as standard initial therapy. In tumors that do not have an activating EGFR mutation, the role of EGFR kinase inhibitors has evolved.

The National Cancer Institute of Canada Clinical Trials Group (NCIC CTG) conducted a trial to compare best supportive care plus erlotinib 150 mg daily or placebo in patients who had failed one or two prior lines of chemotherapy.[26] The response rate was 8.9% with erlotinib and under 1% with placebo. Both PFS and survival favored erlotinib (PFS 2.2 months vs. 1.8 months; overall survival 6.7 months vs. 4.7 months). Multiple subsequent studies compared erlotinib with docetaxel. In the randomized phase III INTEREST trial, patients with previously treated NSCLC were randomized to the EGFR kinase inhibitor gefitinib 250 mg by mouth daily or docetaxel 75 mg/m². This study of 1433 patients did demonstrate noninferiority for overall survival (HR 1.020, 95% CI 0.905–1.150). Median survival was 7.6 months with gefitinib and 8.0 months with docetaxel.

Subsequent studies have been less favorable. In the TAILOR trial, patients with NSCLC who had progression after first-line chemotherapy were registered, and their tumors were genotyped for EGFR mutations.[27] Only patients with wild-type EGFR were enrolled and randomized to erlotinib 150 mg daily or docetaxel 75 mg/m². In this study, chemotherapy was superior to EGFR-directed therapy with a median survival of 8.2 months with docetaxel versus 5.4 months with erlotinib. The DELTA study randomized unselected patients to erlotinib or docetaxel.[28] In an unselected population, erlotinib did not improve outcomes versus docetaxel with a median PFS of 2.0 months versus 3.2 months and a median overall survival of 14.8 months versus 12.2 months. In the subset of EGFR wild-type patients, outcomes favored docetaxel with a median PFS of

1.3 months with erlotinib and 2.9 months with docetaxel and a median overall survival of 9.0 months with erlotinib and 10.1 months with docetaxel. Initial activity of EGFR tyrosine kinase inhibitors in an unselected population was likely driven by the inclusion of tumors harboring sensitizing EGFR mutations. In the absence of an activating EGFR alteration, use of EGFR kinase inhibitors is no longer recommended in the management of pulmonary adenocarcinoma.

Cetuximab is a monoclonal IgG antibody that targets EGFR. The combination of cetuximab plus docetaxel showed promise in a small phase II trial. Patients with previously treated NSCLC received cetuximab (400 mg/m² initially then 250 mg/m² weekly thereafter) with docetaxel 75 mg/m².[29] The objective response rate was 20% including 1 complete response and the median time to disease progression was 104 days. Median overall survival was 7.5 months and 1-year survival rate was 35%. An open-label phase III study was then completed and 939 patients were randomized to receive chemotherapy (docetaxel or pemetrexed) or chemotherapy with cetuximab.[30] The addition of cetuximab to pemetrexed did not improve outcomes with a median PFS of 2.9 months with cetuximab and 2.8 months with pemetrexed alone. Toxicity was much higher with the addition of cetuximab and with no evidence of a PFS or survival benefit, use of cetuximab in this setting is not recommended.

Vascular Endothelial Growth Factor
Bevacizumab, a monoclonal antibody targeting vascular endothelial growth factor (VEGF), improved overall survival in the first-line setting when combined with the doublet of carboplatin plus paclitaxel.[31] VEGF inhibition has been studied in the second-line setting as well. A retrospective analysis of patients who received docetaxel with bevacizumab reported a response rate of 26.7%, although all 15 patients identified experienced grade 3 or 4 neutropenia and 26.7% developed febrile neutropenia.[32] A small retrospective study compared outcomes with second-line pemetrexed monotherapy compared with pemetrexed plus bevacizumab.[33] While the 6-month survival rate favored the bevacizumab cohort (66.7% vs. 56.3%), there was no difference in response rate, time to progression, or overall survival. A prospective phase II study of pemetrexed 500 mg/m² plus bevacizumab 15 mg/kg in the second-line setting demonstrated an overall response rate of 10.4%, although an additional 40% of patients achieved stable disease lasting at least 6 weeks.[34] The median PFS was 4 months and median overall survival was 8.6 months. While the results were interesting, the

study did not meet its primary endpoint. The triplet of pemetrexed 500 mg/m^2 plus oxaliplatin 120 mg/m^2 and bevacizumab 15 mg/kg was studied in 36 patients (34 evaluable) enrolled on a multicenter phase II trial.[35] The reported response rate was 27% with a median PFS of 5.8 months and a median overall survival of 12.5 months. The most promising results stem from a multicenter, randomized phase II study that randomized 120 patients with nonsquamous NSCLC to receive second-line chemotherapy (either docetaxel 75 mg/m^2 or pemetrexed 500 mg/m^2 at the treating physician's discretion), chemotherapy plus bevacizumab 15 mg/kg, or erlotinib, an EGFR tyrosine kinase inhibitor, 150 mg daily plus bevacizumab 15 mg/kg.[36] The primary endpoint of PFS favored the arms with bevacizumab; median PFS was 4.8 months with chemotherapy plus bevacizumab in contrast to 3.0 months with chemotherapy alone. Survival also favored the bevacizumab arms with a median survival of 12.6 months with bevacizumab plus chemotherapy, 13.7 months for bevacizumab plus erlotinib and 8.6 months with chemotherapy. While encouraging, larger studies are still needed to define any role of bevacizumab in the second-line setting.

Ramucirumab is a monoclonal antibody that targets VEGFR-2 that is approved for use in the second-line setting. In the randomized phase III REVEL trial, 1253 patients with advanced NSCLC who had progressed after first-line platinum doublet chemotherapy with or without bevacizumab were randomized to receive docetaxel 75 mg/m^2 with either ramucirumab 10 mg/kg or placebo.[37] Although squamous and nonsquamous histologies were permitted, the majority of patients had adenocarcinoma (74% in the ramucirumab arm, 72% in the placebo arm). Ramucirumab improved overall survival (10.5 months vs. 9.1 months, $P = .023$) as well as PFS (4.5 months vs. 3.0 months, $P < .0001$) and response rate (23% vs. 14%). The subset of patients with nonsquamous NSCLC had a median survival of 11.1 months with ramucirumab compared with 9.7 months with placebo. Ramucirumab was associated with more toxicity including higher rates of grade 3 or higher neutropenia (49% vs. 39%), febrile neutropenia (16% vs. 10%), and any grade bleeding or hemorrhage (29% vs. 15%), although the rate of grade 3 or higher bleeding was the same in both arms (2%). The increased hematologic toxicity did prompt a regional change in the dose of docetaxel from 75 mg/m^2 to 60 mg/m^2 in East Asia.

Vandetanib is a multikinase inhibitor that can target VEGFR, EGFR, and rearranged during transfection (RET). The addition of vandetanib to chemotherapy has been explored in the second-line setting for NSCLC. A randomized phase II study compared docetaxel 75 mg/m^2 alone with docetaxel plus vandetanib 100 mg daily and docetaxel plus vandetanib 300 mg daily.[38] Vandetanib improved PFS with a median PFS of 18.7 weeks with vandetanib 100 mg, 17.0 weeks with vandetanib 300 mg, and 12 weeks for docetaxel. This prompted a phase III study with the 100 mg dose. Patients with NSCLC who progressed after initial chemotherapy were randomized to docetaxel 75 mg/m^2 plus either vandetanib 100 mg daily or placebo.[39] The study included 1391 patients and demonstrated a modest but statistically significant improvement in PFS with vandetanib; median PFS was 4.0 months with vandetanib and 3.2 months in the placebo group. Vandetanib was also studied with pemetrexed. In a 534 patient phase III study, patients received pemetrexed 500 mg/m^2 with either vandetanib 100 mg daily or placebo. There was no significant difference in PFS or overall survival, although the vandetanib combination did offer a higher response rate (19% vs. 8%).

Nintedanib (BIBF 1120) is another small molecule tyrosine kinase inhibitor of proangiogenic receptors VEGFR 1–3, platelet-derived growth factor receptor (PDGFR), and fibroblast growth factor receptor 1–3 (FGFR1-3). The LUME-Lung 1 trial assessed the efficacy and safety of nintedanib with docetaxel in second-line setting.[40] Nintedanib 200 mg or placebo was administered twice daily orally on days 2–21 after receiving docetaxel 75 mg/m^2 on day 1. The study met its primary endpoint by demonstrating superior PFS with the nintedanib combination compared with docetaxel plus placebo (3.4 months vs. 2.7 months, $P = .0019$). The PFS benefit was greater in tumors with adenocarcinoma histology (4.2 months vs. 1.5 months, $P = .0005$). In patients with adenocarcinoma, overall survival was also superior with nintedanib plus docetaxel (12.6 months vs. 10.3 months, $P = .0349$). Overall, the 2-year survival rate was 25.7% with nintedanib plus docetaxel compared with 19.1% with docetaxel plus placebo. Although tolerable, the addition of nintedanib did increase toxicity over docetaxel alone with higher rates of grade 3 or worse diarrhea (6.6% vs. 2.6%), elevation in ALT (7.8% vs. 0.9%) and elevation in aspartate aminotransferase (AST, 3.4% vs. 0.5%).

The LUME-Lung 2 study of nintedanib plus pemetrexed had a less favorable outcome.[41] Similar to LUME-Lung 1, this trial included NSCLC with one prior line of chemotherapy, but given the pemetrexed backbone, this study was limited to nonsquamous histology. Patients received pemetrexed 500 mg/m^2 on day 1 and either nintedanib 200 mg orally twice daily or placebo on days 2–21 in 3-week cycles. The study was stopped prematurely for futility with enrollment of 713 out of a planned 1300 patients. PFS favored the nintedanib cohort (median 4.4 months vs. 3.6 months), but there was no difference in overall survival (median 12.0 months vs. 12.7 months).

Mitogen-Activated Protein Kinase Kinase

A significant subset of patients with pulmonary adenocarcinoma will harbor a mutation in the Kirsten rat sarcoma viral oncogene homologue (KRAS) gene, which has been challenging to target. As KRAS mutations promote signaling through the mitogen-activated protein kinase kinase (MEK) and extracellular signal–related kinase (ERK) pathways, MEK inhibition was an appealing therapeutic strategy. A randomized phase 2 study compared docetaxel 75 mg/m^2 plus placebo to docetaxel 75 mg/m^2 plus the MEK inhibitor selumetinib 75 mg twice daily in patients with KRAS-mutant NSCLC who had failed first-line chemotherapy.[42] The study randomized 44 patients, and outcomes favored the selumetinib group with superior PFS (5.3 months vs. 2.1 months) and a trend toward an improvement in median overall survival (9.4 months vs. 5.2 months, $P = .21$). The response rate also favored selumetinib (37% vs. 0%). The larger phase II SELECT-2 trial randomized 212 patients with KRAS mutant NSCLC to docetaxel 75 mg/m^2 with either selumetinib or placebo.[43] Unfortunately, the previous results were not replicated as no improvement in PFS was noted. The SELECT-1 trial randomized 510 patients to docetaxel

75 mg/m^2 plus selumetinib or docetaxel 75 mg/m^2 plus placebo.[44] Again, no significant difference in outcomes was noted. Median PFS was 3.9 months with selumetinib and 2.8 months with placebo ($P = .44$), and median overall survival was 8.7 months with selumetinib versus 7.9 months with placebo ($P = .64$).

IMMUNOTHERAPY

The emergence of checkpoint inhibitors has dramatically shifted the treatment paradigms throughout much of oncology, including pulmonary adenocarcinoma. Monoclonal antibodies such as nivolumab, pembrolizumab, and atezolizumab inhibit the interaction of PD-1 with PD-L1 to prevent negative regulation of T-cells and promote an antitumor immune response. Use of pembrolizumab alone or with platinum doublet chemotherapy is an option for many patients with adenocarcinoma as initial therapy. For patients who do not receive pembrolizumab in the first-line setting, there are several immunotherapy agents approved for second-line treatment. While response rates in this setting are modest, checkpoint inhibitors offer the possibility of durable, meaningful responses and the durability of these responses is one of the more appealing features of immunotherapy. While they also are associated with unique and potentially dangerous toxicities, PD-1 and PD-L1 inhibitors have consistently been better tolerated than chemotherapy and are now firmly entrenched as standard second-line therapy for NSCLC (Table 6.1).

TABLE 6.1
Second-Line Checkpoint Inhibitors in NSCLC

Randomized Phase III Study Compared to Docetaxel 75 mg/m^2	Median PFS (months)	RR	Median OS (months)	1-Year OS	D/C due to AE
Nivolumab 3 mg/kg *Checkmate 057* Borghaei, NEJM 2015	**2.3** (vs. 4.2)	**19%** (vs. 12%)	**12.2** (vs. 9.4)	**51%** (vs. 39%)	**5%** (vs. 15%)
Pembrolizumab 2 mg/kg *KEYNOTE-010* Herbst, Lancet 2015	**3.9** (vs. 4.0)	**18%** (vs. 9%)	**10.4** (vs. 8.5)	**43%** (vs. 35%)	**4%** (vs. 10%)
Atezolizumab 1200 mg *OAK* Rittmeyer, Lancet 2016	**2.8** (vs. 4.0)	**14%** (vs. 13%)	**13.8** (vs. 9.6)	**55%** (vs. 41%)	**8%** (vs. 19%)

Results compared to docetaxel 75 mg/m^2. *AE*, adverse event; *D/C*, discontinued therapy; *OS*, overall survival; *PFS*, progression-free survival; *RR*, objective response rate.

Nivolumab

Nivolumab, an IgG4 monoclonal antibody targeting PD-1, was the first checkpoint inhibitor to garner FDA approval for the treatment of NSCLC. In a phase I study of nivolumab, heavily pretreated patients with advanced NSCLC received nivolumab every 2 weeks at doses of 1 mg/kg, 3 mg/kg, or 10 mg/kg.[45] No maximum tolerated dose was noted. Responses were noted in 22 of the 129 patients treated (17%), and the estimated median duration of response was 17.0 months. Median overall survival was 9.9 months. The dose selected for future study was 3 mg/kg, which subsequently was altered to a flat dose of 240 mg. Median survival at the 3 mg/kg dose was 14.9 months. At this dose, the 1-year survival rate was 56%, the 2-year survival rate was 42%, and the 3-year survival rate was an impressive 27%. Nivolumab was associated with toxicity as 71% of patients noted a treatment-related adverse event, although the incidence of grade 3 or 4 treatment-related adverse events was only 14%, most commonly fatigue at 3%. Of note, 3% of patients had treatment-related grade 3 or higher pneumonitis including one case of grade 5 pneumonitis.

While several smaller phase II studies were conducted, a randomized phase III trial was promptly launched that compared nivolumab 3 mg/kg every 2 weeks with standard second-line therapy with docetaxel 75 mg/m^2 every 3 weeks in patients with nonsquamous NSCLC who had progressed after first-line platinum-based chemotherapy.[46] The primary endpoint was overall survival in an unselected population. In the 582 patients randomized to treatment, survival was superior in the nivolumab arm. Median overall survival was 12.2 months with nivolumab and 9.4 months with docetaxel; the hazard ratio for death was 0.73 (95% CI, 0.59–0.89). The 1-year survival rate was 51% with nivolumab and 39% with docetaxel. The 18-month survival rate was 39% in the nivolumab arm and 23% in the docetaxel arm. Objective response rate was 19% with nivolumab and 12% with docetaxel. The median duration of response was 17.2 months in the nivolumab arm and only 5.6 months with docetaxel. PFS was shorter with nivolumab (2.3 months vs. 4.2 months) but PFS rate at 1-year favored nivolumab (19% vs. 8%). In an effort to define the subset of patients deriving the greatest benefit, tumors were tested for PD-L1 expression with the Dako 28-8 IHC assay. Of the 582 patients randomized, 78% had quantifiable PD-L1 expression. Using prespecified expression cutoffs of 1%, 5%, and 10%, nivolumab was associated with superior overall survival independent of PD-L1 expression. At each cutoff, however, response was greater in

tumors expressing PD-L1. The response rate for tumors with <1% expression was 9% compared with 31% in tumors with PD-L1 expression >1%. In addition to superior efficacy, the safety profile favored nivolumab. Patients in the nivolumab arm had a lower incidence of any grade 3 or 4 treatment-related adverse event (10% vs. 54%). Docetaxel was associated with higher rates of grade 3 or 4 neutropenia (27% vs. 0%), febrile neutropenia (10% vs. 0%), and fatigue (5% vs. 1%). Discontinuation of treatment due to treatment-related adverse events was more common with docetaxel (15% vs. 5%). Nivolumab received FDA approval for the treatment of pretreated nonsquamous NSCLC on 10/9/15 independent of PD-L1 expression.

Pembrolizumab

Pembrolizumab is an IgG4 monoclonal antibody targeting PD-1 with a prominent role in the treatment of advanced NSCLC. In the phase I KEYNOTE-001 trial, 495 patients with advanced NSCLC received pembrolizumab monotherapy.[47] Early in its course, the study was amended to require expression of PD-L1 in at least 1% of tumor cells (tumor proportion score of at least 1%) using the proprietary Dako 22C3 IHC assay. In 394 patients who had received prior systemic therapy, the response rate was 18% with a median duration of response of 10 months and a median overall survival of 9.3 months. Among previously treated patients with a PD-L1 tumor proportion score of at least 50%, the response rate was 44%. Among the 824 tissue samples evaluable for PD-L1 analysis, 23.2% of patients had a proportion score of at least 50% and an additional 37.6% had a score between 1% and 49%. Pembrolizumab had a favorable safety profile. Although 70.9% of patients had a treatment-related adverse event, only 9.5% had an event that was grade 3 or higher. Immune-related adverse events that were noted in more than 2% of patients included infusion reactions (3%), hypothyroidism (6.9%), and pneumonitis (3.6%), although grade 3 or greater pneumonitis was noted in only 1.8% of patients. Pembrolizumab was granted FDA approval on 10/2/15 for pretreated NSCLC that expresses PD-L1.

The subsequent randomized trial (KEYNOTE-010) compared two doses of pembrolizumab (2 and 10 mg/kg) with standard docetaxel 75 mg/m^2 in patients with previously treated NSCLC with a PD-L1 proportion score of at least 1%.[48] There were 1034 patients randomized to the three arms, and survival favored pembrolizumab. Median survival was 10.4 months with pembrolizumab 2 mg/kg, 12.7 months with pembrolizumab 10 mg/kg, and 8.5 months with docetaxel.

When compared with docetaxel, pembrolizumab was superior at the 2 mg/kg dose (HR 0.71, 95% CI 0.58−0.88) and at the 10 mg/kg dose (HR 0.61, 95% CI 0.49−0.75). There was no significant difference in PFS between pembrolizumab 2 mg/kg, pembrolizumab 10 mg/kg, or docetaxel (3.9, 4.0, and 4.0 months, respectively), but responses were greater with pembrolizumab (18% at either dose vs. 9% with docetaxel). In the subset of patients with a proportion score of at least 50% (which represented 25% of the study population), the response rate was 29%−30% compared with 8% with docetaxel. In this cohort of patients with high PD-L1, expression survival more strongly favored pembrolizumab over docetaxel: at the 2 mg/kg dose, the HR was 0.54 (95% CI 0.38−0.77) and at the 10 mg/kg dose, the HR was 0.50 (95% CI 0.36−0.70). The median overall survival in these patients was 14.9 months with pembrolizumab 2 mg/kg, 17.3 months at 10 mg/kg, and 8.2 months with docetaxel. There was a significant survival benefit for patients with adenocarcinoma histology with pembrolizumab (pooled analysis) compared with docetaxel (HR 0.63, 95% CI 0.50−0.79). Safety also favored pembrolizumab. Grade 3 or higher treatment-related adverse events were noted in 13% of patients receiving pembrolizumab 2 mg/kg, 16% receiving pembrolizumab 10 mg/kg, and 35% receiving docetaxel. The incidence of pneumonitis was 5% and 4% in the two pembrolizumab arms (2 and 10 mg/kg) and 2% in the docetaxel arm with grade 3 or higher pneumonitis seen in 2% of patients receiving either dose of pembrolizumab and 1% of patients receiving docetaxel. Discontinuation of treatment due to treatment-related adverse event occurred in 4% of patients receiving pembrolizumab 2 mg/kg, 5% with pembrolizumab 10 mg/kg, and 10% of patients receiving docetaxel.

Atezolizumab

Atezolizumab (MPDL3280A) is an IgG1 antagonist antibody targeting PD-L1 that has been engineered to avoid antibody-dependent cell-mediated cytotoxicity. In a phase I study, atezolizumab demonstrated responses across several tumor types including a response rate of 23% in 53 patients with NSCLC and 21% in the 42 patients with nonsquamous histology.[49] There was an association between response and expression of PD-L1, although the assay used to assess PD-L1 expression was different from the ones used above. PD-L1 expression was quantified with the Ventana SP142 IHC assay and included expression of PD-L1 (with different cutoffs) on both tumor cells and tumor-infiltrating immune cells. A randomized phase II study compared atezolizumab 1200 mg with docetaxel 75 mg/m², both given in a 21-day cycle. The study included 287 patients with a primary endpoint of overall survival. Survival favored atezolizumab with a median survival of 12.6 months with atezolizumab and 9.7 months with docetaxel (HR 0.73, 95% CI 0.53−0.99). There was no significant difference in PFS (2.7 months with atezolizumab, 3.0 months with docetaxel) or response rate (15% in both arms), but the duration of response heavily favored atezolizumab (14.3 months vs. 7.2 months). Survival benefit was more pronounced with increasing expression of PD-L1 on tumor cells, tumor-infiltrating immune cells, or both. In the subset of patients with nonsquamous histology, survival was 15.5 months with atezolizumab (95 patients) and 10.9 months with docetaxel (95 patients). Safety again favored the checkpoint inhibitor, with 11% of patients experiencing a treatment-related adverse event with atezolizumab compared with 39% with docetaxel. The most common atezolizumab-related grade 3 events (there were no grade 4 events) were pneumonia (2%) and AST elevation (2%). Atezolizumab was associated with immune-related adverse events including pneumonitis in four patients (3%, one patient with grade 3 pneumonitis), colitis in two patients (1%), and hepatitis in one patient. The incidence of treatment discontinuation was 8% with atezolizumab versus 22% with docetaxel. Atezolizumab was approved by the FDA on 10/18/16 for the treatment of NSCLC following platinum-based chemotherapy independent of PD-L1 expression.

The randomized phase III OAK study also compared atezolizumab 1200 mg with docetaxel 75 mg/m² in patients with NSCLC (any histology, no PD-L1 expression required) who had received 1−2 prior chemotherapy regimens.[50] This large study of 1225 patients had a primary endpoint of overall survival, and survival was improved with atezolizumab, in both the intention to treat population and in the PD-L1 expression subpopulations. Median overall survival was 13.8 months with atezolizumab and 9.6 months with docetaxel (HR 0.73, 95% CI 0.62−0.87). In the subset of patients with any PD-L1 expression (on tumor cells or immune cells), survival favored atezolizumab with a median survival of 15.7 months compared with 10.3 months with docetaxel (HR 0.74, 95% CI 0.58−0.93). In the PD-L1 low or undetectable cohort, survival still favored atezolizumab with a median survival of 12.6 months compared with 8.9 months (HR 0.75, 95% CI 0.59–0.96). Patients with nonsquamous histology also had an improved survival with atezolizumab (HR 0.73, 95% CI 0.60–0.89). There was not a significant difference between atezolizumab and docetaxel in terms of PFS (median 4.0 months vs. 2.8 months, respectively) or response rate (14% vs. 13%), although duration of response strongly favored atezolizumab (16.3 months vs. 6.2 months). Consistent with the above studies, the safety profile favored atezolizumab. Treatment-related adverse events, grade 3 or higher, were noted in 15% of patients receiving atezolizumab and 43% of patients receiving docetaxel. Immune-related adverse events included pneumonitis (1%), colitis (<1%), and hepatitis (<1%). Treatment discontinuation from adverse event occurred in 8% of patients receiving atezolizumab and 19% with docetaxel.

CONCLUSION

Second-line therapy for pulmonary adenocarcinoma is rapidly evolving, largely due to the downstream effect of changes in first-line therapy. As our management of adenocarcinoma increases in sophistication, second-line therapy lends itself less and less to algorithms and flowcharts and requires the judgment and oversight of experienced clinicians. The patterns of success in this disease have been clear—identification of appropriate biomarkers is critical to optimal delivery of care. Certainly this applies to the molecularly defined cohort of patients with adenocarcinoma but presence of an actionable alteration is not adequate—identification of the alteration is needed. Perhaps the strongest recommendation for second-line therapy is to ensure that patients have had appropriate molecular testing at their initial diagnosis and if not, to remedy that promptly. Beyond that, immunotherapy has seized the narrative in the treatment of adenocarcinoma, largely attributed to its potential for durable benefit, but it is increasingly clear that only a minority of patients will achieve this benefit with the available tools. Improvements are needed and are on the horizon in the form of novel agents, rational combinations, and improved predictive markers. Cytotoxic and biologic therapy still has a role in the management of pulmonary adenocarcinoma, and advances in the safe delivery of these agents have increased their relevance. While it is difficult to predict the state of second-line therapy in the coming years, the current trends assure us that it will only continue to improve.

DISCLOSURE STATEMENT

Dr. Patel has no relevant disclosures.

Dr. Liu discloses serving as a consultant or advisor to AstraZeneca, Boehringer Ingelheim, Bristol-Myers Squibb, Celgene, Genentech/Roche, Lilly, Pfizer, Taiho, and Takeda.

REFERENCES

1. Shepherd FA, Dancey J, Ramlau R, et al. Prospective randomized trial of docetaxel versus best supportive care in patients with non-small-cell lung cancer previously treated with platinum-based chemotherapy. *J Clin Oncol.* 2000;18:2095–2103.
2. Fossella FV, DeVore R, Kerr RN, et al. Randomized phase III trial of docetaxel versus vinorelbine or ifosfamide in patients with advanced non-small-cell lung cancer previously treated with platinum-containing chemotherapy regimens. *J Clin Oncol.* 2000;18:2354–2362.
3. Schuette W, Nagel S, Blankenburg T, et al. Phase III study of second-line chemotherapy for advanced non-small-cell lung cancer with weekly compared with 3-weekly docetaxel. *J Clin Oncol.* 2005;23:8389–8395.
4. Gridelli C, Gallo C, Di Maio M, et al. A randomised clinical trial of two docetaxel regimens (weekly *vs* 3 week) in the second-line treatment of non-small-cell lung cancer. The DISTAL 01 study. *Br J Cancer.* 2004;91:1996–2004.
5. Tomasini P, Barlesi F, Mascaux C, et al. Pemetrexed for advanced stage nonsquamous non-small cell lung cancer: latest evidence about its extended use and outcomes. *Ther Adv Med Oncol.* 2016;8:198–208.
6. Hanna N, Shepherd FA, Fossella FV, et al. Randomized phase III trial of pemetrexed versus docetaxel in patients with non-small-cell lung cancer previously treated with chemotherapy. *J Clin Oncol.* 2004;22:1589–1597.
7. Plunkett W, Huang P, Gandhi V. Preclinical characteristics of gemcitabine. *Anticancer Drugs.* 1995;6(6 suppl):7–13.
8. Crino L, Mosconi AM, Scagliotti G, et al. Gemcitabine as second-line treatment for advanced non-small-cell lung cancer: a Phase II trial. *J Clin Oncol.* 1999;17:2081–2085.
9. Van Kooten M, Traine G, Cinat G, et al. Single-agent gemcitabine in pretreated patients with non-small cell lung cancer: results of a multicentre phase II clinic. *Br J Cancer.* 1999;81:846–849.
10. Georgoulias V, Kouroussis C, Agelidou A, et al. Irinotecan plus gemcitabine vs irinotecan for the second-line treatment of patients with advanced non-small-cell lung cancer pretreated with docetaxel and cisplatin: a multicentre, randomised, phase II study. *Br J Cancer.* 2004;91:482–488.
11. Hainsworth JD, Thompson DS, Greco A. Paclitaxel by 1-hour infusion: an active drug in metastatic non-small-cell lung cancer. *J Clin Oncol.* 1995;13:1609–1614.
12. Buccheri G, Ferrigno D. Cuneo Lung Cancer Study Group. Second-line weekly paclitaxel in patients with inoperable non-small cell lung cancer who fail combination chemotherapy with cisplatin. *Lung Cancer.* 2004;45:227–236.

13. Ramlau R, Gervais R, Krzakowski M, et al. Phase III study comparing oral topotecan to intravenous docetaxel in patients with pretreated advanced non-small-cell lung cancer. *J Clin Oncol.* 2006;24:2800–2807.

14. Totani Y, Saito Y, Hayashi M, et al. A phase II study of S-1 monotherapy as second-line treatment for advanced non-small cell lung cancer. *Cancer Chemother Pharmacol.* 2009; 64:1181–1185.

15. Nokihara H, Lu S, Mok TSK, et al. Randomized controlled trial of S-1 versus docetaxel in patients with non-small cell lung cancer previously treated with platinum-based chemotherapy (East Asia S-1 Trial in Lung Cancer). *Ann Oncol.* 2017;28:2698–2706.

16. Pronzato P, Landucci M, Vaira F, et al. Failure of vinorelbine to produce responses in pretreated non-small cell lung cancer patients. *Anticancer Res.* 1994;14:1413–1415.

17. Pallis AG, Agelaki S, Agelidou A, et al. A randomized phase III study of the docetaxel/carboplatin combination versus docetaxel single-agent as second line treatment for patients with advanced/metastatic non-small cell lung cancer. *BMC Cancer.* 2010;10:633–640.

18. Smit EF, Burgers SA, Biesma B, et al. Randomized phase II and pharmacogenetic study of pemetrexed compared with pemetrexed plus carboplatin in pretreated patients with advanced non-small-cell lung cancer. *J Clin Oncol.* 2009; 27:2038–2045.

19. Ardizzoni A, Tiseo M, Boni L, et al. Pemetrexed versus pemetrexed and carboplatin as second-line chemotherapy in advanced non-small-cell lung cancer: results of the GOIRC 02-2006 randomized phase II study and pooled analysis with the NVALT7 trial. *J Clin Oncol.* 2012;30: 4501–4507.

20. Belvedere O, Follador A, Rossetto C, et al. A randomised phase II study of docetaxel/oxaliplatin and docetaxel in patients with previously treated non-small cell lung cancer: an Alpe-Adria Thoracic Oncology Multidisciplinary group trial (ATOM 019). *Eur J Cancer.* 2011;47:1653–1659.

21. Pectasides D, Pectasides M, Farmakis D, et al. Comparison of docetaxel and docetaxel-irinotecan combination as second-line chemotherapy in advanced non-small-cell lung cancer: a randomized phase II trial. *Ann Oncol.* 2005;16:294–299.

22. Takeda K, Negoro S, Tumura T, et al. Phase III trial of docetaxel plus gemcitabine versus docetaxel in second-line treatment for non-small-cell lung cancer: results of a Japan Clinical Oncology Group trial (JCOG0104). *Ann Oncol.* 2009;20:835–841.

23. Soria JC, Wu YL, Nakagawa K, et al. Gefitinib plus chemotherapy versus placebo plus chemotherapy in EGFR-mutation-positive non-small-cell lung cancer after progression on first-line gefitinib (IMPRESS): a phase 3 randomised trial. *Lancet Oncol.* 2015;16:990–998.

24. Mok TSK, Kim SW, Wu YL, et al. Gefitinib plus chemotherapy versus chemotherapy in epidermal growth factor receptor mutation-positive non-small-cell lung cancer resistant to first-line gefitinib (IMPRESS): overall survival and biomarker analysis. *J Clin Oncol.* 2017;35: 4027–4034.

25. Reck M, Rodriguez-Abreu D, Robinson AG, et al. Pembrolizumab versus chemotherapy for PD-L1 positive non-small-cell lung cancer. *N Engl J Med.* 2016;375: 1823–1833.

26. Shepherd FA, Pereira JR, Ciuleanu T, et al. Erlotinib in previously treated non-small-cell lung cancer. *N Engl J Med.* 2005;353:123–132.

27. Garassino MC, Martelli O, Broggini M, et al. Erlotinib versus docetaxel as second-line treatment of patients with advanced non-small-cell lung cancer and wild-type EGFR tumours (TAILOR): a randomised controlled trial. *Lancet Oncol.* 2013;14:981–988.

28. Kawaguchi T, Ando M, Asami K, et al. Randomized phase III trial of erlotinib versus docetaxel as second- or third-line therapy in patients with advanced non-small-cell lung cancer: docetaxel and erlotinib lung cancer trial (DELTA). *J Clin Oncol.* 2014;32:1902–1908.

29. Kim ES, Mauer AM, William Jr WN, et al. A phase 2 study of cetuximab in combination with docetaxel in chemotherapy-refractory/resistant patients with advanced non small cell lung cancer. *Cancer.* 2009;115: 1713–1722.

30. Kim ES, Neubauer M, Cohn A, et al. Docetaxel or pemetrexed with or without cetuximab in recurrent or progressive non-small-cell lung cancer after platinum-based therapy: a phase 3, open-label, randomised trial. *Lancet Oncol.* 2013;14(13):1326–1336.

31. Sandler A, Gray R, Perry MC, et al. Paclitaxel-carboplatin alone or with bevacizumab for non-small-cell lung cancer. *N Engl J Med.* 2006;355:2542–2550.

32. Kurishima K, Watanabe H, Ishikawa H, et al. A retrospective study of docetaxel and bevacizumab as a second- or later-line chemotherapy for non-small cell lung cancer. *Mol Clin Oncol.* 2017;7:131–134.

33. Weiss GJ, Zeng C, Kelly K, et al. Single-institution experience with pemetrexed and bevacizumab as salvage therapy in advanced non-small-cell lung cancer. *Clin Lung Cancer.* 2007;8:335–338.

34. Adjei AA, Mandrekar SJ, Dy GK, et al. Phase II trial of pemetrexed plus bevacizumab for second-line therapy of patients with advanced non-small-cell lung cancer: NCCTG and SWOG study N0426. *J Clin Oncol.* 2010;28: 614–619.

35. Heist RS, Fidias P, Huberman M, et al. A phase II study of oxaliplatin, pemetrexed, and bevacizumab in previously treated advanced non-small cell lung cancer. *J Thorac Oncol.* 2008;3:1153–1158.

36. Herbst RS, O'Neill VJ, Fehrenbacher L, et al. Phase II study of efficacy and safety of bevacizumab in combination with chemotherapy or erlotinib compared with chemotherapy alone for treatment of recurrent or refractory non-small-cell lung cancer. *J Clin Oncol.* 2007;25:4743–4750.

37. Garon EB, Ciuleanu TE, Arrieta O, et al. Ramucirumab plus docetaxel versus placebo plus docetaxel for second-line treatment of stage IV non-small-cell lung cancer after disease progression on platinum-based therapy (REVEL): a multicentre, double-blind, randomised phase 3 trial. *Lancet.* 2014;384:665–673.

38. Heymach JV, Johnson BE, Prager D, et al. Randomized, placebo-controlled phase II study of vandetanib plus docetaxel in previously treated non small-cell lung cancer. *J Clin Oncol.* 2007;25:4270−4277.

39. Herbst RS, Sun Y, Eberhardt WEE, et al. Vandetanib plus docetaxel versus docetaxel as second-line treatment for patients with advanced non-small-cell lung cancer (ZODIAC): a double-blind, randomised, phase 3 trial. *Lancet Oncol.* 2010;11:619−626.

40. Reck M, Kaiser R, Mellemgaard A, et al. Docetaxel plus nintedanib versus docetaxel plus placebo in patients with previously treated non-small-cell lung cancer (LUME-Lung 1): a phase 3, double-blind, randomised controlled trial. *Lancet Oncol.* 2014;15:143−155.

41. Hanna NH, Kaiser R, Sullivan RN, et al. Nintedanib plus pemetrexed versus placebo plus pemetrexed in patients with relapsed or refractory, advanced non-small cell lung cancer (LUME-Lung 2): a randomized, double-blind, phase III trial. *Lung Cancer.* 2016;102:65−73.

42. Janne PA, Shaw AT, Pereira JR, et al. Selumetinib plus docetaxel for KRAS-mutant advanced non-small-cell lung cancer: a randomised, multicentre, placebo-controlled, phase 2 study. *Lancet Oncol.* 2013;14:38−47.

43. Soria JC, Fulop A, Maciel C, et al. SELECT-2: a phase II, double-blind, randomised, placebo-controlled study to assess the efficacy of selumetinib plus docetaxel as a second-line treatment for patients with advanced or metastatic non-small cell lung cancer. *Ann Oncol.* 2017;28: 3028−3036.

44. Janne PA, van den Heuvel MM, Barlesi F, et al. Selumetinib plus docetaxel compared with docetaxel alone and progression-free survival in patients with KRAS-mutant advanced non-small cell lung cancer. The SELECT-1 randomized clinical trial. *JAMA.* 2017;317(18):1844−1853.

45. Gettinger SN, Horn L, Gandhi L, et al. Overall survival and long-term safety of nivolumab (anti-programmed death 1 antibody, BMS_936558, ONO-4538) in patients with previously treated advanced non-small cell lung cancer. *J Clin Oncol.* 2015;33:2004−2012.

46. Borghaei H, Paz-Ares L, Horn L, et al. Nivolumab versus docetaxel in advanced nonsquamous non-small-cell lung cancer. *N Engl J Med.* 2015;373:1627−1639.

47. Garon EB, Rizvi NA, Hui R, et al. Pembrolizumab for the treatment of non-small-cell lung cancer. *N Engl J Med.* 2015;372:2018−2028.

48. Herbst RS, Baas P, Kim DW, et al. Pembrolizumab versus docetaxel for previously treated, PD-L1 positive, advanced non-small-cell lung cancer (KEYNOTE-010): a randomised controlled trial. *Lancet.* 2016;387:1540−1550.

49. Herbst RS, Soria JC, Kowanetz M, et al. Predictive correlates of response to the anti-PD-L1 antibody MPDL3280A in cancer patients. *Nature.* 2014;515:563−567.

50. Rittmeyer A, Barlesi F, Waterkamp D, et al. Atezolizumab versus docetaxel in patients with previously treated non-small-cell lung cancer (OAK): a phase 3, open-label, multicentre randomised controlled trial. *Lancet.* 2017;389: 255−265.

Epidermal Growth Factor Receptor–Mutant Non–Small-Cell Lung Cancer

NICOLAS MARCOUX, MD, FRCPC • LECIA V. SEQUIST, MD, MPH

The discovery of epidermal growth factor receptor (EGFR) mutations in lung cancer has revolutionized the field of thoracic oncology by leading to the development of the first targeted therapies in non–small-cell lung cancer (NSCLC). Far from resting on these significant past accomplishments, EGFR-related research is thriving and remains one of the most exciting and fast-moving topics surrounding lung cancer. Before discussing the current state of EGFR-mutant NSCLC and its treatment, it is essential to look back at the findings and research that led us to where we are now.

Although the use of targeted therapies for EGFR-mutant lung cancer is relatively recent, the discovery of EGFR and its ligands is several decades old. In 1962, Nobel Prize winner Dr Stanley Cohen described and isolated a protein capable of accelerating the development of incisors and eyelids when injected in newborn mice.[1] Initially named "tooth-lid factor" for that reason, subsequent observation that these effects were due to epidermal cell proliferation prompted the name epidermal growth factor (EGF). Almost two decades later, in 1980, further research from Cohen et al. showed that EGF phosphorylates tyrosine residues from membrane proteins[2] on a human epidermoid carcinoma cell line.

Also in 1980 a team from the National Cancer Institute described a transforming growth factor (TGF),[3] later named TGF-α, after identification of a polypeptide competing with EGF for a yet poorly understood receptor. TGF-α would become the second member of the EGF family of ligands. A few decades later, we now know the EGF family comprises 11 ligands, seven of which can interact with the receptor now known as EGFR (ErbB1).[4]

Our understanding of the structure of this elusive receptor greatly improved in 1984 with the successful cloning of the 1210 amino acid EGFR protein[5] and description of its receptor, transmembrane and cytoplasmic components. It was also shown that there is a 95% homology between the cytoplasmic portion of EGFR (including the ATP binding site and the tyrosine residue) and the retroviral protein v-ErbB which induces malignant transformation in chicken. This discovery again proved of the role of EGFR in oncogenesis.

Quickly, attempts at using EGFR as a therapeutic target were made. In 1992 while research on other members of the ErbB family of proteins and their dimerization process was still very active, it was shown that monoclonal antibodies directed against EGFR could inhibit phosphorylation and reduce cell growth in prostatic carcinoma models.[6] A few years later, with initial results presented at the annual AACR conference in 1997 an EGFR-specific tyrosine kinase inhibitor (TKI) known as CP-358, 774 showed antitumor effects in mice.[7] Few people in the audience could have imagined that this drug, now known as erlotinib, would be part of a class of drugs that revolutionized treatment of lung cancer.

EPIDEMIOLOGY

For unknown reasons, frequency of EGFR mutations in patients with metastatic NSCLC varies according to race.[8] For example, in whites, estimated prevalence in adenocarcinomas varies between 7% and 17%, reported as high as 35% in never smokers.[9] However, Asian series frequently estimate prevalence around 30%–40%, even reaching 66.3% in a report of 239 consecutive adenocarcinomas from a Shanghai hospital.[10] Data in blacks are more limited, with estimations ranging from 2% to 19% in reports where the proportion of adenocarcinomas varied. In a study evaluating

1150 patients with NSCLC from Latin America,[11] frequency of EGFR mutations was 33.2%. Although it varied from 19.3% in Argentina to 67% in Peru, clinical characteristics were variable among countries, and some form of selection bias may have played a role. A mutation prevalence of 30.4% in 207 patients with NSCLC from Brazil[12] tends to support these numbers. A large systematic review of 151 worldwide studies (33,162 patients of whom 9749 had an EGFR mutation)[13] provides an estimate of prevalence by country and region, again showing the highest prevalence in Asia and South America.

Clinical characteristics correlated with EGFR-mutant lung cancer were first identified indirectly from EGFR TKI studies in the early 2000s targeting an unselected metastatic NSCLC population. Indeed, the following clinical subgroups repeatedly showed increased benefit to EGFR TKIs in those initial studies: female sex, Asians, never smokers, and adenocarcinoma histology.[14-18] Additionally, as the EGFR TKI gefitinib was nearing FDA approval in 2003, an expanded access program allowed a large number of patients to be treated on a compassionate basis. A subset of such patients had dramatic responses to the drug and from in-depth study of their tumors, the discovery of EGFR mutations emerged. The oncogene-addicted biology triggered by these mutations provides the molecular underpinning of the previously noted excellent responses in some groups of patients.[19-21]

EGFR mutations clinically present as one of the several genetic alterations clustered in the tyrosine kinase domain of EGFR. The most frequent EGFR-activating mutations are exon 19 deletion mutations, clustered in the LREA region of exon 19 and representing approximately half of all EGFR-mutant cases.[18] The next most common activating mutation is the single point mutation L858R in exon 21, representing about 40% of cases. The third most common mutation at diagnosis, exon 20 insertion, is only present in 3%–4% of patients. This mutation, covered later, is unique in that it imparts an oncogene-addicted biology but leads to a conformation of the receptor that is unfavorable for many of the available EGFR TKIs. For that reason it is often thought of as inherently resistant to currently available TKIs. Several other less common, but recurrent, activating mutations have also been described.[22]

EGFR-mutant lung cancer can develop at any age, with a median slightly higher than 60 years in most studies and rare cases reported in children and adolescents.[23] This median age at diagnosis is slightly lower than that seen in unselected NSCLC (approximately 70 years).[24]

DIAGNOSIS

The significant benefits of first-line EGFR-targeted therapy among patients with EGFR mutation-positive advanced adenocarcinoma require rapid determination of mutation status at the time of diagnosis, ideally before initiation of therapy. In such patients, testing for anaplastic lymphoma kinase (ALK), ROS1, BRAF, MET, and other genetic alterations should also be performed as similar benefits have been seen with targeted therapies in these patients. The most time and tissue-efficient way to test for these key abnormalities is by testing them all simultaneously through a genotyping panel.[25] While many allele-specific *polymerase chain reaction* (PCR) and next-generation sequencing (NGS)−based genotyping assays exist, clinicians should select an assay that at minimum includes identification of the following EGFR mutations: exon 19 deletions, G719X, L861Q, L858R, S768I, T790M, and exon 20 insertions. While NGS-based assays are usually more comprehensive, their turnaround time remains slower than that of PCR-based techniques.

Such testing is more controversial in patients with a squamous cell lung cancer (SCC) diagnosis as EGFR mutations (and other targetable oncogenes) are much more rare in SCC with an estimated prevalence of 2% −3%. However, some histologic variants, notably adenosquamous carcinoma, can be associated more frequently with EGFR mutations, and distinction with pure SCC can be difficult on small biopsies. While NCCN guidelines[26] suggest considering testing in nonsmoking patients with SCC, with the increasing availability of genotyping panels, many centers now elect to genotype all metastatic NSCLC cases. Although some efforts are ongoing to evaluate systematic noninvasive genotyping by *liquid biopsies* (NCT02770014), tissue-based genotyping is usually preferred at diagnosis.

TREATMENT

A chronologic examination of the development of available EGFR-targeted therapies allows for a better understanding of the stepwise therapeutic evolution in the field and the current recommended treatment algorithm. Specific clinical settings, such as central nervous system (CNS) metastases, adjuvant therapy, EGFR exon 20 insertions, and histologic transformations, will be discussed later in this chapter.

First- and Second- Generation EGFR TKIs

The first-generation EGFR TKIs erlotinib and gefitinib have been studied for more than 20 years. These agents compete with ATP for the ATP-binding pocket located in the intracellular domain of EGFR, thus blocking tyrosine phosphorylation and further downstream signaling. Reversibility of this action is characteristic of first-generation drugs. Historically, erlotinib and gefitinib were first studied in an unselected metastatic NSCLC population after failure of first-line chemotherapy because no biomarker for selection had yet been discovered. After encouraging results from the phase II IDEAL trial,[16] the ISEL phase III study[15] failed to show a survival advantage to gefitinib compared with placebo as a second- or third-line therapy. However, a preplanned analysis revealed significantly improved survival in the never-smoking and Asian subgroups, a recurrent theme in these early TKI era trials.

Using erlotinib the very similar phase III BR21[14] study showed a survival benefit versus placebo in the second or third line among unselected NSCLC. Although response rate to erlotinib was only 8.9% and median progression-free survival (PFS) was improved by only 0.4 months, median overall survival (OS) was significantly improved by 2 months.

In their seminal 2004 New England Journal of Medicine article,[19] Lynch et al. sequenced tissue sampled at diagnosis from nine patients who had a clinically significant response to gefitinib after a median of two prior lines of therapy. In eight of these patients, EGFR-activating mutations in the kinase domain (exon 19 deletion, L858R, G719C, and L861Q) were detected. Conversely none was present in seven patients who did not respond to gefitinib and in 95 primary tumors and 108 cancer-derived cell lines from various tumor types. Two other groups found similar findings that same year.[20,21]

After these publications, the EGFR field began to shift toward using EGFR TKIs preferentially in populations selected for EGFR mutations, and gradually genotype-directed targeted therapies entered the first-line setting. The evolution was gradual because at that time, the notion of using a biomarker to direct therapy options was still new and many felt it was impractical. The IPASS trial[27,28] was the first randomized trial to suggest that biomarker-directed therapy was the best strategy, and practice standards began to include genotyping in 2009 after IPASS was published. The entire trial (1217 patients) was composed of Asian never- or very light—smoking, treatment-naïve adenocarcinoma patients, and they were randomized to first-line gefitinib or carboplatin-paclitaxel with noninferiority of PFS as the primary endpoint. Although gefitinib PFS exceeded the noninferiority threshold and was shown to be superior to chemotherapy in the whole study population,

there were marked variations in outcomes depending on EGFR mutational status. The PFS advantage for gefitinib was strongest among those with EGFR-mutant tumors (hazard ratio [HR] 0.48, 95% confidence interval [CI] 0.36—0.54), while those who had the clinical phenotype of an EGFR-TKI responder but lacked the genetic biomarker had significantly greater benefit from chemotherapy (HR 2.85, 95% CI 2.05—3.98), with a median PFS on gefitinib of only 1.5 months. Follow-up randomized studies that included only EGFR-mutant patients similarly showed a consistent PFS, response, and quality of life benefit compared with first-line chemotherapy.[29—33]

Skeptics wondered if the results from these trials would translate outside of Asian countries. The EUR-TAC[34] trial that only included patients with EGFR mutations compared erlotinib with cytotoxic chemotherapy in the first-line setting and in a predominantly white population. Erlotinib led to significantly superior median PFS (9.7 vs. 5.2 months), and while toxicity patterns were different, severe treatment-related adverse events were more frequent with chemotherapy (20% vs. 6%).

The second-generation EGFR TKIs afatinib and dacomitinib were designed for greater inhibition of EGFR through a covalent irreversible bond with the ATP-binding pocket on the receptor itself. Second-generation EGFR TKIs also have a wider spectrum of activity, inhibiting ErbB2 (Human epidermal growth factor receptor 2 [HER2]) and ErbB4 as well as the resistance gatekeeper mutation T790M. Preclinical work suggested that the T790M-specific activity would make second-generation drugs the treatment of choice for T790M-mediated acquired resistance to first-generation drugs; however, the narrow therapeutic window between T790M inhibition and EGFR wild-type inhibition prohibited clinical dose escalation to levels that could be active against T790M.[35,36] Therefore the second-generation drugs can be best thought of as slightly more potent drugs for treatment-naïve EGFR patients.

Afatinib was compared with chemotherapy in EGFR-mutant NSCLC in the first-line setting in two large randomized trials: one was conducted in an international population (LUX-Lung 3)[37] and one was conducted in China only (LUX-Lung 6).[38] Although the comparator arm was cisplatin-pemetrexed in the former and cisplatin-gemcitabine in the latter, both studies showed significant PFS and response rate benefits favoring afatinib. Adverse events were generally more frequent than what is expected with first-generation TKIs, although they usually did not lead to treatment discontinuation, and patient-reported outcomes still benefited afatinib.[39] For example, diarrhea and rash of any grade were noted in 95% and 89% of patients, respectively, in the LUX-Lung-3 trial. Rates of stomatitis and paronychia were also significant. The increased adverse events with afatinib are likely from slightly more potent inhibition of wild-type EGFR. In turn the PFS obtained with afatinib in these trials was also slightly longer than that in analogous trials with first-generation EGFR TKIs. For example, median PFS was 13.6 months with afatinib in the Lux-Lung 3 trial among exon 19 deletions and L858R mutations and 9.7 months with erlotinib in EURTAC in the same mutation subgroups.

Most data related to EGFR TKI activity in less common EGFR mutations come from a combined analysis of three afatinib studies: the Lux-Lung 2, 3, and 6 trials.[22] Because these trials all included TKI-naïve patients and allowed enrollment of any EGFR mutation, the authors were able to compile the outcomes for de novo T790M, exon 20 insertions (discussed later in this chapter), and the point mutations G719X, L861Q, and S768I. Unsurprisingly response rate to afatinib in the first two subgroups was low at 15% and 9%, respectively, and PFS was less than 3 months. However, there was significant activity in the patients with less common point mutations, with a response rate of 71% and a median PFS of 10.7 months, similar to results seen with afatinib in exon 19 deletions and L858R mutations. Based on these data, afatinib became the first EGFR TKI approved for G719X, S768I, and L861Q. Despite more limited data, first-generation TKIs also have a role with less common point mutations: in a retrospective study of 161 patients with G719X, L861Q, or S768I treated with first-generation TKIs, response rate was 42% and median PFS was 7.7 months.[40]

Two randomized studies have compared first- and second-generation TKIs to each other in the first-line setting. LUX-Lung 7[41,42] was a phase IIB trial comparing afatinib and gefitinib, which showed a borderline improvement in PFS (HR = 0.74, 95% CI 0.57–0.95) and response rate (72.5% vs. 56%) with afatinib. No difference in OS was seen. The ARCHER 1050 trial[43,44] compared first-line dacomitinib to gefitinib and showed a significant improvement in median PFS (14.7 vs. 9.2 months; HR 0.59, 95% CI 0.47–0.74) and OS (34.1 vs. 26.8 months; HR 0.76, 95% CI 0.58–0.99). This compound, currently not approved by the FDA, also proved more toxic than gefitinib, with more grade ≥3 rash and diarrhea (14% vs. 1% and 8% vs. 1%, respectively) and 66% of patients requiring a dose reduction.

ACQUIRED RESISTANCE TO FIRST- AND SECOND-GENERATION TKIS AND THE DEVELOPMENT OF THIRD-GENERATION EGFR TKIS

Understanding the resistance mechanisms causing failure of EGFR TKIs is fundamental to the development and rational use of current and future therapies. The most frequent cause of acquired resistance to first- and second-generation EGFR TKIs is the EGFR T790M mutation, present in around 60% of cases. This substitution of a threonine with a methionine affects the ATP-binding pocket by increasing the affinity for ATP to the detriment of TKIs, thus limiting their inhibitory action.[45] This resistance mechanism can sometimes be associated with EGFR amplification.[46] The other (much less common) major mechanism of resistance to first- and second-generation drugs is the development of signaling bypass tracks that allow for continuation of growth signaling in tumor cells, despite continuous inhibition of EGFR. MET and HER2 amplifications are the most frequent alterations in this category, as well as point mutations in BRAF and PIK3CA.

In some cases, resistance is accompanied by more profound changes in cell function. Epithelial–mesenchymal transition (EMT) and histologic transformation, either to squamous cell carcinoma or small cell neuroendocrine carcinoma (discussed later), have been described. For example, it has been established that small-cell transformed clones lose expression of the EGFR protein (while maintaining the initial EGFR mutation) and thus become intrinsically resistant to EGFR TKIs.[47] In an elegant experiment analyzing clonal subpopulations, it has also been shown[48] that the clone leading to small-cell transformation may develop before initiation of TKI therapy and remain quiescent for months to years. Alterations in RB1 and TP53 may facilitate the emergence of such clones.

The frequency of major resistance alterations in various case series is shown in Table 7.1. Of note a minority of patients develop more than one mechanism of resistance at progression. In about 15%–20% of cases no explanation for resistance is identified, despite comprehensive genotyping.

It is in this context of acquired resistance that the role of *liquid biopsies*, especially cell-free DNA (cfDNA) assays, is getting more established. A study evaluated plasma T790M detection by BEAMing PCR and compared its predictive value with tissue-based genotyping at progression on prior TKI.[54] T790M-positive patients had similar outcomes with third-generation TKI osimertinib (discussed next), regardless of the

TABLE 7.1
Resistance Alterations in First- and Second-Generation EGFR TKI

Case Series	# pts	T790M	EGFR Amp.	MET Amp.	HER2 Amp.	SCLCt	PIK3CA	BRAF
Yu HA et al. [49]	155	62%	NR	5%	13%	3%	0%	0%
Sequist LV et al.[46]	37	49%	8%	5%	NR	14%	5%	0%
Arcila ME et al. [50]	99	68%	NR	11%	NR	2%	NR	NR
Ohashi K et al. [51]	195	NR	NR	NR	NR	NR	NR	1%
Takezawa K et al. [52]	26	65%	NR	NR	12%	0%	NR	NR
Piotrowska Z et al.[53]	221	59%	19%	5%	NR	3%	2%	1%

 # pts, number of patients; *Amp.*, amplification; *EGFR*, epidermal growth factor receptor; *HER2*, human epidermal growth factor receptor 2; *NR*, not reported; *SCLCt*, small cell lung cancer transformation; *TKI*, tyrosine kinase inhibitor.

technique used to identify the mutation, with a response rate of 62%–63% and a median PFS of 9.7 months in both groups. Sensitivity of the plasma-based assay was, however, imperfect at 70%; patients with T790M positivity only in tissue had a high response rate (69%) and median PFS (16.5 months), confirming the continued relevance of tissue-based genotyping. Conversely 31% of patients with no T790M in tissue had positive plasma testing. It is hypothesized that the T790M might be a minority subclone in these cases rather than the result being falsely positive. Activity of osimertinib was more limited in this group, with response rate and median PFS of 28% and 4.2 months, respectively.

Another important point made by this article is the significance of detecting the original EGFR-activating mutation in plasma T790M negative samples. Cases where neither mutation was identified in blood implies a *non-shedding* tumor, thus making the result nonrevealing. This subgroup had a robust 64% response rate and median PFS of 15.2 months, much higher than expected in a truly T790M negative cohort, implying that some underlying tumors were T790M positive. On the contrary, plasma samples with detectable EGFR-activating mutations but negative for T790M are much more likely to be accurate, as evidenced by a lower response rate of 38% and shorter PFS of 4.4 months.

First these results support the strategy of testing for resistance point mutation blood-based assays, limiting tissue testing in patients with negative results. However, the importance of T790M testing is likely to diminish in the next few years due to widespread adoption of first-line osimertinib not expected to lead to this type of resistance mutation. It is currently unknown if these results are generalizable to other resistance mechanisms such as MET amplification or EGFR C797S. Importantly

the rare but significant resistance mechanism of small-cell transformation is currently not detectable by cfDNA assays.

Because approximately 60% of patients with acquired resistance to first- or second-generation TKI develop the T790M *gatekeeper* resistance mutation, there has been great interest in developing therapeutics targeting T790M. We discussed earlier that second-generation EGFR TKIs were initially thought to be a solution for this problem but were soon found to be impractical because of the narrow therapeutic index between wild-type and T790M inhibition. A combination of afatinib and the EGFR monoclonal antibody cetuximab was studied to combat T790M. In a phase Ib study[55] of 126 heavily pretreated EGFR-mutant patients with acquired resistance to first-generation TKIs, response rate was 29% and surprisingly was similar in both T790M-positive and negative-cases. The median PFS was 4.7 months (95% CI: 4.3–6.4). The major limitation of this regimen was toxicity, with grade ≥3 rash and diarrhea noted in 20% and 6% of patients in this trial, respectively. Hypomagnesemia, related to cetuximab through inhibition of TRMP6 ion channel in the kidney, was also found in 23% of patients but was rarely severe.

The third-generation TKIs entered the clinical trial scene in 2012. They were generally designed to overcome T790M, maintain activity against the founder EGFR mutation, and spare the wild-type form of the protein, thus limiting toxicity. Several experimental third-generation TKIs were studied and some are still under investigation, but many have discontinued clinical development. Here we will focus on osimertinib, the only FDA-approved third-generation EGFR TKI.

The phase I-II AURA[56] study of osimertinib began as a dose-finding first-in-human study and expanded to test efficacy of osimertinib in EGFR-mutant patients previously treated with a first- or second-generation EGFR TKI. The study confirmed the safety of osimertinib, without observing any dose-limiting toxicities with doses up to 240 mg daily, three times the currently approved dosage. In this early trial, response rate and PFS both favored patients whose tumor was tested positive for T790M, although 21% of patients without T790M detected on a resistance biopsy still responded, likely related in part to heterogeneity of resistance mechanisms within patients. After AURA, most subsequent osimertinib trials have required T790M positivity for enrollment. One notable exception is the BLOOM trial, specifically looking at activity in patients with leptomeningeal disease, discussed later in this chapter.

These initial results in previously treated patients led to the phase III AURA3 trial[57] comparing osimertinib 80 mg daily with platinum-pemetrexed in T790M-positive NSCLC after progression on first-line EGFR TKIs. Osimertinib proved superior both for PFS (10.1 vs. 4.4 months, HR = 0.30, 95% CI: 0.23−0.41) and response rate (71% vs. 31%; odds ratio 5.39, $P < .001$). The magnitude of benefit was maintained in patients with CNS metastases. Adverse events were numerically similar in both arms, but grade $\geq$3 events felt to be drug-related were rare with osimertinib compared with chemotherapy (6% vs. 34%).

Sparing of wild-type EGFR (confirmed clinically by low rates of adverse events), central nervous activity, and the ability to target a frequent resistance mechanism while remaining active against the original activating mutation all constituted reasons to study third-generation TKIs in previously untreated patients. Results from the first-line phase I expansion cohort from the AURA trial were published.[58] In the 80-mg daily-dose cohort (the currently FDA-approved dosage in the second-line setting) the reported median PFS of more than 22 months was unprecedented. Furthermore, no patient developed the T790M mutation at progression, although the group studied for resistance mechanisms was small.

This promising level of activity led to phase III FLAURA study[59] comparing osimertinib with either gefitinib or erlotinib in 994 treatment-naïve EGFR-mutant patients (with either exon 19 deletion or L858R mutation). Osimertinib demonstrated improved PFS (median 18.9 vs. 10.2 months, HR = 0.46, 95% CI: 0.37−0.57), with a similar response rate (80% vs. 76%; odds ratio 1.27, $P = .24$). OS data are currently immature, but an early analysis showed a strong trend favoring osimertinib. Interestingly median PFS2 (the time to progression on second-line therapy) among FLAURA patients randomized to the first-generation TKI arm

was 20.0 months, suggesting that second-line therapy can provide significant benefit. Forty-six percent of patients in this arm of the study received TKI-based second-line therapy; however, the "sequencing strategy" has some important limits as 17% of patients who received first-generation TKIs as first-line therapy died without receiving any subsequent therapy. Although little is known about these patients, it is well recognized that unexpected events or patient preference can prevent delivery of second-line therapy in real-world practice and this, many argue, is rationale to use the most effective therapy upfront.

The frequency of most adverse events in FLAURA was relatively similar between the arms, although grade $\geq$3 toxicities were lower with osimertinib. Rashes, liver function tests perturbations, and alopecia were all more frequent with first-generation drugs. However, stomatitis, dyspnea, headaches, fever, and QT interval prolongation were more common with osimertinib. While rates of dose reductions and interruptions were similar, there was less permanent discontinuation of osimertinib because of adverse events (13% vs. 18%).

Although little is currently known about combining a third-generation TKI with other therapies, it has been shown preclinically that the acquisition of the C797S resistance mutation in *trans* to T790M can be responsive to a combination of erlotinib and osimertinib.[60] Unfortunately the majority of patients with the T790M mutation develop C797S in *cis*, a mutational combination for which no targeted therapy is currently available.

CYTOTOXIC CHEMOTHERAPY

In addition to targeted therapies, it is important to discuss the data specific to EGFR-mutant patients related to cytotoxic chemotherapy. Most EGFR-mutant lung cancers being adenocarcinomas, the first chemotherapy used is usually a platinum doublet in which the nonplatinum component is pemetrexed. This preferential use is based on a phase III trial[61] showing significantly improved OS for cisplatin-pemetrexed regimen compared with cisplatin-gemcitabine. Impact of EGFR mutational status was not analyzed in this trial.

Briefly maintenance pemetrexed is recommended after response or stable disease after four to six cycles of doublet chemotherapy[62,63] as it improves PFS and OS in patients with nonsquamous histology. This maintenance phase is well tolerated, with discontinuation due to adverse events in only 5% of patients. The choice of platinum agent used (cisplatin vs. carboplatin) in metastatic lung cancer is controversial.[64] However, this decision should not be influenced by EGFR mutational status.

Historically in first-line trials where chemotherapy was the comparator arm, meaningful response rates and median PFS with use of platinum doublets were noted. For example, cisplatin-pemetrexed led to a median PFS of 6.9 months in Lux Lung 3[37] and carboplatin-paclitaxel was associated with a 47% response rate in the EGFR-mutant subgroup of IPASS.[27] However, in the current era most patients with EGFR-mutant NSCLC receiving chemotherapy have received prior TKI therapy. In those pretreated patients, the most recent data on efficacy of platinum doublet chemotherapy come from the AURA3 study.[57] In this trial, response rate and median PFS for platinum-pemetrexed were at 31% and 4.4 months, respectively. Unfortunately the paucity of data in the post–third-generation TKI setting limits conclusions about chemotherapy efficacy after these agents.

Because of data suggesting that up to 25% of EGFR patients could have a disease "flare"[65] if EGFR TKI was discontinued even in the face of radiographic progression, a strategy of continuing EGFR TKI beyond progression and adding in chemotherapy was popular in the 2010 era. This strategy was formally[66] evaluated in the phase III IMPRESS trial, in which patients progressing on first-line gefitinib were randomized to continue gefitinib with cisplatin-pemetrexed chemotherapy or discontinue it and switch to placebo plus chemotherapy. Much to the surprise of many experts the gefitinib with chemo arm failed to show a PFS advantage. Updated data also show a potential detrimental effect on OS in the continuation arm, further arguing against this strategy. However, there are still a subset of patients who have disease flare off TKIs, and for such patients, many recommend continuing TKI with chemotherapy, although there are no clear data about this strategy.

Results from the phase III NEJ009 trial comparing carboplatin-pemetrexed-gefitinib with single-agent gefitinib as first-line therapy[67] revealed a significant prolongation of median PFS (20.9 vs. 11.2 months, HR = 0.49, 95% CI: 0.39–0.70) and OS (52.2 vs. 38.8 months, HR = 0.70, 95% CI: 0.52–0.93). Survival after progression on the randomized assignment of first-line treatment was not different between arms, suggesting that the PFS advantage of chemotherapy with gefitinib was the driving force behind the OS advantage seen in this trial. Toxicity was additive, with 65% of patients receiving the triplet having at least one grade ≥3 toxicity, but rates of discontinuation due to adverse events were similar and low in both arms.

Finally the antiangiogenic agent bevacizumab has also been studied in combination with erlotinib, notably in a Japanese phase II study,[68] demonstrating a significant median PFS benefit of 16 months compared with 9 months (HR 0.54, 95% CI: 0.36–0.79). However, an update[69] showed no OS improvement in this study, although an important caveat is that it was not initially designed to follow up patients until death. A smaller but statistically significant median PFS benefit of 3.3 months (HR: 0.61; 95% CI: 0.42–0.88) was found in a confirmatory phase III trial NEJ 026.[70] A similar US-based trial (NCT01532089) is currently ongoing.

IMMUNE THERAPY
The oncologic revolution brought forward by the arrival of checkpoint inhibitors in the last 10 years has deeply influenced the current treatment algorithm of lung cancer. Unfortunately results have been underwhelming in the setting of targetable mutations such as EGFR, regardless of programmed death ligand 1 (PD-L1) status. The reasons behind the discrepancy with the favorable results observed in EGFR/ALK wild-type tumors are incompletely understood, but low mutational burden is often cited as a major culprit. Furthermore, a single-center retrospective study[71] looked at PD L1 expression in 68 EGFR-mutant cancers. PD L1 positivity (≥1% by monoclonal antibody E1L3N) was noted in 24% of EGFR-positive cases, numerically lower than that found in KRAS mutants (35%). CD8+ tumor-infiltrating lymphocytes were also more frequent in KRAS-mutant cases (grade 2–3 by immunohistochemistry 21.8% vs. 4.2%). Use of pembrolizumab in TKI-naïve EGFR-mutant NSCLC has been attempted in prospective phase II trial,[72] which was closed early due to the lack of efficacy. The only tumor response on this trial was noted in a patient in whom the identification of an EGFR mutation was erroneous (the patient was actually EGFR wild type), and two early deaths within 6 months of enrollment (including the one attributed to pneumonitis) were noted.

Limited checkpoint inhibitor efficacy was also noted in later lines of therapy among EGFR mutants. Nivolumab, pembrolizumab, and atezolizumab have all been compared with docetaxel in phase III trials after progression on platinum-based chemotherapy. In these trials, respectively, CheckMate-057,[73] KEYNOTE-010[74] and OAK,[75] most of the 8%–14% of patients with an activating EGFR mutation had received prior TKI therapy in addition to platinum-based chemotherapy. Although small subgroup size limited statistical significance, the benefit of immunotherapy compared with docetaxel was markedly reduced in EGFR mutants. Notably in the OAK and CHECKMATE-057 trials, HR for OS numerically favored the docetaxel arm in contrast to the overall population (HR for OS 1.24 vs. 0.73 and 1.18 vs. 0.75, respectively).

Patients with EGFR-mutant tumors were not eligible for the KEYNOTE-024[76] trial comparing pembrolizumab with standard first-line doublet chemotherapy in patients with PD L1 staining $\geq$50%. The same exclusion applied to cohort G of KEYNOTE-021[77] and KEYNOTE-189,[78] both evaluating the efficacy of pembrolizumab in addition to carboplatin and pemetrexed in the first-line setting. Despite this, the FDA approval of the triplet in previously untreated patients does not mention any restriction related to mutational status.

The ATLANTIC trial[79] evaluated the efficacy of durvalumab in patients who had received at least two prior lines of therapy, including platinum-based chemotherapy and TKIs when indicated. One subgroup of this trial specifically contained ALK- or EGFR-mutant NSCLC, and although enrollment was initially allowed regardless of PD-L1 status, it was later restricted to patients with $\geq$25% tumor cells positive for PD-L1. Of the 28 evaluable patients from this subgroup with PD-L1 <25% (enrolled before the PD-L1 status amendment), only one patient with an EGFR-mutant tumor had a partial response. In the 64 evaluable patients with EGFR-mutant tumors and PD-L1 $\geq$25%, nine patients (14%) responded, and disease control rate at 6 months was 23%. Interestingly eight of these nine responders had a PD-L1 level of $\geq$90%. While these patients might benefit from durvalumab, they unfortunately represent a very small minority of EGFR-mutant NSCLC.

Two exceptions can be noted to the largely unsatisfactory results of checkpoint inhibitors in EGFR-mutant lung cancer. In the locally advanced setting the PACIFIC trial[80] showed an 11.2-month benefit in median PFS with the addition of 1 year of anti—PD-L1 agent durvalumab after chemoradiation for stage III NSCLC. All subgroups, including EGFR mutants and nonsmokers tended to benefit from durvalumab addition. Indeed, although the EGFR subgroup was very small (6% of the study population) and had a large CI, the HR for relapse or death still numerically favored immune therapy (0.76, as compared with 0.55 for the overall population). Interestingly the same is true for the slightly larger nonsmoking subgroup with a statistically significant HR of 0.29 favoring durvalumab. The elusive abscopal effect and its modulation by checkpoint inhibitors might contribute to the benefits seen after chemoradiation in the curative setting. Despite this encouraging signal of efficacy, confirmation of these findings in future trials would be ideal considering the small sample size and the repeatedly underwhelming results in the metastatic setting. This is especially true as new and promising TKI-based approaches to stage III EGFR-mutant NSCLC begin to emerge.[81]

In the metastatic setting the phase III IMpower150 trial[82] investigated the role of adding atezolizumab to carboplatin-pemetrexed-bevacizumab and included previously TKI-treated EGFR-mutant tumors (10% of the overall population). The EGFR/ALK-mutated subgroup had a significantly increased median PFS with the triplet (9.7 vs. 6.1 months add HR 0.59 and 95% CI 0.37 to 0.94), but currently published OS results specifically exclude this subgroup.

Using another strategy, combinations of EGFR TKIs with immunotherapy have been tested in hopes of better stimulating immune response and improving efficacy. Unfortunately significant toxicity was reported in some of these trials and importantly decreased excitement about this strategy. For example, one of the arms of the phase Ib TATTON trial combined osimertinib with durvalumab.[83] Interstitial lung disease developed in 13 of 34 patients (38%), five cases being grade 3—4, significantly more often than usual with either osimertinib or durvalumab alone leading to the premature suspension of this part of the trial. Another study evaluating various combination strategies with gefitinib and durvalumab[84] showed rates of elevated alanine aminotransferase of 60%—70% but also a high response rate of 77%—80%. While the use of these types of combinations should currently be discouraged outside of clinical trials, early signals of efficacy certainly justify further research.

ADJUVANT THERAPY

Although the high activity of EGFR TKIs in the metastatic setting has led to research in the adjuvant setting, this strategy cannot currently be recommended outside of a clinical trial. Indeed, because the main goal of therapy in the adjuvant setting is cure and not disease control, proving an OS benefit is essential. This concept must be kept in mind while interpreting the following data.

The largest adjuvant trial related to EGFR is the RADIANT trial[85] that included 931 patients with high EGFR expression. These patients had stage IB-IIIA NSCLC and received 2 years of erlotinib or placebo. No disease-free survival (DFS) advantage was seen, with an HR of 0.9 (95% CI: 0.74—1.10), while rash and diarrhea were noted in 86.4% and 52.2% of patients, respectively. A subgroup analysis of 161 patients with either exon 19 deletion or L858R EGFR mutation revealed a more favorable HR of 0.61 (95% CI:

0.38–0.98), with a median DFS benefit of 17 months favoring erlotinib. However, this study was designed in such a way that subgroup analyses could not be considered statistically positive if the overall study population did not have a positive result. No OS benefit was seen among the EGFR-mutant cohort, but only 35 patients had died at the time of data analysis.

The phase II multicenter SELECT trial,[86] also evaluating adjuvant erlotinib for 2 years in stage I-IIIA, EGFR-mutant NSCLC, showed an impressive 90% 2-year DFS, an improvement compared with historical data. However, these results were immature when last presented at the ASCO 2014 Annual Meeting, and median DFS and OS are currently unknown.

These results were the rationale behind the published ADJUVANT/CTONG1104 trial,[87] conducted exclusively in China. Two hundred twenty-two patients with resected stage II-IIIA, node-positive, EGFR-mutant NSCLC were randomized between gefitinib for 2 years and four cycles of a cisplatin-vinorelbine regimen. Notably only 23% of patients had PET staging, and while around 65% of patients had N2 involvement, no radiotherapy was allowed after surgery. Further complicating the analysis, 4.5% and 20.7% of patients never received study drugs in the gefitinib and chemotherapy arms, respectively. After a median follow-up of 36 months, DFS favored gefitinib (median of 28.7 vs. 18 months, HR 0.60). However, this benefit might attenuate with time as 3-year DFS is similar between the two groups (34% vs. 27%, $P = .37$). Although OS data are immature, numerically more patients died from disease progression with gefitinib (40 vs. 33). As expected, gefitinib was better tolerated than cisplatin-vinorelbine. Despite the authors' intentions to prove a chemotherapy-free adjuvant regimen can be active, adjuvant cytotoxic chemotherapy in such a high-risk population has a well-defined OS benefit,[88] while, as mentioned above, TKIs have yielded limited results. The design of this study, in which only 40% of patients received some form of cytotoxic chemotherapy postoperatively, has been criticized. This approach is not currently recommended.

In contrast to this chemotherapy-free approach the currently accruing ALCHEMIST trial is randomizing EGFR-mutant patients to 2 years of erlotinib or observation after completion of standard adjuvant therapy (chemotherapy and/or radiation). An ALK + arm (crizotinib vs. placebo) and an unmutated arm (nivolumab vs. observation) are also accruing. Hopefully this trial, along with the ongoing ADAURA trial (NCT02511106) evaluating adjuvant osimertinib in a similar population, will once and for all determine the level of benefit associated with adjuvant TKIs in EGFR-mutant NSCLC.

TREATMENT BEYOND PROGRESSION AND OLIGOPROGRESSIVE DISEASE

There are two patterns of progression that should be clinically noted when caring for patients with EGFR-mutant disease because their presence may signal the opportunity to do something other than changing systemic therapy. Slow, indolent progression can sometimes be approached with watchful waiting (termed "treatment beyond progression"), and progression that is limited in anatomic scope (oligoprogression) can often be treated with locally ablative techniques.

As EGFR TKIs became widely used in practice, it was noted by several groups that progression would commonly occur in a more indolent, slow-moving pattern than was historically typical of NSCLC.[89,90] For those with such a pattern of growth who were asymptomatic, treatment beyond progression, or continuing the same TKI until the clinical picture more clearly dictated a change in therapy, became popular. Although difficult to prospectively study, the best data we have are the multicenter phase II ASPIRATION study[91] in which 176 patients were followed up from the start of first-line erlotinib and had a median PFS of 11 months. At that point they were assigned by investigator preference (clinical judgment) to continue erlotinib or change to another therapy. Ninety-three were assigned to continue erlotinib, and median time to clinically relevant progression was 3.9 months. OS was not reported. To date, treatment beyond progression is a strategy that is enthusiastically embraced by some but that has limited evidence basis.

Oligoprogressive disease is a term used when all disease remains under good control with the current therapy except one (or a small number of) metastatic site(s). In EGFR patients, isolated progression in the CNS is a common clinical situation and will be discussed in the following subsection. For oligoprogression outside the CNS there is a growing collection of data. One retrospective single-site study[92] evaluated if locally ablative therapy (LAT) could extend the duration of TKI treatment (erlotinib in EGFR-mutant and crizotinib in ALK-rearranged patients). To be considered for a local approach in this cohort, patients had to have good tolerance to their TKI, Eastern Cooperative Oncology Group performance status of 0–1, no more than four sites of extra-CNS progression, and no evidence of leptomeningeal disease. Of 51 patients who progressed on their TKIs, 25 met these criteria, including 10 who had

CNS oligoprogression only. They received LAT, either radiotherapy or surgery, followed by ongoing treatment beyond progression with the same TKI. Patients usually interrupted their TKI during LAT and restarted soon after completion. Median PFS on the initial TKI course was 9.8 months, and median time from the first progression to the second progression or death was 6.2 months. The 10 patients with CNS-only progression had an even longer median time to the second progression (7.1 months) than those with at least one extra CNS site (4.0 months). A published Chinese retrospective study[93] of 46 patients using a relatively similar definition of oligoprogressive disease showed a comparable median PFS of 7.0 months after LAT. In practice, LAT is frequently limited by local availability or expertise in approaches such as hypofractionated radiation therapy or cryoablation.

CNS METASTASES

Management of CNS metastases in EGFR-mutant lung cancer is a complex issue as multiple factors need to be taken into account when proposing a treatment strategy, including age, the number of metastases, presence of leptomeningeal involvement, and available systemic treatments.

Despite the blood-brain barrier, most EGFR TKIs have some degree of CNS activity. Objective TKI response rates in the CNS are difficult to confirm because of concurrent or recent use of whole brain or stereotaxic radiation therapy in many cases. However, we are accumulating better data on this topic. For example, in a series where 93% of patients with brain metastases at diagnosis received radiation before initiation of systemic therapy, first-generation TKIs were associated with a 1-year CNS progression rate of 5% compared with 24% with chemotherapy. In addition, significantly fewer patients developed CNS progression while on a TKI compared with chemotherapy, 30% and 50%, respectively. In a phase II study using gefitinib without radiation in 41 patients with untreated brain metastases,[94] CNS response rate was 87.8% and median time to progression of CNS lesions was 14.5 months. Similarly although a nonstandard pulse-dosing strategy was used, a small trial showed a response rate to erlotinib of 74% in untreated brain metastases.[95]

Considering this significant CNS activity, TKI therapy is sometimes used in lieu of radiation for patients with small, asymptomatic brain metastases with careful subsequent follow-up. To clarify the optimal radiation approach, a retrospective study[96] was performed on 351 TKI-naïve EGFR patients with brain metastases.

Patients received either stereotactic radiosurgery (SRS) or whole-brain radiation followed by TKI or a third option of upfront TKI alone followed, at intracranial progression, by radiation. In 98% of cases the TKI used was erlotinib. Use of upfront SRS and even whole brain radiation therapy (WBRT) yielded better median OS than upfront TKI (46, 30, and 25 months, respectively). This benefit persisted after controlling for significant covariables, with HR of 0.39 (95% CI: 0.26–0.58) and 0.70 (95% CI: 0.50–0.98) for survival with SBRT and whole-brain radiation, respectively, compared with upfront TKI. However, this study has been heavily criticized for its atypical population (more than 70% had CNS as the only site of visible metastatic disease) and for not assessing the strategy of starting with TKI and performing SRS to any residual sites.

Much of the CNS activity data for EGFR TKIs now must be reconsidered in light of the development of the third-generation TKI osimertinib. The CNS activity of osimertinib was noticeable early in its development. For example, a subgroup analysis of T790M-positive, TKI-pretreated patients with CNS metastases in the AURA3 study revealed a CNS response rate of 70% among those with measurable metastases. Similarly CNS progression events occurred in only 6% of those receiving first-line osimertinib on FLAURA, compared with 15% with first-line gefitinib or erlotinib.

In the poor-prognosis subgroup of patients with leptomeningeal disease the BLOOM[97] study evaluated osimertinib at an increased dose of 160 mg daily in 32 patients, most of whom were not selected based on T790M status. According to preliminary data at 12 weeks all patients evaluated radiologically had either a response or stable disease. Importantly, at 12 weeks, neurological examination had deteriorated from baseline in only 9% of evaluated patients. While there is a lack of a consensus on the optimal treatment approach for EGFR-mutant patients with CNS disease at the time of diagnosis, the increasing number of active therapies undoubtedly constitutes great progress for patients. Close collaboration among neurosurgeons, radiologists, and medical oncologists to answer some of these questions in future studies is essential.

SMALL-CELL LUNG CANCER TRANSFORMATION

Small-cell transformation is a less common but recurrent finding at the time of acquired resistance to EGFR TKIs, developing in 3%–14% of cases. The transformed cancers appear histologically indistinguishable from de novo small cell lung cancer (SCLC), and although the cases maintain the same founder *EGFR* mutation as the prior adenocarcinoma, dependence on EGFR signaling is typically lost.[47] Patients with alterations of TP53 and RB1 at the time of initial diagnosis of adenocarcinoma seem to be at higher risk of transformation.[48] Although such a finding does not currently influence pretransformation therapy, it should lower the threshold to obtain a tissue biopsy at progression.

In a retrospective series of 67 EGFR-mutant patients with SCLC transformation treated in 11 high-volume North American centers in the past 12 years,[98] median time between initial diagnosis of metastatic NSCLC and SCLC transformation was 17.8 months. There were not demographic characteristics that seemed divergent from a general EGFR population. Median OS from initial diagnosis was 31.5 months, similar to what is seen in standard EGFR-mutant NSCLC. However, once SCLC transformation was identified (including in nine patients who had evidence of SCLC from initial diagnosis), median survival was 10.9 months, in line with what is seen in de novo SCLC. While high clinical response rates to platinum etoposide (54%) and taxanes (50%) were noted, these responses were mostly transient. No responses were seen in 17 patients who received checkpoint inhibitors, including the ipilimumab-nivolumab combination.

No data exist concerning prophylactic cranial irradiation in small-cell transformed EGFR lung cancer. Such an approach is currently not recommended.

EXON 20 INSERTION MUTATIONS

Specific discussion of EGFR exon 20 insertion mutations is necessary because although these mutations are "activating", meaning they have an oncogene-addicted behavior, they tend to be resistant to most known EGFR TKIs. Indeed, because of its configuration, the mutant receptor is not conducive to drug binding.[99] These alterations, the third most frequent category of EGFR mutations after exon 19 deletions and L858R, were associated with a response rate of 0% and median PFS of 3 months to first-generation TKIs.[100] As mentioned earlier, efficacy of afatinib in this setting is similarly low.[22]

Although studies are not yet mature, some third-generation TKIs may have more activity against exon 20 insertions than prior drugs. Activity has been reported with poziotinib,[101] AP32788,[102] and osimertinib.[103] Activity in exon 20 insertion patients was also seen with the hsp90 inhibitor luminespib (formerly AUY9922), but this compound is no longer being developed.

Outside of a research setting, standard chemotherapy remains the standard of care in these patients.

TREATMENT OF SELECTED TKI TOXICITIES

Dermatologic side effects of EGFR TKIs are varied, ranging from xerosis to paronychia and rash. The "classical" acneiform rash usually involves areas rich in sebaceous glands, the face being the most frequently affected site. In more severe cases the upper part of the chest and the extremities can also be involved. It usually evolves over a few weeks and tends to wax and wane. It can also be associated with dysesthesia and pruritis.

Limited sun exposure, regular use of SPF ≥15 sunscreen, use of skin emollients, and avoidance of alcohol-based or perfumed skin products are examples of measures that can prevent its apparition.[104] We also recommend, with first- and second-generation TKIs, consideration of prophylaxis with minocycline 100 mg twice a day or other similar antibiotic. Of note, various dosing of minocycline or other agents (especially doxycycline) have also been described in prophylaxis. A metaanalysis of 1073 patients from both randomized and observational studies revealed HR of 0.54 and 0.36 for any rash and grade 2 or 3 rash, respectively, with the use of either doxycycline or minocycline as prophylaxis.[105] This approach is not necessary with third-generation TKIs as rates of severe rash are very low. Treatment of established rash varies by severity, and a consultation with a dermatologist, preferably with experience in treating patients receiving targeted therapy, can be helpful in persistent or severe cases. Although many algorithms exist, they usually have many points in common, allowing general recommendations to be made. In case of grade 1 rash (papulopustular rash covering <10% of the body[106]), topical gel or cream combining low-potency corticosteroid and an antibiotic are recommended. No dose reduction of the TKI is usually necessary. With grade 2, combination of a topical low-potency corticosteroid with oral tetracyclines such as minocycline 100 mg BID is recommended. Again the TKI can usually be maintained at its usual dosage. A rash covering more than 30% of the body, associated with moderate or severe symptoms, limiting self-care or associated with local superinfection requiring specific oral antibiotics is considered grade 3. In addition to topical therapies used for grade 2 rash, the TKI should be withheld, ideally for at least 10 days, although exceedingly long interruptions should be avoided. Some experts also recommend a short course of prednisone 0.5 mg/kg daily for 1 week[104] or even isotretinoin in refractory cases, but collaboration with dermatology is essential in those rare, severe cases. If toxicities improve to grade 2 or lower, the TKI should be reintroduced at 50% of the initial dose, with gradual increase back to the initial dose, if tolerated. In case of life-threatening toxicities, in addition to the aforementioned therapies, permanent discontinuation of the TKI is recommended. TKIs associated with a lower risk of rash, especially osimertinib, could be considered with very close initial follow-up.

Diarrhea is a frequent side effect of EGFR TKIs but is rarely severe. As dehydration can develop quickly in those unusual cases, good communication with patients is vital. Most low-grade toxicities can be managed with dietary changes (especially avoidance of fatty and spicy foods[107]), good hydration and over-the-counter loperamide. Recommendations for loperamide use varies among centers, but an initial dose of 4 mg followed by 2 mg after each loose stool is frequently used, up to the usually maximum recommended dose of 16 mg. Although doses higher than 16 mg can usually be administered safely, patients requiring such doses usually have grade ≥3 diarrhea and require TKI interruption, very close follow-up, and further work up to rule out alternate diagnoses.

SUMMARY OF CURRENT TREATMENT RECOMMENDATIONS

Therapeutic recommendations in EGFR-mutant lung cancer are changing at an ever-faster pace and new data released either near the time or after publication of this textbook might modify the current standard of care.

For limited stage disease, patients are encouraged to participate in randomized clinical trials, such as ALCHEMIST, to help confirm if there are benefits from adjuvant TKI after completion of standard of care therapy.

In most EGFR-mutant patients with stage IV disease, strong consideration should be given to using osimertinib as first-line therapy, if available, considering the significant PFS advantage identified in the FLAURA trial. Use of first- and second-generation TKIs remains appropriate in the first-line setting, especially in countries without access to front-line osimertinib, potentially in combination with chemotherapy based on NEJ009.[67] If a single-agent TKI is preferred, the choice among gefitinib, erlotinib, and afatinib should be individualized, but higher toxicity of afatinib should be taken into account. In return, efficacy with afatinib might be slightly higher in exon 19 deletions and less common in

activating mutations (G719X, L861Q and S768) compared with first-generation drugs.

If the patient progresses on a first- or second-generation TKI, tissue biopsy or plasma-based genotyping should be performed to determine the T790M status. If a *liquid biopsy* is performed and results are negative, reflex tissue testing should be strongly considered. In case of T790M positivity, osimertinib is recommended. If mutational testing is negative, or if there is progression after osimertinib, clinical trials or cytotoxic chemotherapy should be pursued. When technically feasible, biopsy of a progressive site can be considered to rule out small-cell transformation, especially if TP53 and RB1 alterations have been identified.

If progression is limited to a few sites, localized treatment or observation on continued TKI therapy can be appropriate. Discussion in a multidisciplinary setting, such as tumor boards, is essential. The same is true for CNS involvement.

FUTURE DIRECTIONS

Although osimertinib is the recommended first-line TKI currently, little is known about the pattern and frequency of resistance mutations in this setting. It is suspected that as it is the case in second-line osimertinib resistance, the C797S mutation and MET amplification will be frequent. Currently no experimental agents specifically target C797S. As C797S leads to resistance to all irreversible EGFR TKIs, it can be hypothesized that the C797S/T790 wild-type genotype expected with first-line osimertinib would remain sensitive to first-generation TKIs. However, such a sequence of treatment successfully causing tumor response in patients has not yet been described.

Data are showing promise for patients developing acquired resistance via MET amplification. Various case reports[108,109] have shown activity of EGFR TKI and crizotinib combinations in this setting. Preliminary data from the phase IB expansion cohort of the TATTON trial,[110] combining osimertinib with MET inhibitor savolitinib in MET amplified, EGFR-mutant patients, revealed response rates of 20% and 42% in third-generation TKI-pretreated and naïve patients, respectively.

How to allow EGFR-mutant patients to benefit from immune therapies also remains a major area of unmet need in the EGFR field. As it is becoming clear that conventional checkpoint inhibitor therapy have limited single-agent efficacy in EGFR-mutant lung cancers, combination regimens, cell-based therapy, antibody-drug conjugates, and vaccines are currently under evaluation.

The development of noninvasive diagnostic techniques will also improve patient care and understanding of resistance mechanisms. The landscape of EGFR C797S mutations using an NGS-based plasma assay has been presented,[111] which allows the important distinction between the *cis* and *trans* configuration. In another study, although mainly in an EGFR wild-type population, a blood tumor mutational burden assay, analyzing single nucleotide variants in 394 genes, was predictive of atezolizumab activity in pretreated NSCLC.[112] The development of such assays will certainly allow better understanding of the molecular complexity and genetic landscape of pretreated EGFR patients without having to subject them to invasive maneuvers.

REFERENCES

1. Cohen S. Isolation of a mouse submaxillary gland protein accelerating incisor eruption and eyelid opening in the new-born animal. *J Biol Chem*. May 1, 1962;237(5): 1555–1562.
2. Ushiro H, Cohen S. Identification of phosphotyrosine as a product of epidermal growth factor-activated protein kinase in A-431 cell membranes. *J Biol Chem*. September 25, 1980;255(18):8363–8365.
3. Roberts AB, Lamb LC, Newton DL, et al. Transforming growth factors: isolation of polypeptides from virally and chemically transformed cells by acid/ethanol extraction. *Proc Natl Acad Sci USA*. June 1, 1980;77(6): 3494–3498.
4. Yarden Y, Pines G. The ERBB network: at last, cancer therapy meets systems biology. *Nat Rev Cancer*. August 1, 2012;12(8):553–563.
5. Ullrich A, Coussens L, Hayflick JS, et al. Human epidermal growth factor receptor cDNA sequence and aberrant expression of the amplified gene in A431 epidermoid carcinoma cells. *Nature*. May 31, 1984;309(5967): 418–425.
6. Fong CJ, Sherwood ER, Mendelsohn J, et al. Epidermal growth factor receptor monoclonal antibody inhibits constitutive receptor phosphorylation, reduces autonomous growth, and sensitizes androgen-independent prostatic carcinoma cells to tumor necrosis factor α. *Cancer Res*. November 1, 1992;52(21):5887–5892.
7. Pollack VA, Savage DM, Baker DA, et al. Inhibition of epidermal growth factor receptor-associated tyrosine phosphorylation in human carcinomas with CP-358,774: dynamics of receptor inhibition in situ and antitumor effects in athymic mice. *J Pharmacol Exp Ther*. November 1, 1999;291(2):739–748.
8. El-Telbany A, Ma PC. Cancer genes in lung cancer: racial disparities: are there any? *Genes Cancer*. July 2012; 3(7–8):467–480.
9. Sekine I, Yamamoto N, Nishio K, et al. Emerging ethnic differences in lung cancer therapy. *Br J Cancer*. 2008; 99(11):1757–1762.
10. Gao B, Sun Y, Zhang J, Ren Y, et al. Spectrum of LKB1, EGFR, and KRAS mutations in Chinese lung adenocarcinomas. *J Thorac Oncol*. August 31, 2010;5(8):1130–1135.
11. Arrieta O, Cardona AF, Bramuglia GF, et al. Genotyping non-small cell lung cancer (NSCLC) in Latin America. *J Thorac Oncol*. November 30, 2011;6(11):1955–1959.
12. Bacchi CE, Ciol H, Queiroga EM, et al. Epidermal growth factor receptor and KRAS mutations in Brazilian lung cancer patients. *Clinics*. 2012;67(5):419–424.
13. Midha A, Dearden S, McCormack R. EGFR mutation incidence in non-small-cell lung cancer of adenocarcinoma histology: a systematic review and global map by ethnicity (mutMapII). *Am J Cancer Res*. 2015;5(9):2892.
14. Shepherd FA, Rodrigues Pereira J, Ciuleanu T, et al. Erlotinib in previously treated non–small-cell lung cancer. *N Engl J Med*. July 14, 2005;353(2):123–132.
15. Thatcher N, Chang A, Parikh P, et al. Gefitinib plus best supportive care in previously treated patients with refractory advanced non-small-cell lung cancer: results from a randomised, placebo-controlled, multicentre study (Iressa Survival Evaluation in Lung Cancer). *Lancet*. November 4, 2005;366(9496):1527–1537.
16. Fukuoka M, Yano S, Giaccone G, et al. Multi-institutional randomized phase II trial of gefitinib for previously treated patients with advanced non–small-cell lung cancer. *J Clin Oncol*. June 15, 2003;21(12):2237–2246.
17. Kris MG, Natale RB, Herbst RS, et al. Efficacy of gefitinib, an inhibitor of the epidermal growth factor receptor tyrosine kinase, in symptomatic patients with non–small cell lung cancer: a randomized trial. *Jama*. October 22, 2003; 290(16):2149–2158.
18. Zhang YL, Yuan JQ, Wang KF, et al. The prevalence of EGFR mutation in patients with non-small cell lung cancer: a systematic review and meta-analysis. *Oncotarget*. November 29, 2016;7(48):78985.
19. Lynch TJ, Bell DW, Sordella R, et al. Activating mutations in the epidermal growth factor receptor underlying responsiveness of non–small-cell lung cancer to gefitinib. *N Engl J Med*. May 20, 2004;350(21):2129–2139.
20. Paez JG, Jänne PA, Lee JC, et al. EGFR mutations in lung cancer: correlation with clinical response to gefitinib therapy. *Science*. June 4, 2004;304(5676):1497–1500.
21. Pao W, Miller V, Zakowski M, et al. EGF receptor gene mutations are common in lung cancers from "never smokers" and are associated with sensitivity of tumors to gefitinib and erlotinib. *Proc Natl Acad Sci USA*. September 7, 2004;101(36):13306–13311.
22. Yang JC, Sequist LV, Geater SL, et al. Clinical activity of afatinib in patients with advanced non-small-cell lung cancer harbouring uncommon EGFR mutations: a combined post-hoc analysis of LUX-Lung 2, LUX-Lung 3, and LUX-Lung 6. *Lancet Oncol*. July 31, 2015;16(7): 830–838.
23. Kayton ML, He M, Zakowski MF, et al. Primary lung adenocarcinomas in children and adolescents treated for pediatric malignancies. *J Thorac Oncol*. November 30, 2010;5(11):1764–1771.

24. American Cancer Society. *Key Statistics for Lung Cancer [Internet]*; 2017 [cited January 3rd 2018]. Available from: https://www.cancer.org/cancer/non-small-cell-lung-cancer/about/key-statistics.html24.

25. Kalemkerian GP, Narula N, Kennedy EB, et al. Molecular testing guideline for the selection of patients with lung cancer for treatment with targeted tyrosine kinase inhibitors: American Society of Clinical Oncology endorsement of the College of American Pathologists/International Association for the Study of Lung Cancer/Association for Molecular Pathology clinical practice guideline update. *J Clin Oncol*. February 5, 2018;36(9):911−919.

26. National Comprehensive Cancer Network. Non-Small Cell Lung Cancer (version 4.2018). https://www.nccn.org/professionals/physician_gls/pdf/nscl.pdf26.

27. Mok TS, Wu YL, Thongprasert S, et al. Gefitinib or carboplatin−paclitaxel in pulmonary adenocarcinoma. *N Engl J Med*. September 3, 2009;361(10):947−957.

28. Fukuoka M, Wu YL, Thongprasert S, et al. Biomarker analyses and final overall survival results from a phase III, randomized, open-label, first-line study of gefitinib versus carboplatin/paclitaxel in clinically selected patients with advanced non−small-cell lung cancer in Asia (IPASS). *J Clin Oncol*. June 13, 2011;29(21):2866−2874.

29. Maemondo M, Inoue A, Kobayashi K, et al. Gefitinib or chemotherapy for non−small-cell lung cancer with mutated EGFR. *N Engl J Med*. June 24, 2010;362(25):2380−2388.

30. Mitsudomi T, Morita S, Yatabe Y, et al. Gefitinib versus cisplatin plus docetaxel in patients with non-small-cell lung cancer harbouring mutations of the epidermal growth factor receptor (WJTOG3405): an open label, randomised phase 3 trial. *Lancet Oncol*. February 1, 2010;11(2):121−128.

31. Zhou C, Wu YL, Chen G, et al. Erlotinib versus chemotherapy as first-line treatment for patients with advanced EGFR mutation-positive non-small-cell lung cancer (OPTIMAL, CTONG-0802): a multicentre, open-label, randomised, phase 3 study. *Lancet Oncol*. August 31, 2011;12(8):735−742.

32. Chen G, Feng J, Zhou C, et al. Quality of life (QoL) analyses from OPTIMAL (CTONG-0802), a phase III, randomised, open-label study of first-line erlotinib versus chemotherapy in patients with advanced EGFR mutation-positive non-small-cell lung cancer (NSCLC). *Ann Oncol*. March 1, 2013;24(6):1615−1622.

33. Wu YL, Zhou C, Liam CK, et al. First-line erlotinib versus gemcitabine/cisplatin in patients with advanced EGFR mutation-positive non-small-cell lung cancer: analyses from the phase III, randomized, open-label, ENSURE study. *Ann Oncol*. June 23, 2015;26(9):1883−1889.

34. Rosell R, Carcereny E, Gervais R, et al. Erlotinib versus standard chemotherapy as first-line treatment for European patients with advanced EGFR mutation-positive non-small-cell lung cancer (EURTAC): a multicentre, open-label, randomised phase 3 trial. *Lancet Oncol*. March 31, 2012;13(3):239−246.

35. Sequist LV, Besse B, Lynch TJ, et al. Neratinib, an irreversible pan-ErbB receptor tyrosine kinase inhibitor: results of a phase II trial in patients with advanced non−small-cell lung cancer. *J Clin Oncol*. May 17, 2010;28(18):3076−3083.

36. Miller VA, Hirsh V, Cadranel J, et al. Afatinib versus placebo for patients with advanced, metastatic non-small-cell lung cancer after failure of erlotinib, gefitinib, or both, and one or two lines of chemotherapy (LUX-Lung 1): a phase 2b/3 randomised trial. *Lancet Oncol*. May 1, 2012;13(5):528−538.

37. Sequist LV, Yang JC, Yamamoto N, et al. Phase III study of afatinib or cisplatin plus pemetrexed in patients with metastatic lung adenocarcinoma with EGFR mutations. *J Clin Oncol*. July 1, 2013;31(27):3327−3334.

38. Wu YL, Zhou C, Hu CP, et al. Afatinib versus cisplatin plus gemcitabine for first-line treatment of Asian patients with advanced non-small-cell lung cancer harbouring EGFR mutations (LUX-Lung 6): an open-label, randomised phase 3 trial. *Lancet Oncol*. February 28, 2014;15(2):213−222.

39. Yang JC, Hirsh V, Schuler M, et al. Symptom control and quality of life in LUX-Lung 3: a phase III study of afatinib or cisplatin/pemetrexed in patients with advanced lung adenocarcinoma with EGFR mutations. *J Clin Oncol*. September 20, 2013;31(27):3342−3350.

40. Chiu CH, Yang CT, Shih JY, et al. Epidermal growth factor receptor tyrosine kinase inhibitor treatment response in advanced lung adenocarcinomas with G719X/L861Q/S768I mutations. *J Thorac Oncol*. May 1, 2015;10(5):793−799.

41. Park K, Tan EH, O'Byrne K, et al. Afatinib versus gefitinib as first-line treatment of patients with EGFR mutation-positive non-small-cell lung cancer (LUX-Lung 7): a phase 2B, open-label, randomised controlled trial. *Lancet Oncol*. May 31, 2016;17(5):577−589.

42. Paz-Ares L, Tan EH, O'byrne K, et al. Afatinib versus gefitinib in patients with EGFR mutation-positive advanced non-small-cell lung cancer: overall survival data from the phase IIb LUX-Lung 7 trial. *Ann Oncol*. February 1, 2017;28(2):270−277.

43. Wu YL, Cheng Y, Zhou X, et al. Dacomitinib versus gefitinib as first-line treatment for patients with EGFR-mutation-positive non-small-cell lung cancer (ARCHER 1050): a randomised, open-label, phase 3 trial. *Lancet Oncol*. November 1, 2017;18(11):1454−1466.

44. Mok TS, Cheng Y, Zhou X, et al. Improvement in overall survival in a randomized study that compared dacomitinib with gefitinib in patients with advanced non−small-cell lung cancer and EGFR-activating mutations. *Lancet Oncol*. 2017 Nov;18(11):1454−1466. https://doi.org/10.1016/S1470-2045(17)30608-3. Epub 2017 Sep 25.

45. Yun CH, Mengwasser KE, Toms AV, et al. The T790M mutation in EGFR kinase causes drug resistance by increasing the affinity for ATP. *Proc Natl Acad Sci USA*. February 12, 2008;105(6):2070−2075.

46. Sequist LV, Waltman BA, Dias-Santagata D, et al. Genotypic and histological evolution of lung cancers acquiring resistance to EGFR inhibitors. *Sci Transl Med*. March 23, 2011;3(75):75ra26.

47. Niederst MJ, Sequist LV, Poirier JT, et al. RB loss in resistant EGFR mutant lung adenocarcinomas that transform to small-cell lung cancer. *Nat Commun*. March 11, 2015;6:6377.

48. Lee JK, Lee J, Kim S, et al. Clonal history and genetic predictors of transformation into small-cell carcinomas from lung adenocarcinomas. *J Clin Oncol*. May 12, 2017; 35(26):3065–3074.

49. Yu H, Arcila ME, Rekhtman N, et al. Analysis of mechanisms of acquired resistance to EGFR TKI therapy in 155 patients with EGFR-mutant lung cancers. *Clin Cancer Res*. 2013;19(8):2240–2247.

50. Arcila ME, Oxnard GR, Nafa K, et al. Rebiopsy of lung cancer patients with acquired resistance to EGFR inhibitors and enhanced detection of the T790M mutation using a locked nucleic acid-based assay. *Clin Cancer Res*. March 1, 2011;17(5):1169–1180.

51. Ohashi K, Sequist LV, Arcila ME, et al. Lung cancers with acquired resistance to EGFR inhibitors occasionally harbor BRAF gene mutations but lack mutations in KRAS, NRAS, or MEK1. *Proc Natl Acad Sci USA*. July 31, 2012; 109(31):E2127–E2133.

52. Takezawa K, Pirazzoli V, Arcila ME, et al. HER2 amplification: a potential mechanism of acquired resistance to EGFR inhibition in EGFR-mutant lung cancers that lack the second-site EGFR T790M mutation. *Cancer Discov*. October 1, 2012;2(10):922–933.

53. Piotrowska Z, Stirling K, Heist R, et al. OA 07.05 serial biopsies in patients with EGFR-mutant NSCLC highlight the spatial and temporal heterogeneity of resistance mechanisms. *J Thorac Oncol*. November 1, 2017;12(11): S1762.

54. Oxnard GR, Thress KS, Alden RS, et al. Association between plasma genotyping and outcomes of treatment with osimertinib (AZD9291) in advanced non–small-cell lung cancer. *J Clin Oncol*. June 27, 2016;34(28):3375–3382.

55. Janjigian YY, Smit EF, Groen HJ, et al. Dual inhibition of EGFR with afatinib and cetuximab in kinase inhibitor–resistant EGFR-mutant lung cancer with and without T790M mutations. *Cancer Discov*. September 1, 2014; 4(9):1036–1045.

56. Jänne PA, Yang JC, Kim DW, et al. AZD9291 in EGFR inhibitor–resistant non–small-cell lung cancer. *N Engl J Med*. April 30, 2015;372(18):1689–1699.

57. Mok TS, Wu YL, Ahn MJ, et al. Osimertinib or platinum–pemetrexed in EGFR T790M–positive lung cancer. *N Engl J Med*. February 16, 2017;376(7):629–640.

58. Ramalingam SS, Yang JC, Lee CK, et al. Osimertinib as first-line treatment of EGFR mutation–positive advanced non–small-cell lung cancer. *N Engl J Med*. 2018 Jan 11;378(2):113–125. https://doi.org/10.1056/NEJMoa1713137. Epub 2017 Nov 18.

59. Soria JC, Ohe Y, Vansteenkiste J, et al. Osimertinib in untreated EGFR-mutated advanced non–small-cell lung cancer. *N Engl J Med*. January 11, 2018;378(2):113–125.

60. Wang Z, Yang JJ, Huang J, et al. Lung adenocarcinoma harboring EGFR T790M and in trans C797S responds to combination therapy of first-and third-generation EGFR TKIs and shifts allelic configuration at resistance. *J Thorac Oncol*. November 30, 2017;12(11):1723–1727.

61. Scagliotti GV, Parikh P, Von Pawel J, et al. Phase III study comparing cisplatin plus gemcitabine with cisplatin plus pemetrexed in chemotherapy-naive patients with advanced-stage non–small-cell lung cancer. *J Clin Oncol*. July 20, 2008;26(21):3543–3551.

62. Ciuleanu T, Brodowicz T, Zielinski C, et al. Maintenance pemetrexed plus best supportive care versus placebo plus best supportive care for non-small-cell lung cancer: a randomised, double-blind, phase 3 study. *Lancet*. October 30, 2009;374(9699):1432–1440.

63. Paz-Ares LG, de Marinis F, Dediu M, et al. PARAMOUNT: final overall survival results of the phase III study of maintenance pemetrexed versus placebo immediately after induction treatment with pemetrexed plus cisplatin for advanced nonsquamous non–small-cell lung cancer. *J Clin Oncol*. July 8, 2013;31(23):2895–2902.

64. de Castria TB, da Silva EM, Gois AF, et al. Cisplatin versus carboplatin in combination with third-generation drugs for advanced non-small cell lung cancer. *Cochrange Database Syst Rev*. 2013;8:CD009256.

65. Chaft JE, Oxnard GR, Sima CS, et al. Disease flare after tyrosine kinase inhibitor discontinuation in patients with EGFR-mutant lung cancer and acquired resistance to erlotinib or gefitinib: implications for clinical trial design. *Clin Cancer Res*. October 1, 2011;17(19):6298–6303.

66. Soria JC, Wu YL, Nakagawa K, et al. Gefitinib plus chemotherapy versus placebo plus chemotherapy in EGFR-mutation-positive non-small-cell lung cancer after progression on first-line gefitinib (IMPRESS): a phase 3 randomised trial. *Lancet Oncol*. August 31, 2015;16(8): 990–998.

67. Nakamura A, Inoue A, Satoshi M, et al. Phase III study comparing gefitinib monotherapy (G) to combination therapy with gefitinib, carboplatin, and pemetrexed (GCP) for untreated patients (pts) with advanced non-small cell lung cancer (NSCLC) with EGFR mutations (NEJ009). *J Clin Oncol*. 2018;36(suppl; abstr 9005).

68. Seto T, Kato T, Nishio M, et al. Erlotinib alone or with bevacizumab as first-line therapy in patients with advanced non-squamous non-small-cell lung cancer harbouring EGFR mutations (JO25567): an open-label, randomised, multicentre, phase 2 study. *Lancet Oncol*. October 31, 2014;15(11):1236–1244.

69. Yamamoto N, Seto T, Nishio M, et al. Erlotinib plus bevacizumab (EB) versus erlotinib alone (E) as first-line treatment for advanced EGFR mutation–positive non-squamous non–small-cell lung cancer (NSCLC): survival follow-up results of JO25567. *J Clin Oncol*. 2018; 36(suppl; abstr 9007).

70. Furuya N, Fukuhara T, Saito H, et al. Phase III study comparing bevacizumab plus erlotinib to erlotinib in patients with untreated NSCLC harboring activating EGFR mutations: NEJ026. *J Clin Oncol*. 2018;36(suppl; abstr 9006).

71. Gainor JF, Shaw AT, Sequist LV, et al. EGFR mutations and ALK rearrangements are associated with low response rates to PD-1 pathway blockade in non-small cell lung cancer (NSCLC): a retrospective analysis. *Clin Cancer Res.* 2016;22(18):4585–4593.

72. Lisberg AE, Cummings AL, Goldman JW, et al. A phase II study of pembrolizumab in EGFR-mutant, PD-L1+, tyrosine kinase inhibitor (TKI) naïve patients with advanced NSCLC. *J Clin Oncol.* 2018;36(suppl; abstr 9014).

73. Borghaei H, Paz-Ares L, Horn L, et al. Nivolumab versus docetaxel in advanced nonsquamous non–small-cell lung cancer. *N Engl J Med.* October 22, 2015;373(17):1627–1639.

74. Herbst RS, Baas P, Kim DW, et al. Pembrolizumab versus docetaxel for previously treated, PD-L1-positive, advanced non-small-cell lung cancer (KEYNOTE-010): a randomised controlled trial. *Lancet.* April 15, 2016;387(10027):1540–1550.

75. Rittmeyer A, Barlesi F, Waterkamp D, et al. Atezolizumab versus docetaxel in patients with previously treated non-small-cell lung cancer (OAK): a phase 3, open-label, multicentre randomised controlled trial. *Lancet.* January 27, 2017;389(10066):255–265.

76. Reck M, Rodríguez-Abreu D, Robinson AG, et al. Pembrolizumab versus chemotherapy for PD-L1–positive non–small-cell lung cancer. *N Engl J Med.* November 10, 2016;375(19):1823–1833.

77. Langer CJ, Gadgeel SM, Borghaei H, et al. Carboplatin and pemetrexed with or without pembrolizumab for advanced, non-squamous non-small-cell lung cancer: a randomised, phase 2 cohort of the open-label KEYNOTE-021 study. *Lancet Oncol.* November 1, 2016;17(11):1497–1508.

78. Gandhi L, Rodríguez-Abreu D, Gadgeel S, et al. Pembrolizumab plus chemotherapy in metastatic non–small-cell lung cancer. *N Engl J Med.* 2018;378:2078–2092.

79. Garassino MC, Cho BC, Kim JH, et al. Durvalumab as third-line or later treatment for advanced non-small-cell lung cancer (ATLANTIC): an open-label, single-arm, phase 2 study. *Lancet Oncol.* April 1, 2018;19(4):521–536.

80. Antonia SJ, Villegas A, Daniel D, et al. Durvalumab after chemoradiotherapy in stage III non–small-cell lung cancer. *N Engl J Med.* November 16, 2017;377(20):1919–1929.

81. Sequist LV, Willers H, Lanuti M, et al. The ASCENT trial: a phase II study of neoadjuvant afatinib, chemoradiation and surgery for stage III EGFR mutation-positive NSCLC. *J Clin Oncol.* 2018;36(suppl; abstr 8544).

82. Socinski MA, Jotte RM, Cappuzzo F, et al. Atezolizumab for first-line treatment of metastatic nonsquamous NSCLC. *N Engl J Med.* 2018;378:2288–2301.

83. Ahn MJ, Yang J, Yu H, et al. 136O: osimertinib combined with durvalumab in EGFR-mutant non-small cell lung cancer: results from the TATTON phase Ib trial. *J Thorac Oncol.* April 1, 2016;11(4):S115.

84. Gibbons DL, Chow LQ, Kim DW, et al. 57O Efficacy, safety and tolerability of MEDI4736 (durvalumab [D]), a human IgG1 anti-programmed cell death-ligand-1 (PD-L1) antibody, combined with gefitinib (G): a phase I expansion in TKI-naive patients (pts) with EGFR mutant NSCLC. *J Thorac Oncol.* April 1, 2016;11(4):S79.

85. Kelly K, Altorki NK, Eberhardt WE, et al. Adjuvant erlotinib versus placebo in patients with stage IB-IIIA non–small-cell lung cancer (RADIANT): a randomized, double-blind, phase III trial. *J Clin Oncol.* August 31, 2015;33(34):4007–4014.

86. Pennell NA, Neal JW, Chaft JE, et al. SELECT: a multicenter phase II trial of adjuvant erlotinib in resected early-stage EGFR mutation-positive NSCLC. *J Clin Oncol.* 2014;5s(suppl; abstr 7514):32.

87. Zhong WZ, Wang Q, Mao WM, et al. Gefitinib versus vinorelbine plus cisplatin as adjuvant treatment for stage II–IIIA (N1–N2) EGFR-mutant NSCLC (ADJUVANT/CTONG1104): a randomised, open-label, phase 3 study. *Lancet Oncol.* 2018;19(1):139–148.

88. Pisters KM, Evans WK, Azzoli CG, et al. Cancer Care Ontario and American Society of Clinical Oncology adjuvant chemotherapy and adjuvant radiation therapy for stages I-IIIA resectable non–small-cell lung cancer guideline. *J Clin Oncol.* December 1, 2007;25(34):5506–5518.

89. Lo PC, Dahlberg SE, Nishino M, et al. Delay of treatment change after objective progression on first-line erlotinib in epidermal growth factor receptor-mutant lung cancer. *Cancer.* August 1, 2015;121(15):2570–2577.

90. Li W, Ren S, Li J, et al. T790M mutation is associated with better efficacy of treatment beyond progression with EGFR-TKI in advanced NSCLC patients. *Lung Cancer.* June 1, 2014;84(3):295–300.

91. Park K, Yu CJ, Kim SW, et al. First-line erlotinib therapy until and beyond response evaluation criteria in solid tumors progression in Asian patients with epidermal growth factor receptor mutation–positive non–small-cell lung cancer: the ASPIRATION study. *JAMA Oncol.* March 1, 2016;2(3):305–312.

92. Weickhardt AJ, Scheier B, Burke JM, et al. Local ablative therapy of oligoprogressive disease prolongs disease control by tyrosine kinase inhibitors in oncogene-addicted non–small-cell lung cancer. *J Thorac Oncol.* December 31, 2012;7(12):1807–1814.

93. Qiu B, Liang Y, Li Q, et al. Local therapy for oligoprogressive disease in patients with advanced stage non–small-cell lung cancer harboring epidermal growth factor receptor mutation. *Clin Lung Cancer.* April 12, 2017;18(6):e369–e373.

94. Iuchi T, Shingyoji M, Sakaida T, et al. Phase II trial of gefitinib alone without radiation therapy for Japanese patients with brain metastases from EGFR-mutant lung adenocarcinoma. *Lung Cancer.* November 30, 2013; 82(2):282–287.
95. Kris MG, Arbour KC, Riely GJ, et al. Pulse-continuous dose erlotinib as initial targeted therapy for patients with EGFR-mutant lung cancers with untreated brain metastases. *J Clin Oncol.* May 20, 2017;35(15suppl): 9039.
96. Magnuson WJ, Lester-Coll NH, Wu AJ, et al. Management of brain metastases in tyrosine kinase inhibitor–naïve epidermal growth factor receptor–mutant non–small-cell lung cancer: a retrospective multi-institutional analysis. *J Clin Oncol.* January 23, 2017;35(10):1070–1077.
97. Yang JC, Cho BC, Kim DW, et al. Osimertinib for patients (pts) with leptomeningeal metastases (LM) from EGFR-mutant non-small cell lung cancer (NSCLC): updated results from the BLOOM study. *J Clin Oncol.* 2017; 35(Suppl). abstr 2020.
98. Marcoux N, Gettinger SN, O'Kane GM, et al. Outcomes of EGFR-mutant lung adenocarcinomas (AC) that transform to small cell lung cancer (SCLC). *J Clin Oncol.* 2018;36(suppl; abstr 8573).
99. Robichaux JP, Elamin YY, Tan Z, et al. Mechanisms and clinical activity of an EGFR and HER2 exon 20–selective kinase inhibitor in non–small cell lung cancer. *Nat Med.* May 2018;24(5):638.
100. Tu HY, Ke EE, Yang JJ, et al. A comprehensive review of uncommon EGFR mutations in patients with non-small cell lung cancer. *Lung Cancer.* December 1, 2017;114: 96–102.
101. Elamin Y, Robichaux J, Lam V, et al. OA 12.01 the preclinical and clinical activity of poziotinib, a potent, selective inhibitor of EGFR exon 20 mutant NSCLC. *J Thorac Oncol.* November 1, 2017;12(11):S1776.
102. Doebele RC, Riely GJ, Spira AI, et al. First report of safety, PK, and preliminary antitumor activity of the oral EGFR/HER2 exon 20 inhibitor TAK-788 (AP32788) in non–small cell lung cancer (NSCLC). *J Clin Oncol.* May 20, 2018;36(15_suppl):9015.
103. Piotrowska Z, Fintelmann F, Sequist LV. Response to osimertinib in an EGFR exon 20 insertion-positive lung adenocarcinoma. *J Thorac Oncol.* 2018 [in press].
104. Lacouture ME, Balagula Y. *Acneiform Eruption Secondary to Epidermal Growth Factor Receptor (EGFR) Inhibitors [internet]*; 2017 (cited January 3rd 2018). Available from: https://www.uptodate.com/contents/acneiform-eruption-secondary-to-epidermal-growth-factor-receptor-egfr-inhibitors?source=see_link#H52639369104.
105. Petrelli F, Borgonovo K, Cabiddu M, et al. Antibiotic prophylaxis for skin toxicity induced by anti-EGFR agents: a systematic review and meta-analysis. *Br J Dermatol.* May 1, 2016;175(6):1166–1174.
106. NCI, NIH, DHHS. *National Cancer Institute Common Terminology Criteria for Adverse Events V4. 0.* NIH publication 09-7473. May 29, 2009.
107. Melosky B, Hirsh V. Management of common toxicities in metastatic NSCLC related to anti-lung cancer therapies with EGFR–TKIs. *Front Oncol.* September 16, 2014;4:238.
108. Gainor JF, Niederst MJ, Lennerz JK, et al. Dramatic response to combination erlotinib and crizotinib in a patient with advanced, EGFR-mutant lung cancer harboring de novo MET amplification. *J Thorac Oncol.* July 1, 2016; 11(7):e83–e85.
109. York ER, Varella-Garcia M, Bang TJ, et al. Tolerable and effective combination of full-dose crizotinib and osimertinib targeting met amplification sequentially emerging after T790M positivity in EGFR-mutant non–small cell lung cancer. *J Thorac Oncol.* July 1, 2017;12(7):e85–e88.
110. Ahn M, Han J, Sequist L, et al. OA 09.03 TATTON Ph Ib expansion cohort: osimertinib plus savolitinib for pts with EGFR-mutant met-amplified NSCLC after progression on prior EGFR-TKI. *J Thorac Oncol.* November 1, 2017;12(11):S1768.
111. Piotrowska Z, Nagy R, Fairclough S, et al. OA 09.01 characterizing the genomic landscape of EGFR C797S in lung cancer using ctDNA next-generation sequencing. *J Thorac Oncol.* November 1, 2017;12(11):S1767.
112. Gandara DR, Kowanetz M, Mok TS, et al. 1295OBlood-based biomarkers for cancer immunotherapy: tumor mutational burden in blood (bTMB) is associated with improved atezolizumab (atezo) efficacy in 2L+ NSCLC (POPLAR and OAK). *Ann Oncol.* September 1, 2017; 28(suppl_5).

CHAPTER 8

Approach to Anaplastic Lymphoma Kinase (ALK) Gene Rearranged Non—Small Cell Lung Cancer (NSCLC)

SHIRISH GADGEEL, MD

INTRODUCTION

One of the major advances in the management of lung cancer is the identification of genetic alterations that are the primary drivers of the oncogenic phenotype and which could be targeted for clinical benefit. This is especially true in lung adenocarcinomas, where it is possible to identify such "driver" genetic alterations in majority of the tumors.

Anaplastic lymphoma kinase (ALK) belongs to the insulin receptor superfamily of tyrosine kinases. In adults, ALK expression is restricted to only certain body parts, including testes and neural tissues. Soda et al., identified a novel fusion gene EML4 (echinoderm microtubule-associated protein-like 4)-ALK, arising from an inversion on the short arm of chromosome 2, as a driver genetic alteration in non—small cell lung cancer (NSCLC).[1] The resulting chimeric protein leads to constitutive activation of ALK tyrosine kinase resulting in an oncogenic phenotype. Although the break point in the ALK gene is consistent in these gene rearrangements, different break points in the EML4 gene have been detected resulting in variants of the chimeric protein.[2] The different variants maybe associated with different tumor biology and different responses to ALK tyrosine kinase inhibitors (TKIs). Rarely other genes may partner with ALK to form novel fusion genes resulting in activation of ALK. These include KIF5B and TFG.[3,4]

CLINICAL FEATURES OF ANAPLASTIC LYMPHOMA KINASE POSITIVE NON—SMALL CELL LUNG CANCER

ALK gene rearrangement occurs in 2%—4% of NSCLCs.[5,6] Despite the low percentage of NSCLCs with this genetic alteration, it is estimated that 6000 new cases of ALK positive NSCLC are diagnosed each year in the United States. Although the initial case that lead to the discovery of ALK gene rearrangements in NSCLC was a smoker, ALK gene rearrangements are more commonly detected in tumors of patients who are never or light smokers. Several reports have shown that the median age of patients with ALK gene rearrangement tends to be younger at 50—55 years.[5,6] The incidence of ALK positive NSCLC may not differ among the different regions of the world nor does it differ among the sexes.

TESTING FOR ANAPLASTIC LYMPHOMA KINASE

Fluorescence in situ hybridization (FISH) was the first test used to detect ALK gene rearrangement.[7] It utilizes DNA probes to the 3′ and 5′ of the ALK gene. In tumors without ALK rearrangement fusion the test shows fusion of the two signals or signals that are in close proximity of each other. However, in tumors with ALK gene rearrangement the signals from the two probes are separated. Immunohistochemistry (IHC) is a more readily available test and can be used to detect ALK positive NSCLC. Recently released guidelines by the IASLC (International Association for the Study of Lung Cancer) state that IHC can be considered as an alternative test to ALK FISH testing.[8] It is important to note that patients in the randomized phase III ALEX trial were selected based on ALK IHC testing, performed at a central laboratory.

Some have raised concerns about the ALK tests. Cabillic et al. showed that there was significant discordance between FISH and IHC when they conducted parallel testing on the same samples.[9] Of the 3244 cases, 150 were found to be ALK positive by FISH and/or positive by IHC, but only 80 of those samples were found to be positive by both FISH and IHC. They concluded that one-fourth of ALK positive samples would have been missed had only single FISH or IHC testing been employed. Others have shown far less discordance between the two tests.[8] Nonetheless, it is important that in appropriate patients a second test should be considered if the first test was negative for ALK gene rearrangement.

Reverse transcription polymerase chain reactions (RT-PCR) and next-generation sequencing (NGS) panels are also being used to detect for targetable gene alterations, including ALK gene rearrangement. RT-PCR is highly specific for most fusions but not sensitive to assess all fusions and patients with negative results may need to be tested with a different, more sensitive method.[8] The IASLC guidelines do recommend using multiplexed genetic sequencing panels including NGS testing over conducting single gene tests.

APPROACH TO ADVANCED-STAGE ANAPLASTIC LYMPHOMA KINASE PATIENT

Since the discovery of ALK rearrangement as a driver genetic alteration in NSCLC in 2007, therapy for ALK positive NSCLC patients has evolved significantly. Initial trials demonstrated that using an ALK TKI provided improved clinical benefit compared with chemotherapy both in treatment naïve and recurrent ALK patients. Subsequent trials have now shown that next-generation ALK TKIs can provide benefit in crizotinib-treated patients and provide better clinical benefit than crizotinib in treatment naïve patients. It is important to review the data from these trials to gain a proper perspective on the management of advanced ALK positive NSCLC patients.

CRIZOTINIB

Crizotinib is an oral inhibitor of ALK, ROS1, and c-Met tyrosine kinases. Based on its known activity against ALK, NSCLC patients known to have tumors with ALK

gene rearrangement were enrolled in an expansion cohort of a phase I study.[10] The response rate with crizotinib in this expansion cohort was 61%, and the median progression-free survival (PFS) was 10 months.

Following the phase I trial, crizotinib was evaluated in two separate phase III trials. In PROFILE 1007, crizotinib demonstrated superior efficacy to pemetrexed or docetaxel in ALK positive NSCLC patients previously treated with platinum-based chemotherapy.[11] In PROFILE 1014, treatment naïve advanced ALK positive NSCLC patients were randomized to crizotinib alone or to the combination of pemetrexed with carboplatin or cisplatin.[12] In this study, crizotinib significantly improved PFS compared with chemotherapy, with a median of 10.9 months compared with 7.0 months with chemotherapy (HR-0.45, $P < .001$). Recently, Mok et al. presented long-term outcomes of this study[13] (Tables 8.1 and 8.3). The 4-year survival rate in patients treated with crizotinib was 56.6% compared with 49.1% among patients treated with chemotherapy, HR 0.76, $P = .0978$. Among the patients randomized to crizotinib, 57 patients received another ALK inhibitor as the next therapy. The median survival of these patients exceeded 5 years.

NEXT-GENERATION ALK INHIBITORS IN CRIZOTINIB-TREATED PATIENTS

Despite the superior clinical benefit with crizotinib, the median PFS with this drug is approximately 8−11 months. Broadly, three distinct mechanisms of resistance to targeted agents have been recognized.[14] These are genetic alterations in the target gene, activation of bypass tracks or phenotypic change in the tumor such as epithelial mesenchymal transition, and finally progression at sites of limited penetration such as the central nervous system (CNS). All three mechanisms of resistance have been observed with crizotinib. Genetic alterations in the ALK gene as a resistance mechanism has been observed in about 30% of crizotinib-treated patients, with the most common point mutations being L1196M and G1269A.[15]

TABLE 8.1 Long-Term Outcomes With Front-Line ALK Inhibitors					
Trial	Phase	Drug	N	PFS 4-year Rate	OS 4-year Rate
PROFILE 1014[14]	III	Crizotinib	172[a]	—	56.6%
AF-001 JP[21]	I/II	Alectinib	46	52%	70%

[a] Patients randomized to receive crizotinib in PROFILE 1014 trial.

ALK, anaplastic lymphoma kinase; *OS*, overall survival; *PFS*, progression-free survival.

TABLE 8.2
Efficacy of Approved ALK Drugs in Crizotinib-Refractory Patients

Design/Assessment	Ceritinib[20] N = 163	Alectinib[21] N = 138	Brigatinib[22] N = 110
	Phase I/II Investigator/BIRC	Phase 2 BIRC	Phase 2 Investigator
PS 2	12%	9%	8%
Brain metastases	60%	61%	67%
Previous Rx	56% (≥3 prior)	80% (≥2 prior)	74% (≥2 prior)
ORR	56% (49–64)	50% (41–59)	55% (45–64)
Central nervous system response	36% N = 28	57% N = 35	67% N = 12
Median Progression-free survival	6.9 m (5.6–8.7)	8.9 (5.6–11.3)	16.7 (11.6-NR)

TABLE 8.3
Randomized Phase III Trials Evaluating Front-Line ALK Inhibitor

Trial	N	Experimental Arm	PFS Median	Standard Arm	PFS Median	Hazard Ratio
PROFILE 1014	343	Crizotinib	10.9 mo	Cisplatin/Carboplatin Pemetrexed	7.0 mo	0.45 (95% CI 0.35–0.60)
JALEX	207	Alectinib	NR[a]	Crizotinib	10.2 mo	0.34 (99.7% CI 0.17–0.71)
ALEX	303	Alectinib	NR[a]	Crizotinib	11.2 mo	0.47 (95% CI 0.34–0.65)
ASCEND-4	376	Ceritinib	16.6 months	Cisplatin/Carboplatin Pemetrexed	8.1 mo	0.55 (95% CI 0.42–0.73)

[a] Not reached.
PFS, progression-free survival.

CNS is an important site of recurrence in crizotinib-treated patients. In a retrospective analysis of two clinical trials of crizotinib, 72% of patients who had previously been treated for brain metastases had progression in the CNS. Among patients who did not have evidence of brain metastases at baseline, 20% developed brain metastases while on therapy.[16] There are data to suggest that crizotinib may not penetrate the blood–brain barrier sufficiently.[17]

Next-generation drugs were evaluated in ALK positive crizotinib-treated NSCLC patients. In preclinical studies, these drugs demonstrated more potent inhibition of ALK and could inhibit many of the ALK mutations that were observed in tumors refractory to crizotinib.[18,19] In the United States, three drugs are approved for the treatment of crizotinib-treated ALK positive NSCLC patients (Table 8.2). The response rates with these drugs in phase II studies were 50%–55%, median PFS ranged from 7 to 16 months.[20–22] In addition, each of these drugs demonstrated activity against CNS metastases. These drugs differ in their toxicity profiles. Gastrointestinal (GI) symptoms are common with ceritinib. Myalgias, fatigue, and constipation have been observed with alectinib. Patients treated with brigatinib may experience pulmonary symptoms in the first week of therapy. To minimize the possibility of these symptoms, brigatinib is initiated at a dose of 90 mg daily, and if there are no significant pulmonary symptoms, the daily dose is increased to 180 mg. Two phase III trials have evaluated next-generation ALK TKIs in crizotinib-treated patients, one with ceritinib and the other with alectinib. Both trials demonstrated superior efficacy with these ALK inhibitors compared with chemotherapy.[23,24] These data strongly suggest that ALK inhibitor is the most appropriate therapy for patients with disease progression following treatment with crizotinib.

Other drugs have demonstrated activity in patients previously treated with crizotinib. These include lorlatinib and ensartinib.[25,26] The clinical activity of each of these drugs is similar to the activity observed with the three approved drugs.

Defining molecular mechanisms of resistance in crizotinib-treated tumors prior to starting a next-generation ALK TKI is not necessary because clinical activity with next-generation ALK TKIs in crizotinib-treated patients was observed without identifying the specific mechanism of resistance. The activity of the different next generation ALK inhibitors against resistant ALK mutations is variable. It is possible that in the future choice of next ALK inhibitor may be dictated by the specific resistant ALK mutation identified in a patient's tumor.

NEXT-GENERATION ALK TKIS AS FRONT-LINE THERAPY

Based on the activity of the next-generation ALK inhibitors in crizotinib-treated patients and their activity against CNS metastases, there was interest in evaluating these agents as front-line therapy.

ALECTINIB

Alectinib was the first ALK inhibitor to be compared against crizotinib as front-line therapy. Three separate trials have evaluated the activity of alectinib as front-line therapy.

AF-001JP

AF-001JP was a phase I/II study conducted exclusively in Japan.[27] Advanced ALK positive NSCLC patients who had never received a prior ALK inhibitor were enrolled on the trial. In the phase I portion of the study, 24 patients were treated at doses of 20–300 mg twice daily. No dose-limiting toxicities or grade 4 adverse events were observed. Dose was not escalated beyond 300 mg BID due to limitations in Japan on the quantity of an additive present in alectinib capsules. Of the 46 patients enrolled in the phase II portion of the study, 98% of the patients had received at least one chemotherapy regimen. At a minimum follow-up of 4.5 years and the median duration of therapy with alectinib of 46 months, the 4-year PFS rate and OS rates were 52% and 70%, respectively[28] (Table 8.1). The median PFS in patients with brain metastases was 38 months. The most common adverse events observed were increase in blood bilirubin, liver enzymes, and blood creatinine; constipation; dysgeusia; and rash. The most common grade 3 AE was neutropenia. No grade 4 or 5 toxicities were observed.

JALEX (TABLE 8.3)

Following AF-001JP, a randomized phase III study was conducted in Japan comparing alectinib with crizotinib.[29] Patient's tumors were first screened for ALK by IHC, and if positive, ALK rearrangement was confirmed by FISH or patient's tumor had to be positive for ALK rearrangement by RT-PCR. Patients who had received one prior chemotherapy regimen were allowed. Patients with asymptomatic or treated brain metastases were also allowed. However, the study did not stratify patients according to baseline brain metastases status. This resulted in an imbalance between the two arms, with 30% of patients randomized to crizotinib having brain metastases compared with only 16% in patients randomized to alectinib. The primary endpoint of the study was PFS, as assessed by independent review committee. The study enrolled 207 patients, 103 were randomized to alectinib.

At the second planned interim analysis, alectinib demonstrated significantly superior PFS compared with crizotinib, with a median survival that not been reached compared with 10.2 months with crizotinib (HR 0.34, 99.7% CI 0.17–0.71, $P < .0001$). The response rates with alectinib and crizotinib were 92% and 79%, respectively. Benefits were observed across all subsets including patients with brain metastases (HR 0.08) and patients who had received prior chemotherapy (HR 0.39). Grade 3/4 adverse events were less common with alectinib, 26% compared with crizotinib, 52%.

ALEX (TABLE 8.3)

A trial similar to the JALEX trial, called the ALEX trial, was conducted worldwide.[30] There were some differences between the study designs of the ALEX and JALEX trials. ALEX trial only allowed patients who were treatment naïve. Patients were eligible for the study only if their tumors were positive for ALK by IHC conducted at a central laboratory. Tumors were collected to assess ALK rearrangement by FISH, but such confirmation was not required for study eligibility. Patients with asymptomatic or treated brain metastases were eligible for the study, but in the ALEX trial, patients were stratified according to presence or absence of brain metastases at baseline. Patients randomized to alectinib were treated at a dose of 600 mg bid. This dose was based on a prior phase I study conducted in the United States because the Japanese restrictions on additives in the alectinib capsules are not applicable in the rest of the world.[31] The primary endpoint of ALEX was investigator-assessed PFS.

The study enrolled 303 patients, 152 of whom were randomized to alectinib. Alectinib demonstrated significantly superior PFS compared with crizotinib, with a median PFS that had not been reached with alectinib and was 11.2 months with crizotinib (HR 0.47, 95% CI 0.34–0.65, $P < .001$). The response rates with alectinib and crizotinib were 83% and 76%, respectively. Efficacy in the CNS was prospectively assessed in this trial. All patients underwent baseline scans, and all patients irrespective of whether they had brain metastases or not underwent repeat brain imaging every 8 weeks while on the study. Alectinib significantly improved PFS both in patients with (HR 0.40, $P < .0001$) and without CNS metastases (HR 0.51, $P = .0024$).[26] In addition, PFS was significantly improved in patients with brain metastases irrespective of whether patients had received prior brain radiation therapy or not.[32] Time to CNS progression was also superior with alectinib both in patients with and without baseline metastases. In patients who did not have brain metastases, 31% of the crizotinib-treated patients developed progression in the brain at 1 year compared with only 4.6% of the patients treated with alectinib (HR 0.14, $P < .0001$). These data suggest that alectinib may delay the occurrence of new brain metastases even in patients who do not have baseline brain metastases. Anemia, myalgias, photosensitivity, increased bilirubin, and increased weight were more commonly observed in alectinib-treated patients. Nausea, diarrhea, and vomiting were more common among crizotinib-treated patients. The rates of grade 3/4 toxicities (41% vs. 50%) and drug discontinuation (11% vs. 13%) due to toxicities were similar between the alectinib- and crizotinib-treated patients.

SUMMARY OF ALEX AND JALEX

The only two trials that have directly compared one ALK TKI to another and have reported results are ALEX and JALEX. In both trials, alectinib significantly improved PFS compared with crizotinib (Table 8.2). In both ALEX and JALEX outcomes with crizotinib were comparable to the results observed with crizotinib in the PROFILE 1014 trial. The benefits with alectinib in JALEX (HR 0.34) and in ALEX trial (HR 0.47) were similar. In addition, both trials showed that alectinib was effective in patients with brain metastases. Finally, the adverse event profile with alectinib in both trials was favorable compared with crizotinib.

Based on the results of these trials, alectinib has now been accepted as a standard of care for treatment naïve

advanced ALK positive NSCLC patients by the NCCN guidelines and was approved both by the US FDA and the European regulatory agency EMEA.

CERITINIB

The phase III ASCEND-4 trial evaluated ceritinib as first-line therapy for ALK-rearranged NSCLC patients compared with platinum-pemetrexed chemotherapy[33] (Table 8.3). This study demonstrated improved PFS (HR 0.55, $P < .00001$) with median PFS of 16.6 months in ceritinib-treated patients and 8.1 months in chemotherapy-treated patients. The efficacy appeared to differ based on the presence of brain metastases at baseline. The median PFS in patients without baseline brain metastases was 26.3 months for ceritinib compared with 8.3 months for chemotherapy (HR 0.48). In contrast, in patients with baseline brain metastases, the median PFS was 10.7 months for ceritinib and 6.7 months for chemotherapy (HR0 0.70). This suggests that the benefit with ceritinib in patients with brain metastases maybe limited.

Another concern with ceritinib is that a high proportion of patients can experience adverse events, particularly GI toxicities. These toxicities did appear to impact drug delivery in the ASCEND-4 trial as suggested by a median dose intensity of 78.4%. Due to the high toxicity rate observed with ceritinib at the approved dose of 750 mg daily on an empty stomach, ASCEND-8 evaluated the safety and efficacy of two lower doses 450 and 600 mg daily given following a low-fat meal.[34] The study enrolled 267 patients, of which 121 patients were treatment naïve and were randomized to each of the three arms. The pharmacokinetic analysis demonstrated that the 450 mg dose with low-fat meal provided the highest drug exposure with lowest number of patients requiring dose reductions. In addition, the response rates were very similar between the three arms, ranging from 70% to 78%. Although, the grade 3/4 GI toxicities were lower at the 450 mg dose, 50% of the patients developed all-grade diarrhea. Based on these data, ceritinib at 450 mg with low-fat meal could be another option for either front-line therapy or in patients previously treated with crizotinib.

OTHER DRUGS

There is limited data available on other next-generation drugs as first ALK inhibitor. As part of a phase I/II study, 30 patients with ALK positive NSCLC who had no prior exposure to an ALK inhibitor were treated with lorlatinib.[25] The response rate was 90% with a median PFS that had not been reached. Eight ALK inhibitor naïve patients were treated with brigatinib in a phase I/II trial. The response rate in these eight patients was 100%, with a median PFS of 34 months.[33] Promising results have also been reported with ensartinib.[26] Ongoing phase III studies will define the role of these agents as front-line ALK inhibitor.

RESISTANCE TO NEXT-GENERATION ALK INHIBITORS

Limited data are available on mechanisms of resistance to next-generation ALK inhibitors and almost all the data are in patients who received these agents following treatment with crizotinib. As is true with other TKIs, target alteration, activation of alternative signaling pathways, and phenotypic changes in the tumor have been observed in tumors resistant to next-generation ALK inhibitors. Gainor et al. showed in an analysis of 83 ALK-positive patients that target alteration with ALK is much more commonly observed in tumors following next-generation ALK inhibitors than in tumors of patients treated with crizotinib.[35] The most common mutation observed was G1202R, a mutation in the solvent-exposed region of ALK, resulting in steric hindrance to most ALK inhibitors. It is unclear if the same mechanisms of resistance or in the same proportions will be observed in tumors of patients treated with next-generation ALK inhibitor as the first ALK inhibitor.

SEQUENCE OF ALK INHIBITORS (FIGS. 8.1 AND 8.2)

Based on the results of ALEX and JALEX, the standard of care for the management of treatment naïve ALK positive NSCLC has changed to alectinib. An important issue to consider before making a switch in the standard of care is whether the outcomes of starting with alectinib compared with starting with crizotinib followed by alectinib are superior. Although there are no prospective data to address this issue, it appears that the median PFS observed in the JALEX and the ALEX trials with alectinib is superior to the expected combined median PFS with crizotinib followed by alectinib of 18–20 months. Whether this superior efficacy observed with alectinib will necessarily translate into improved survival is unclear and may never be known because there are several other ALK inhibitors available. Ceritinib is also approved for front-line therapy, but due to limited activity in patients with CNS metastases and toxicities associated with the drug it is not commonly used as front-line therapy.

Data regarding therapy for patients with disease progression following next-generation ALK TKI as front-line is limited. Lorlatinib is known to inhibit several of the resistant mutations, including G1202R, a common mutation observed in tumors resistant to next-generation ALK inhibitors. In a phase II study, the agent demonstrated a response rate of approximately 37% in patients who had received a next-generation ALK TKI.[25] Preclinical data suggest that the activity of lorlatinib following next-generation ALK inhibitors maybe superior in patients with tumors that have ALK-related mechanisms of resistance than in patients with tumors that have non-ALK-dependent resistance mechanisms.[25] Preliminary clinical data support this preclinical observation. Lorlatinib is currently not approved but is likely to be approved in the United States in the coming months. Ensartinib has also demonstrated activity in this patient population. Among 19 response evaluable patients, 5 (26%) achieved a partial response and 6 (32%) achieved stable disease.[36]

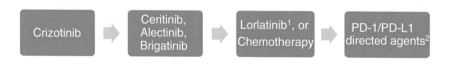

In patients with limited metastatic sites (≤ 3sites) at diagnosis or at progression local ablative therapy with continuation of systemic therapy can be considered.

1. Lorlatinib has received FDA breakthrough designation but not yet approved.
2. PD-1 directed agents should be considered before systemic chemotherapy only if patient's tumor is PD-L1 high. Otherwise after chemotherapy.

FIG. 8.1 Treatment schema with crizotinib as front-line therapy.

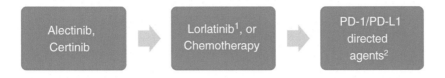

In patients with limited metastatic sites (≤ 3sites) at diagnosis or at progression local ablative therapy with continuation of systemic therapy can be considered.

1. Lorlatinib has received FDA breakthrough designation but not yet approved.
2. PD-1 directed agents should be considered before systemic chemotherapy only if patient's tumor is PD-L1 high. Otherwise after chemotherapy.

FIG. 8.2 Treatment schema with next-generation ALK inhibitor as front-line therapy.

NON-ALK-DIRECTED THERAPY

Many ALK patients eventually require non-ALK-directed therapy. The most common treatment utilized in this situation is chemotherapy. In ASCEND-4 and PROFILE-1014, platinum-pemetrexed combination in treatment naïve patients demonstrated a median PFS of 7–8 months. There are no prospective data with platinum-pemetrexed combination chemotherapy following treatment with ALK TKIs. The expectation is that this combination will provide similar benefit after ALK TKIs as in treatment naïve ALK positive NSCLC patients.

In recent years, immune checkpoint inhibitors have demonstrated clinical benefit in patients with recurrent NSCLC. However, the activity of these agents in ALK positive NSCLC patients has been disappointing. In the ATLANTIC trial, no responses were observed with durvalumab, a PD-L1 inhibitor in 15 ALK positive NSCLC patients.[37] Similarly, in a retrospective analysis from a single institution, Gainor et al., reported no responses in six ALK positive NSCLC patients.[38] In the same study, they found that proportion of ALK tumors with PD-L1 expression was no different from ALK wild-type NSCLCs. Despite PD-L1 expression, many EGFR and ALK tumors lacked CD8 infiltration in the tumor microenvironment. This disconnect between PD-L1 expression and relative lack of CD8 T cells may explain the limited clinical benefit observed with immune checkpoint inhibitors. Another marker that can predict for clinical benefit with these agents is tumor mutational burden (TMB). In a retrospective analysis, patients with tumors that had TMB-derived durable clinical benefit.[39] There were only two ALK positive patients in this series. Among EGFR patients, most tumors had low TMB and did not derive significant benefit. It is

expected that TMB profile of ALK tumors is similar to EGFR tumors and could also explain the low clinical benefit rate with immune checkpoint inhibitors in these patients. Based on the available data, chemotherapy is preferred over immune checkpoint inhibitors following therapy with ALK TKIs.

It is also important to note that studies that have evaluated immune checkpoint inhibitors as front-line either alone or in combination with other agents excluded patients with ALK gene rearranged NSCLC.[40] Therefore, in patients with ALK gene rearranged NSCLC, ALK TKI should be the front-line therapy even if the tumor PD-L1 expression is high. Recently, the results of the IMPOWER 150 trial demonstrated superior PFS with the addition of atezolizumab to the combination of carboplatin, paclitaxel, and bevacizumab. In this trial, patients with ALK rearranged or EGFR mutation positive NSCLC were eligible following treatment with TKIs.[41] In a subset analysis, improved clinical benefit was also observed in EGFR/ALK patients who received atezolizumab. If the atezolizumab combination is approved by regulatory authorities, this combination could be a therapeutic option for ALK positive NSCLC patients following ALK TKI therapy.

CENTRAL NERVOUS SYSTEM METASTASES

CNS is one of the major metastatic sites in advanced ALK positive NSCLC and is also a common site of disease progression. Recent trials suggest that at diagnosis, about 33%–39% of ALK positive NSCLC patients have evidence of CNS metastases.[30,33] The percentage of CNS metastases may be even higher at diagnosis because patients with symptomatic CNS metastases were excluded from these trials. Response rates in the CNS with agents such as alectinib were similar to overall response rates. Based on these data, patients with asymptomatic CNS metastases are treated with ALK TKIs rather than with CNS radiation therapy and ALK TKIs.

In patients who have disease progression in the CNS, with a drug like crizotinib, switch to a drug with activity in the brain is a consideration. Even in patients who develop progression in the CNS following a next-generation ALK TKI lorlatinib has demonstrated activity in the CNS.[25] CNS radiation therapy remains an option in these patients, but an important goal is to avoid whole brain radiation which can result in cognitive impairment.

MANAGEMENT OF PATIENTS WITH OLIGOMETASTATIC DISEASE

It is well recognized that some stage IV NSCLC patients have only few sites of metastases. The term oligometastatic cancer was first introduced by Hellman and Weichselbaum.[42] The definition of oligometastatic disease has varied. Most series have considered it to be less than four or five sites that can be treated by local ablative therapy. Patients may have oligometastatic disease at diagnosis or may be converted to an oligometastatic state with systemic therapy and finally may develop oligometastatic progression. There are data to suggest that integration of local ablative therapy in such patients may prolong disease control.

Limited data have shown that in ALK patients with oligometastatic progression, treatment of the sites with local ablative therapy followed by continuation of ALK TKI may prolong disease control.[43] This should be a consideration in patients who have limited disease progression while receiving an ALK TKI, particularly if the patient has derived prolonged control on the TKI before developing oligometastatic progression.

Local ablative therapy can also be considered as consolidation therapy in oligometastatic patients. Recently, the first randomized phase II study of oligometastatic NSCLC was reported. Patients with ≤3 metastatic sites following systemic therapy were randomized to local ablative therapy followed by continuation of systemic therapy or maintenance systemic therapy alone.[44] In this study of only 49 patients, improved PFS and improved time to new site of failure were observed in patients who received local ablative therapy. Future studies with larger patient numbers will need to be conducted for this approach to be considered as standard of care.

EARLY-STAGE AND LOCALLY ADVANCED ALK POSITIVE NSCLC

There is a desire to incorporate targeted therapy in the management of earlier stages of NSCLC. However, to date there is no evidence that addition of targeted therapy to standard of care management of earlier stages of ALK positive NSCLC provides superior clinical outcomes. Currently, the ALCHEMIST trial sponsored by NCI is evaluating the presence of ALK gene rearrangement in early-stage NSCLC patients (NCT02194738). A companion trial is evaluating the role of adjuvant crizotinib in ALK positive NSCLC patients following surgery and adjuvant chemotherapy (NCT02201992). The accrual to this arm of the study has been slow. It is possible that tumor biology of ALK gene rearrangements dictates that it is more commonly present with advanced-stage lung cancer. It is also possible that since these patients tend to be younger, the diagnosis of lung cancer is delayed in these patients.

Based on the clinical observation that complete responses are very uncommon with ALK TKIs, there is a perception that these drugs are unable to eradicate every last cancer cell. Therefore adjuvant use of ALK TKIs may improve disease-free survival but may not necessarily improve overall survival, an important objective of adjuvant therapy. Based on lack of data and concerns that ALK TKIs may not eradicate the disease adjuvant ALK TKI in an early-stage ALK positive NSCLC is not considered standard of care.

FUTURE DIRECTIONS

Over the last 10 years the therapy for ALK positive NSCLC has evolved considerably. Clinical trials have established ALK TKI as the standard of care for frontline therapy of advanced ALK positive NSCLC patients, and there are several ALK TKIs available that can provide clinical benefit in patients previously treated with a different AL inhibitor. Despite these advances the current therapy of ALK positive NSCLC is not based on detailed understanding of the patient's tumor and is largely empiric. Further improvements in the outcomes of ALK positive NSCLC patients are likely to occur with smart selection of combination treatments based on a comprehensive analysis of the molecular profile of the patient's tumor.[35] Another challenge is to develop immunotherapy that can be effective in this patient population and integration of such immunotherapy with targeted therapy.

REFERENCES

1. Soda M, Choi YL, Enomoto M, et al. Identification of the transforming EML4-ALK fusion gene in non-small-cell lung cancer. *Nature.* 2007;448:561−566.
2. Lin JJ, Zhu VW, Yoda S, et al. Impact of EML4-ALK variant on resistance mechanisms and clinical outcomes in ALK-positive lung cancer. *J Clin Oncol.* 2018;36:1119−1206.
3. Takeuchi K, Choi YL, Togashi Y, et al. KIF5B-ALK, a novel fusion oncokinase identified by an immunohistochemistry-based diagnostic system for ALK-positive lung cancer. *Clin Cancer Res.* 2009;15:3143−3149.
4. Rikova K, Guo A, Zeng Q, et al. Global survey of phospho-tyrosine signaling identifies oncogenic kinases in lung cancer. *Cell.* 2007;131:1190−1203.
5. Shaw AT, Yeap BY, Mino-Kenudson M, et al. Clinical features and outcome of patients with non-small-cell lung cancer who harbor EML4-ALK. *J Clin Oncol.* 2009;27(26):4247−4253.
6. Rodig SJ, Mino-Kenudson M, Dacic S, et al. Unique clinicopathologic features characterize ALK-rearranged lung adenocarcinoma in the western population. *Clin Cancer Res.* 2009;15:5216−5223.
7. Shaw AT, Solomon B, Kenudson MM. Crizotinib and testing for ALK. *J Natl Compr Canc Netw.* 2011;9:1335−1341.
8. Lindeman NI, Cagle PT, Aisner DL, et al. Updated molecular testing guideline for the selection of lung cancer patients for treatment with targeted tyrosine kinase inhibitors: guideline from the College of American Pathologists, the International Association for the Study of Lung Cancer, and the Association for Molecular Pathology. *J Thorac Oncol.* 2018;142:321−346.
9. Cabillic F, Gros A, Dugay F, et al. Parallel FISH and immunohistochemical studies of ALK status in 3244 non-small-cell lung cancers reveal major discordances. *J Thorac Oncol.* 2014;9:295−306.
10. Kwak EL, Bang YJ, Camidge DR, et al. Anaplastic lymphoma kinase inhibition in non-small-cell lung cancer. *N Engl J Med.* 2010;363:1693−1703.
11. Shaw AT, Kim DW, Nakagawa K, et al. Crizotinib versus chemotherapy in advanced ALK-positive lung cancer. *N Engl J Med.* 2013;368:2385−2394.
12. Solomon BJ, Mok T, Kim DW, et al. First line crizotinib versus chemotherapy in ALK-positive lung cancer. *N Engl J Med.* 2014;371:2167−2177.
13. Mok TS, Kim D, Wu Y, et al. Overall survival for first line crizotinib versus chemotherapy in ALK+ lung cancer: updated results from PROFILE 1014. *Ann Oncol.* 2017;28(suppl 5):605−649. abstract LBA50.
14. Camidge DR, Pao W, Sequist LV. Acquired resistance to TKIs in solid tumors: learning from lung cancer. *Nat Rev Clin Oncol.* 2014;11:473−481.
15. Awad MM, Shaw AT. ALK inhibitors in non-small cell lung cancer: crizotinib and beyond. *Clin Adv Hematol Oncol.* 2014;12:429−439.
16. Costa DB, Shaw AT, Ou S-HI, et al. Clinical experience with crizotinib in patients with advanced alk-rearranged non-small-cell lung cancer and brain metastases. *J Clin Oncol.* 2015;33:1881−1888.
17. Costa DB, Kobayashi S, Pandya SS, et al. CSF concentration of the anaplastic lymphoma kinase inhibitor crizotinib. *J Clin Oncol.* 2011;29:e443−445.
18. Kodama T, Tsukaguchi T, Yoshida M, et al. Selective ALK inhibitor alectinib with potent antitumor activity in models of crizotinib resistance. *Cancer Lett.* 2014;351:215−221.
19. Kinoshita K, Asoh K, Furuichi N, et al. Design and synthesis of a highly selective and orally active and potent anaplastic lymphoma kinase inhibitor (CH5424802). *Bioorg Med Chem.* 2012;20:1271−1280.
20. Yang JC, Ou SI, De Petris L, et al. Pooled systemic efficacy and safety data from the pivotal phase II studies (NP28673 and NP28761) of alectinib in ALK-positive non-small cell lung cancer. *J Thorac Oncol.* 2017;12:1552−1560.
21. Shaw AT, Kim D-W, Mehra R, et al. Ceritinib in ALK-rearranged non-small-cell lung cancer. *N Engl J Med.* 2014;370:1189−1197.
22. Ahn M, Camidge DR, Tiseo M, et al. Brigatinib in crizotinib-refractory ALK+ NSCLC: updated efficacy and safety results from ALTA, a randomised phase 2 trial. *J Thorac Oncol.* 2017;12(suppl 2):S1755−S1756. abstract OA 05.05.
23. Shaw AT, Kim TM, Crino L, et al. Ceritinib versus chemotherapy in patients with ALK-rearranged non-small-cell lung cancer previously given chemotherapy and crizotinib (ASCEND-5): a randomised, controlled, open-label, phase 3 trial. *Lancet Oncol.* 2017;18:874−886.
24. Wolf J, Mazieres J, Oh I, et al. Primary results from the phase III ALUR study of alectinib versus chemotherapy in previously treated alk+ non-small-cell lung cancer. *Ann Oncol.* 2017;28(suppl 5). abstract 12990_PR.
25. Solomon B, Shaw A, Ou S, et al. Phase 2 study of lorlatinib in patients with advanced ALK$^+$/ROS$^+$ non-small-cell lung cancer. *J Thorac Oncol.* 2017;12(suppl 2):11. abstract OA 05.06.
26. Horn L, Infante JR, Reckamp KL, et al. Ensartinib (X-396) in ALK-positive non-small cell lung cancer: results from a first-in-human phase I/II, multicenter study. *Clin Cancer Res.* 2018;24(12):2771−2779.
27. Tamura T, Kiura K, Seto T, et al. Three-year follow-up of an alectinib phase I/II study in ALK-positive non-small cell lung cancer: AF-001 JP. *J Clin Oncol.* 2017;35:1515−1521.
28. Nishio M, Kiura K, Seto T, et al. Final result of phase I/II study (AF-001JP) of alectinib, a selective CNS-active ALK inhibitor, in ALK+NSCLC patients. *J Thorac Oncol.* 2017;12(suppl 2):S1757. abstract OA 05.08.
29. Hida T, Nokihara H, Kondo M, et al. Alectinib versus crizotinib in patients with ALK positive non-small-cell lung cancer (J-ALEX): an open-label, randomized phase 3 trial. *Lancet.* 2017;390:29−39.

30. Peters S, Camidge DR, Shaw AT, et al. Alectinib versus crizotinib in untreated ALK-positive non-small-cell lung cancer. *N Engl J Med.* 2017;377:829–838.

31. Gadgeel SM, Gandhi L, Riely GJ, et al. Safety and activity of alectinib against systemic disease and brain metastases in patients with crizotinib-resistant ALK-rearranged non-small-cell lung cancer (AF-002 JG): results from the dose finding portion of a phase 1/2 study. *Lancet Oncol.* 2014; 15:1119–1128.

32. Gadgeel S, Peters S, Mok T, et al. Alectinib vs crizotinib in treatment naïve ALK+ NSCLC: CNS efficacy results from the ALEX trial. *Ann Oncol.* 2017;28(suppl 5). abstract 12980_PR.

33. Soria JC, Tan DSW, Chiari R, et al. First-line ceritinib versus platinum-based chemotherapy in advanced ALK-rearranged non-small-cell lung cancer (ASCEND-4): a randomized, open-label, phase 3 study. *Lancet.* 2017;389: 917–929.

34. Cho B, Obermannova R, Bearz A, et al. Efficacy and updated safety of ceritinib (450 mg or 600 mg) with low-fat meal vs 750 mg fasted in ALK+ metastatic NSCLC. *J Thorac Oncol.* 2017;12(11 suppl 2):S1757. abstract OA 05.07.

35. Gainor JF, Dardaei L, Yoda S, et al. Molecular mechanisms of resistance to first- and second-generation ALK inhibitors in ALK-rearranged lung cancer. *Cancer Discov.* 2016;6: 1118–1133.

36. Horn L, Leal TA, Oxnard G, et al. Activity of ensartinib after second generation anaplatic lymphoma kinase (ALK) tyrosine kinase inhibitors (TKI). *J Thorac Oncol.* 2017;12: S1556. abstract OA03.08.

37. Garassino MC, Cho BC, Kim JH, et al. Durvalumab as third line or later treatment for advanced non-small cell lung cancer (ATLANTIC): an open-label, single-arm, phase 2 study. *Lancet Oncol.* 2018;19:521–536.

38. Gainor J, Shaw AT, Sequist LV, et al. EGFR mutations and ALK rearrangements are associated with low response rates to PD-1 pathway blockade in non-small cell lung cancer. *Clin Cancer Res.* 2016;22:4585–4593.

39. Rizvi H, Sanchez-Vega F, La K, et al. Molecular determinants of response to anti-programmed cell death (PD)-1 and anti-programmed death-ligand 1 (PD-L1) blockade in patients with non-small-cell lung cancer profiled with targeted next-generation sequencing. *J Clin Oncol.* 2018; 36:633–641.

40. Gandhi L, Delvys Rodríguez-Abreu MD, Gadgeel S, et al. Pembrolizumab plus chemotherapy in metastatic non-small-cell lung cancer. *N Engl J Med.* 2018;378: 2078–2092.

41. Reck M, Socinski M, Capuzzo F, et al. Primary PFS and safety analyses of a randomised phase III study of carboplatin + paclitaxel ± bevacizumab, with or without atezolizumab in 1L non-squamous metastatic nsclc. (IMPOWER 150). *Ann Oncol.* 2017;28(suppl 11). abstract LBA1_PR.

42. Hellman S, Weichselbaum RR. Oligometastases. *J Clin Oncol.* 1995;13:8–10.

43. Gan GN, Weickhardt AJ, Scheier B, et al. Stereotactic radiation therapy can safely and durably control sites of extra-central nervous system oligoprogressive disease in anaplastic lymphoma kinase-positive lung cancer patients receiving crizotinib. *Int J Radiat Oncol Biol Phys.* 2014;88: 892–898.

44. Gomez DR, Blumenschein GR, Lee JJ, et al. Local consolidative therapy versus maintenance therapy or observation for patients with oligometastatic non-small-cell lung cancer without progression after first-line systemic therapy: a multicentre, randomised, controlled, phase 2 study. *Lancet Oncol.* 2016;17:1672–1682.

Targeted Therapy in Non—Small-Cell Lung Cancer (Beyond Epidermal Growth Factor Receptor and Anaplastic Lymphoma Kinase)

EMILY DICKINSON • DAN ZHAO, MD, PHD • KAREN L. RECKAMP, MD, MS

INTRODUCTION

Lung cancer is the most common cause of cancer-related death in both men and women in the United States, accounting for more deaths each year than breast, colon, prostate, and pancreatic cancers combined. Over 200,000 new cases of lung cancer were estimated in 2017, representing 14% of all new cancer cases.[1] The 5-year survival remains low because most patients are diagnosed with advanced stage disease. Approximately 80% of lung cancers are related to carcinogens in tobacco smoke, but understanding the molecular basis of lung cancer in "never smokers" is improving. Lung cancer is a heterogeneous genomic disease defined by molecular pathways that mediate oncogenesis, which are often driven by genetic alterations, and targeted therapies are available to modulate these pathways and improve patient outcomes.[2]

Genetic alterations in non—small-cell lung cancer (NSCLC) have led the field of oncology in our understanding of driver oncogenes and the potential of targeted therapy alter the course of the disease. Activating mutations in the *epidermal growth factor receptor* (*EGFR*) gene have been associated with improved progression-free survival (PFS) when patients are treated with EGFR tyrosine kinase inhibitor (TKI) therapy.[3] The use of clinical characteristics such as smoking status, ethnicity, and tumor histology was found to be associated with *EGFR* mutation, but only the genetic data accurately informed the appropriate treatment for patients. From this knowledge our understanding of additional mutations and gene alterations in NSCLC and other cancers has grown, and the number of targeted therapies approved for NSCLC grows each year. New genetic alterations have been described with potential therapeutic interventions, and more than 60% of patients with the adenocarcinoma subtype of NSCLC have a defined molecular alteration.[4] Targetable alterations beyond *EGFR* and *anaplastic lymphoma kinase* (*ALK*) demonstrate the complexities within the disease called lung cancer, and precision therapy is necessary to extend the survival for patients.

ROS1

ROS1 is made up of a glycoprotein-rich extracellular domain, a transmembrane domain, and an intracellular tyrosine kinase and is located on chromosome 6. A ligand for ROS1 has not been identified. *ROS1* gene rearrangements were initially defined in glioblastoma and now are recognized in a number of malignancies, including NSCLC.[5] In NSCLC, *ROS1* fusions occur in 1%—2%, and multiple fusion partners have been identified, but all involve ROS1 break points that conserve the tyrosine kinase domain. Potent oncogenic transformation occurs through constitutive kinase activation.

Patients with *ROS1* fusions are similar to those with *ALK* gene rearrangement, associated with younger age, never smoking history, Asian ethnicity, advanced stage, and adenocarcinoma subtype, although ROS1 has also been seen in large cell and squamous cell histologies.[6] Both ROS1 and ALK share significant homology within their tyrosine kinase domains, and preclinical studies revealed significant activity of crizotinib in cell lines with *ROS1* rearrangements.

A single-arm phase II trial that investigated crizotinib in 50 patients with *ROS1* gene rearrangement revealed an objective response rate (ORR) of 72% (95% confidence interval [CI], 58%–84%), and a median PFS of 19.2 months (95% CI, 14.4 months to not reached).[7] A second study of 30 patients with *ROS1* gene rearrangement revealed an ORR of 80% and a median PFS of 9.1 months.[8] Both of these trials are small but demonstrate significant activity of crizotinib in patients NSCLC with *ROS1* rearrangements. Ceritinib is a more selective inhibitor of *ALK*, and preclinical studies demonstrated activity in *ROS1* NSCLC. An open-label, phase II trial was performed in 32 patients with advanced NSCLC with ROS1 gene rearrangement, and 30 were crizotinib naïve.[9] The ORR was 62% (95% CI, 45%–77%), and a median PFS was 9.3 months (95% CI, 0–22 months), indicating clinical activity.

Resistance can also occur, and a patient with a *CD74-ROS1* rearrangement treated with crizotinib subsequently developed a point mutation G2032R, leading to resistance.[10] Preclinical data suggest that the multitargeted TKI cabozantinib can overcome this resistance in NSCLC.[11] Furthermore, a resistance D2033N mutation was reported in a patient with *CD74-ROS1* rearrangement, and the patient experienced rapid clinical and radiographic response to treatment with cabozantinib.[12] Further work is needed to understand and overcome resistance in *ROS1*-rearranged NSCLC.

BRAF

The *BRAF* proto-oncogene encodes for a serine/threonine protein kinase that leads to signaling through the mitogen-activated protein kinase (MAPK) pathway. *BRAF* mutations, mainly V600E, were initially described as driver mutations in melanoma, and subsequently mutant *BRAF* was shown to mediate oncogenesis in lung adenocarcinoma.[13] *BRAF* mutations are detected in approximately 2%–3% of adenocarcinoma of the lung and are more frequently detected in patients with a history of tobacco use, and approximately 50%–75% of the *BRAF* mutations are the *BRAF* V600E mutation seen in melanoma.[4,14,15]

Similar to the activity seen in *BRAF* V600E–mutated melanoma, vemurafenib[16] and dabrafenib[17] have demonstrated efficacy in patients with metastatic NSCLC who harbor a *BRAF* V600E mutation.[18] A phase II trial investigated dabrafenib in 84 patients with metastatic *BRAF* V600E–mutant NSCLC.[19] The ORR was 33% (95% CI, 23%–45%), and the median overall survival

(OS) was 12.7 months (95% CI, 7.3–16.9 months). Owing to previously described MAPK/extracellular signal–regulated kinase (MEK) dependency in *BRAF* cells[20] and the activity of BRAF inhibitors in combination with MEK inhibitors seen in *BRAF* V600E melanoma, the combination of dabrafenib and trametinib was investigated in a single-arm phase II trial in 59 patients with *BRAF* V600E–mutant NSCLC.[21] The ORR was 63.2% (95% CI, 49.3%–75.6%) and PFS was 9.7 months (95% CI, 6.9–19.6 months). These data led to the Food and Drug Administration approval of the combination therapy for patients with NSCLC with a *BRAF* V600E mutation.

MESENCHYMAL–EPITHELIAL TRANSITION

Mesenchymal–epithelial transition (MET) is a proto-oncogene of a transmembrane receptor tyrosine kinase and binds to the ligand scatter factor/hepatocyte growth factor, which actives the MAPK, phosphoinositide 3-kinase/AKT, signal transducer and activator of transcription proteins, and nuclear factor kappa B signaling cascades, thus promoting proliferation, blocking apoptosis, and increasing cell motility.[22-25] MET pathway alterations are found in multiple cancers, including lung cancer. Mechanisms by which MET leads to tumor growth include protein overexpression and phosphorylation, gene amplification, rearrangement, and mutations.[26]

Overexpression of MET is found in 35%–72% of the NSCLC, and p-MET can be found in 67% of the NSCLC, while amplification of *MET* is seen in approximately 2%–5% of newly diagnosed adenocarcinoma.[27,28] *MET* gene copy number is a negative prognosis factor in surgically resected NSCLC, with OS of 25.5 months for patients with MET ≥5 copies/cell compared with 47.5 months for patients with MET<5 copies/cell (*P* = .0045).[27] *MET* gene rearrangement is uncommon, but the kinase fusion *KIF5B-MET* has been reported in lung adenocarcinoma.[29]

MET exon 14 alterations are a diverse group of alterations that drive tumorigenesis and are found in approximately 4% of lung adenocarcinomas.[28] The alteration is more common in older patients, with a median age of 73 years, and patients are less likely to be heavy smokers.[30] The mutations lead to exon 14 skipping, impaired receptor degradation, and oncogenic transformation.[31,32] Exon 14 encodes the juxtamembrane domain of the protein, which is the binding site for E3 ubiquitin ligase for protein degradation. *MET* exon 14 alterations have been shown to interrupt the mRNA splicing process before transcription into a protein, which controls gene regulation and leads to dysregulation of protein synthesis. The alterations in *MET* exon 14 vary widely, with base substitutions and deletions that alter the branch point of intron 13, the splice site of intron 13, or the ending splice site of intron 14.[33]

Currently there are multiple MET inhibitors under investigation, including small molecule multitargeted TKIs, such as cabozantinib, crizotinib, glesatinib, merestinib, and S49076, and others with increased MET specificity, such as savolitinib, tepotinib, capmatinib, SAR125844, sitravatinib, AMG 337, and tivantinib. Monoclonal antibodies have also been studied in patients with MET-driven tumors. Crizotinib is a dual MET and ALK inhibitor that has demonstrated responses in *MET*-amplified and *MET*-mutated NSCLC.[34,35] In addition, tumor response to crizotinib and cabozantinib has been reported in patients with lung adenocarcinoma with exon 14 alterations.[36] Overexpression or phosphorylation of MET has not been consistently predictive of response to MET inhibitors, based on multiple trials. Targeting the MET pathway appears promising; however, alterations and responses to targeted therapy have been varied, so identification of the appropriate biomarkers and cut points is needed in future investigation.

It has been reported that *MET* amplification can increase to 5%–22% after treatment with EGFR TKI therapy (erlotinib and gefitinib).[37] Amplification of *MET* has also been shown to be an alternative mechanism of resistance to EGFR TKIs in patients with EGFR mutation–positive NSCLC, leading to ERBB3 signaling.[38] Combination of MET and EGFR TKI therapy is being studied as a treatment option for patients with resistant *EGFR*–mutant NSCLC.

RET

RET is a receptor tyrosine kinase that mediates neural crest development, and alterations in *RET* have been described in thyroid and lung cancers, among others. *RET* fusions were first described in NSCLC in 2012 and occur in approximately 1%–2% of patients.[39-42] The fusions are more likely to be found in patients who have minimal to no history of smoking, younger age (≤60 years), and more poorly differentiated histology.[39] The most common fusion partner is *KIF5B*, and gene rearrangement leads to ligand-independent dimerization and downstream growth pathway activation.[41] In a study of patients undergoing next-generation sequencing, *RET* gene status was evaluated in more than 4800 patients with diverse malignancies and

occurred in 1.8%, with the majority of cases having coexisting, actionable genomic alterations.[43]

Cabozantinib is a multitargeted TKI that also has activity against RET.[44] A phase II trial enrolled 26 patients with *RET*-rearranged lung adenocarcinoma and found a 28% ORR (95% CI, 12%–49%) with a median PFS of 5.5 months (95% CI, 3.8–8.4 months) and median OS 9.9 months (95% CI, 8.1 to not reached months).[45] A phase II study investigating vandetanib in 19 *RET* fusion–positive patients was performed.[46] The ORR was 53% (95% CI, 28%–77%), and the median PFS was 4.7 months (95% CI, 2.8–8.5 months). These trials suggest activity of the inhibitors in *RET*-rearranged NSCLC but for most, responses are short lived.

A global registry described treatment of 165 patients with *RET*-rearranged NSCLC, of which 53 had been treated with one or more RET inhibitors.[47] The ORR for cabozantinib, sunitinib, and vandetanib was 37%, 22%, and 18%, respectively; and tumor responses were also seen with lenvatinib and nintedanib. In this population a median PFS of 2.3 months (95% CI, 1.6–5.0 months) and a median OS of 6.8 months (95% CI, 3.9–14.3 months) were observed. The response rate to multitargeted TKI therapy has been modest, and RET-specific inhibitors are currently being evaluated in the clinic.

HUMAN EPIDERMAL GROWTH FACTOR RECEPTOR 2

Human epidermal growth factor receptor 2 (HER2) is activated through homodimerization or heterodimerization with EGFR or HER3 to interact with downstream signaling pathways resulting in tumorigenesis.[48] *HER2* amplification is infrequently found, and exon 20 insertion mutations in *HER2* are seen in about 2% of NSCLC.[49] The mutation has been observed primarily in female patients, nonsmokers, and those with adenocarcinoma histology.[50] Small series and case reports of treatment with HER2 inhibitors (trastuzumab)[51] and pan-HER inhibitors (afatinib, lapatinib, dacomitinib)[52-55] have shown some tumor regression and disease control.

A retrospective study across European centers evaluated patients treated with chemotherapy or HER2-targeted therapy, and 101 patients were assessed.[56] Patients received a median number of three lines of therapy for advanced NSCLC. The median OS was 24 months for all patients, regardless of therapy received. For patients who received conventional chemotherapy without HER2-directed therapy, the

ORR was 43.5% for first-line and 10% for second-line therapy, and PFS was 6 months for first-line and 4.3 months for second-line therapy. Sixty-five patients received HER2-targeted therapy (trastuzumab, neratinib, afatinib, lapatinib, ado-trastuzumab emtansine [T-DM1]), and ORR was highest for those who received trastuzumab with or without chemotherapy or T-DM1 at 50.9% with PFS 4.8 months. The largest prospective study in patients with *HER2* aberrations in NSCLC was performed with dacomitinib.[57] In this phase II trial, 30 patients with HER2-mutant or HER2-amplified tumors were enrolled, and 26 had mutation. Dacomitinib treatment resulted in an ORR of 12% (95% CI, 2% −30%). In the four patients with HER2 amplification, no responses were observed. Additional studies are investigating T-DM1 and pertuzumab/trastuzumab combination therapy in patients with HER2-altered NSCLC with mixed results. The appropriate biomarker for selection remains elusive in this group of patients, and mutation may be most predictive of response to HER2-directed therapy.

NEUROTROPHIN TYROSINE RECEPTOR KINASE−MUTATED NSCLC

Tropomyosin-related kinase (TRK) is a receptor tyrosine kinase family of neurotrophin receptors found in multiple tissues.[58] The genetic family is involved in neuronal synapse development and memory. Three members of the family are proto-oncogenes encoded by neurotrophin tyrosine kinase receptor *(NTRK) 1, NTRK2,* and *NTRK3.* Neural growth factor is the ligand for TRKA; brain deprived growth factor is the ligand for TRKB; neurotrophin 3 is the ligand for TRKC. The binding of these ligands activates several cellular pathways, including MAPK and AKT.[59] *NTRK* fusions occur in all three genes across multiple malignancies, and were first described in colon cancer.[60] The gene rearrangements result in the activation of the cellular pathways leading to cell proliferation, differentiation, and survival. *NTRK* rearrangements have been identified in multiple types of cancer, including lung cancer,[61] and the prevalence of *NTRK* fusions in NSCLC is <1%.

Doeble et al. described the first patient with *NTRK* fusion to demonstrate tumor regression with a selective TRK inhibitor, larotrectinib (LOXO-101). The patient with soft tissue sarcoma was enrolled in the phase I trial and was found to have an *LMNA-NTRK1* gene fusion encoding an LMNA-TRKA fusion oncoprotein and experienced tumor reduction and clinical symptom improvement within 4 weeks.[62] Preclinical models showed inhibition of the tumor growth in vitro and in vivo. A phase I trial investigated larotrectinib in patients with *NTRK* fusions across tumor types in both pediatric and adult patients.[63] Fifty-five patients were enrolled (43 adult and 12 pediatric), and the most common fusions seen were *NTRK3* (n = 29), followed by *NTRK1* (n = 25) and *NTRK2* (n = 1), with 14 unique fusion partners. Patients with 13 tumor types were treated, and the ORR was 78% (95% CI, 64%−89%), and the median duration of response had not been reached at the time of presentation. Because this is a rare event in many tumor types, screening tests for TRK by immunohistochemistry have been developed for a more rapid assessment.[64] Additional TRK inhibitors are under investigation in the clinic and have demonstrated tumor responses.

CONCLUSIONS

Clinical studies and molecular genotyping have delineated the heterogeneity of lung tumorigenesis and the inadequacy of the concept of "one size fits all" in diagnosis and therapy. The establishment of predictive genomic "drivers" has led to improvements in therapy for patients. Molecular selection clearly identifies specific populations that derive enhanced benefit from targeted treatment and provide insight into our understanding of potential resistance to therapy. Despite the progress that has been made, work is necessary to untangle the complex causes for primary and secondary resistance to therapy to make a dramatic impact on treatment for more individuals with lung cancer. Furthermore, our knowledge of signaling pathways in lung cancer must acknowledge interactions within the tumor microenvironment and the importance of immune modulation. Evaluation of combination treatment in select populations involving targeted therapy, immunotherapy, and/or chemotherapy may bring optimal treatment to patients.

REFERENCES

1. Siegel RL, Miller KD, Jemal A. Cancer Statistics, 2017. *CA A Cancer Journal Clinicians.* January 2017;67(1):7−30.
2. Govindan R, Ding L, Griffith M, et al. Genomic landscape of non-small cell lung cancer in smokers and never-smokers. *Cell.* September 14, 2012;150(6):1121−1134.
3. Mok TS, Wu YL, Thongprasert S, et al. Gefitinib or carboplatin-paclitaxel in pulmonary adenocarcinoma. *N Engl J Med.* September 3, 2009;361(10):947−957.

4. Kris MG, Johnson BE, Berry LD, et al. Using multiplexed assays of oncogenic drivers in lung cancers to select targeted drugs. *JAMA The Journal Am Med Assoc.* May 21, 2014;311(19):1998–2006.

5. Rikova K, Guo A, Zeng Q, et al. Global survey of phosphotyrosine signaling identifies oncogenic kinases in lung cancer. *Cell.* December 14, 2007;131(6):1190–1203.

6. Bergethon K, Shaw AT, Ignatius Ou SH, et al. ROS1 rearrangements define a unique molecular Class of lung cancers. *J Clin Oncol.* Mar 10, 2012;30(8):863–870.

7. Shaw AT, Solomon BJ. Crizotinib in ROS1-rearranged non-small-cell lung cancer. *N Engl J Med.* February 12, 2015;372(7):683–684.

8. Mazieres J, Zalcman G, Crino L, et al. Crizotinib therapy for advanced lung adenocarcinoma and a ROS1 rearrangement: results from the EUROS1 cohort. *J Clin Oncol.* March 20, 2015;33(9):992–999.

9. Lim SM, Kim HR, Lee JS, et al. Open-label, Multicenter, phase II study of ceritinib in patients with non-small-cell lung cancer harboring ROS1 rearrangement. *J Clin Oncol.* August 10, 2017;35(23):2613–2618.

10. Awad MM, Katayama R, McTigue M, et al. Acquired resistance to crizotinib from a mutation in CD74-ROS1. *N Engl J Med.* June 20, 2013;368(25):2395–2401.

11. Katayama R, Kobayashi Y, Friboulet L, et al. Cabozantinib overcomes crizotinib resistance in ROS1 fusion-positive cancer. *Clin Cancer Research An Official Journal Am Assoc Cancer Res.* JaSn 1 2015;21(1):166–174.

12. Drilon A, Somwar R, Wagner JP, et al. A Novel crizotinib-resistant Solvent-Front mutation responsive to cabozantinib therapy in a patient with ROS1-rearranged lung cancer. *Clin Cancer Research An Official Journal Am Assoc Cancer Res.* May 15, 2016;22(10):2351–2358.

13. Davies H, Bignell GR, Cox C, et al. Mutations of the BRAF gene in human cancer. *Nature.* June 27, 2002;417(6892):949–954.

14. Paik PK, Arcila ME, Fara M, et al. Clinical characteristics of patients with lung adenocarcinomas harboring BRAF mutations. *J Clin Oncol.* May 20, 2011;29(15):2046–2051.

15. Litvak AM, Paik PK, Woo KM, et al. Clinical characteristics and course of 63 patients with BRAF mutant lung cancers. *J Thoracic Oncology Official Publication Int Assoc Study Lung Cancer.* November 2014;9(11):1669–1674.

16. Gautschi O, Pauli C, Strobel K, et al. A patient with BRAF V600E lung adenocarcinoma responding to vemurafenib. *J Thoracic Oncology Official Publication Int Assoc Study Lung Cancer.* October 2012;7(10):e23–24.

17. Rudin CM, Hong K, Streit M. Molecular characterization of acquired resistance to the BRAF inhibitor dabrafenib in a patient with BRAF-mutant non-small-cell lung cancer. *J Thoracic Oncology Official Publication Int Assoc Study Lung Cancer.* May 2013;8(5):e41–42.

18. Hyman DM, Puzanov I, Subbiah V, et al. Vemurafenib in multiple Nonmelanoma cancers with BRAF V600 mutations. *N Engl J Med.* August 20, 2015;373(8):726–736.

19. Planchard D, Kim TM, Mazieres J, et al. Dabrafenib in patients with BRAF(V600E)-positive advanced non-small-cell lung cancer: a single-arm, multicentre, open-label, phase 2 trial. *The Lancet Oncol.* May 2016;17(5):642–650.

20. Solit DB, Garraway LA, Pratilas CA, et al. BRAF mutation predicts sensitivity to MEK inhibition. *Nature.* January 19, 2006;439(7074):358–362.

21. Planchard D, Besse B, Groen HJM, et al. Dabrafenib plus trametinib in patients with previously treated BRAF(V600E)-mutant metastatic non-small cell lung cancer: an open-label, multicentre phase 2 trial. *The Lancet Oncol.* July 2016;17(7):984–993.

22. Cooper CS, Park M, Blair DG, et al. Molecular cloning of a new transforming gene from a chemically transformed human cell line. *Nature.* September 6-11, 1984;311(5981):29–33.

23. Giordano S, Ponzetto C, Di Renzo MF, Cooper CS, Comoglio PM. Tyrosine kinase receptor indistinguishable from the c-met protein. *Nature.* May 11, 1989;339(6220):155–156.

24. Bottaro DP, Rubin JS, Faletto DL, et al. Identification of the hepatocyte growth factor receptor as the c-met proto-oncogene product. *Science.* February 15, 1991;251(4995):802–804.

25. Ponzetto C, Bardelli A, Zhen Z, et al. A multifunctional docking site mediates signaling and transformation by the hepatocyte growth factor/scatter factor receptor family. *Cell.* April 22, 1994;77(2):261–271.

26. Sadiq AA, Salgia R. MET as a possible target for non-small-cell lung cancer. *J Clin Oncol.* March 10, 2013;31(8):1089–1096.

27. Cappuzzo F, Marchetti A, Skokan M, et al. Increased MET gene copy number negatively affects survival of surgically resected non-small-cell lung cancer patients. *J Clin Oncol.* April 1, 2009;27(10):1667–1674.

28. Cancer Genome Atlas Research N. Comprehensive molecular profiling of lung adenocarcinoma. *Nature.* July 31, 2014;511(7511):543–550.

29. Stransky N, Cerami E, Schalm S, Kim JL, Lengauer C. The landscape of kinase fusions in cancer. *Nat Communications.* September 10, 2014;5:4846.

30. Awad MM, Oxnard GR, Jackman DM, et al. MET exon 14 mutations in non-small-cell lung cancer are associated with advanced age and stage-dependent MET genomic amplification and c-met overexpression. *J Clin Oncol.* March 1, 2016;34(7):721–730.

31. Awad MM. Impaired c-met receptor degradation mediated by MET exon 14 mutations in non-small-cell lung cancer. *J Clin Oncol.* March 10, 2016;34(8):879–881.

32. Drilon A. MET exon 14 alterations in lung cancer: exon skipping extends Half-Life. *Clin Cancer Research An Official Journal Am Assoc Cancer Res.* June 15, 2016;22(12):2832–2834.

33. Frampton GM, Ali SM, Rosenzweig M, et al. Activation of MET via diverse exon 14 splicing alterations occurs in multiple tumor types and confers clinical sensitivity to MET inhibitors. *Cancer Discovery.* August 2015;5(8):850–859.

34. Ou SH, Kwak EL, Siwak-Tapp C, et al. Activity of crizotinib (PF02341066), a dual mesenchymal-epithelial transition (MET) and anaplastic lymphoma kinase (ALK) inhibitor, in a non-small cell lung cancer patient with de novo MET amplification. *J Thoracic Oncology Official Publication Int Assoc Study Lung Cancer*. May 2011;6(5):942−946.

35. Mendenhall MA, Goldman JW. MET-mutated NSCLC with major response to crizotinib. *J Thoracic Oncology Official Publication Int Assoc Study Lung Cancer*. May 2015;10(5):e33−34.

36. Paik PK, Drilon A, Fan PD, et al. Response to MET inhibitors in patients with stage IV lung adenocarcinomas harboring MET mutations causing exon 14 skipping. *Cancer Discovery*. August 2015;5(8):842−849.

37. Bean J, Brennan C, Shih JY, et al. MET amplification occurs with or without T790M mutations in EGFR mutant lung tumors with acquired resistance to gefitinib or erlotinib. *Proc Natl Acad Sci U. S. A.* December 26, 2007;104(52):20932−20937.

38. Engelman JA, Zejnullahu K, Mitsudomi T, et al. MET amplification leads to gefitinib resistance in lung cancer by activating ERBB3 signaling. *Science*. May 18, 2007;316(5827):1039−1043.

39. Wang R, Hu H, Pan Y, et al. RET fusions define a unique molecular and clinicopathologic subtype of non-small-cell lung cancer. *J Clin Oncol*. December 10, 2012;30(35):4352−4359.

40. Li F, Feng Y, Fang R, et al. Identification of RET gene fusion by exon array analyses in "pan-negative" lung cancer from never smokers. *Cell Research*. May 2012;22(5):928−931.

41. Kohno T, Ichikawa H, Totoki Y, et al. KIF5B-RET fusions in lung adenocarcinoma. *Nat Medicine*. February 12, 2012;18(3):375−377.

42. Takeuchi K, Soda M, Togashi Y, et al. RET, ROS1 and ALK fusions in lung cancer. *Nat Medicine*. February 12, 2012;18(3):378−381.

43. Kato S, Subbiah V, Marchlik E, Elkin SK, Carter JL, Kurzrock R. RET aberrations in diverse cancers: next-generation sequencing of 4,871 patients. *Clin Cancer Research An Official Journal Am Assoc Cancer Res*. April 15, 2017;23(8):1988−1997.

44. Drilon A, Wang L, Hasanovic A, et al. Response to Cabozantinib in patients with RET fusion-positive lung adenocarcinomas. *Cancer Discovery*. June 2013;3(6):630−635.

45. Drilon A, Rekhtman N, Arcila M, et al. Cabozantinib in patients with advanced RET-rearranged non-small-cell lung cancer: an open-label, single-centre, phase 2, single-arm trial. *The Lancet Oncol*. December 2016;17(12):1653−1660.

46. Yoh K, Seto T, Satouchi M, et al. Vandetanib in patients with previously treated RET-rearranged advanced non-small-cell lung cancer (LURET): an open-label, multicentre phase 2 trial. *The Lancet Respir Medicine*. January 2017;5(1):42−50.

47. Gautschi O, Milia J, Filleron T, et al. Targeting RET in patients with RET-rearranged lung cancers: results from the global, Multicenter RET registry. *J Clin Oncol*. May 1, 2017;35(13):1403−1410.

48. Yarden Y, Sliwkowski MX. Untangling the ErbB signalling network. *Nat Reviews. Mol Cell Biology*. February 2001;2(2):127−137.

49. Shigematsu H, Takahashi T, Nomura M, et al. Somatic mutations of the HER2 kinase domain in lung adenocarcinomas. *Cancer Res*. March 1, 2005;65(5):1642−1646.

50. Mazieres J, Peters S, Lepage B, et al. Lung cancer that harbors an HER2 mutation: epidemiologic characteristics and therapeutic perspectives. *J Clin Oncol*. June 1, 2013;31(16):1997−2003.

51. Cappuzzo F, Bemis L, Varella-Garcia M. HER2 mutation and response to trastuzumab therapy in non-small-cell lung cancer. *N Engl J Med*. June 15, 2006;354(24):2619−2621.

52. De Greve J, Teugels E, Geers C, et al. Clinical activity of afatinib (BIBW 2992) in patients with lung adenocarcinoma with mutations in the kinase domain of HER2/neu. *Lung Cancer*. April 2012;76(1):123−127.

53. Kelly RJ, Carter CA, Giaccone G. HER2 mutations in non-small-cell lung cancer can be continually targeted. *J Clin Oncol*. September 10, 2012;30(26):3318−3319.

54. Lopez-Chavez A, Thomas A, Rajan A, et al. Molecular profiling and targeted therapy for advanced thoracic malignancies: a biomarker-derived, multiarm, multihistology phase II basket trial. *J Clin Oncol*. March 20, 2015;33(9):1000−1007.

55. Park CK, Hur JY, Choi CM, et al. Efficacy of afatinib in a previously-treated patient with non-small cell lung cancer harboring HER2 mutation: case report. *J Korean Medical Science*. January 1, 2018;33(1):e7.

56. Mazieres J, Barlesi F, Filleron T, et al. Lung cancer patients with HER2 mutations treated with chemotherapy and HER2-targeted drugs: results from the European EUHER2 cohort. *Ann Oncology Official Journal Eur Soc Med Oncol*. February 2016;27(2):281−286.

57. Kris MG, Camidge DR, Giaccone G, et al. Targeting HER2 aberrations as actionable drivers in lung cancers: phase II trial of the pan-HER tyrosine kinase inhibitor dacomitinib in patients with HER2-mutant or amplified tumors. *Ann Oncology Official Journal Eur Soc Med Oncol*. July 2015;26(7):1421−1427.

58. Nakagawara A. Trk receptor tyrosine kinases: a bridge between cancer and neural development. *Cancer Letters*. August 28, 2001;169(2):107−114.

59. Vaishnavi A, Le AT, Doebele RC. TRKing down an old oncogene in a new era of targeted therapy. *Cancer Discovery*. January 2015;5(1):25−34.

60. Martin-Zanca D, Hughes SH, Barbacid M. A human oncogene formed by the fusion of truncated tropomyosin and protein tyrosine kinase sequences. *Nature*. Feb 27-Mar 5 1986;319(6056):743−748.

61. Vaishnavi A, Capelletti M, Le AT, et al. Oncogenic and drug-sensitive NTRK1 rearrangements in lung cancer. *Nat Medicine.* November 2013;19(11):1469–1472.
62. Doebele RC, Davis LE, Vaishnavi A, et al. An oncogenic NTRK fusion in a patient with soft-tissue sarcoma with response to the tropomyosin-related kinase inhibitor LOXO-101. *Cancer Discovery.* October 2015;5(10): 1049–1057.
63. Hyman DM, Laetsch TW, Kummar S, et al. The efficacy of larotrectinib (LOXO-101), a selective tropomyosin receptor kinase (TRK) inhibitor, in adult and pediatric TRK fusion cancers. *J Clin Oncol.* 2017;35. suppl; abstr LBA2501.
64. Hechtman JF, Benayed R, Hyman DM, et al. Pan-trk immunohistochemistry is an Efficient and Reliable screen for the detection of NTRK fusions. *The Am Journal Surgical Pathology.* November 2017;41(11):1547–1551.

Treatment of Pulmonary Adenocarcinoma With Immune Checkpoint Inhibitors

RINA HUI, MBBS, PHD • MICHAEL MILLWARD, MBBS, MA

INTRODUCTION

The paradigm change in cancer treatment that unfolded with the successful development of immune checkpoint inhibitors in many tumor types has been most apparent in the treatment of melanoma and non–small cell lung cancer (NSCLC). Fundamental to this has been the recognition that cancer patients may develop a T cell–mediated immune response to cancer neoantigens and that successful eradication of cancer can be achieved by inhibiting specific negative regulators of the immune response that are activated by tumor cells in the microenvironment surrounding the cancer or more distant sites. The first such negative regulator, CLTA-4 (cytotoxic T lymphocyte–associated protein 4) inhibited by the antibody ipilimumab resulted in regulatory approval of this drug for metastatic melanoma in 2011 and for adjuvant therapy of high-risk stage III melanoma in 2015. However, CTLA-4 inhibitors did not achieve phase III success in NSCLC[1] or any other tumor type as a single agent or in combination with nonimmune-based therapies.

In contrast, the second negative regulator, namely, PD-1 (programmed cell death 1) and its chief ligand PD-L1 have each been targeted by multiple antibodies that have resulted in regulatory approval for NSCLC, melanoma, and multiple other tumor types as single agents. From clinical trials across NSCLC and other solid cancers, some common themes have emerged: (1) responses to immune checkpoint inhibitors occur in some but not all patients with advanced cancers; (2) responses are usually much more durable than obtained with systemic chemotherapy leading to a pronounced "tail" in progression-free and overall survival curves; (3) responses can occur in patients who have progressed on or after systemic chemotherapy; (4) responses may be preceded by radiologic evidence

of disease worsening including the appearance of new metastatic sites (now referred to as pseudoprogression); (5) responses are more likely in patients with features that are also predictive of benefit from chemotherapy or drugs targeting specific mutations (good performance status, lesser disease burden measured by radiologic summation of lesions or markers such as lactic dehydrogenase [LDH]) and (6) benefit from PD-1/PD-L1 targeting drugs can be variably predicted in different tumor types by expression of PD-L1 on tumor cells and/or immune cells in tumor biopsies; and (7) a spectrum of toxicities referred to as immune-related adverse events (ir-AEs) can affect many different organs most commonly the skin, gastrointestinal tract, lung, and endocrine system.

The current place of PD-1/PD-L1 checkpoint inhibitors in pulmonary adenocarcinoma therapy will be discussed in this chapter. A large majority of clinical trials have been done on "NSCLC" with stratification by histology (squamous cell carcinoma vs. nonsquamous). Trials involving only squamous cell carcinoma of the lung will not be discussed. Following this, we will highlight major ongoing trials that will provide hopefully the "second wave" of positive results extending the potential benefits of immunotherapy to the majority of NSCLC patients.

PREVIOUSLY TREATED ADVANCED NON–SMALL CELL LUNG CANCER

Antitumor activity following administration of the anti-PD1 immune checkpoint inhibitor nivolumab in heavily pretreated NSCLC was first published in 2012.[2] Subsequently, other phase I studies of drugs targeting the PD-1/PD-L1 checkpoint including anti-PD1 agent pembrolizumab and anti-PDL-1 agents atezolizumab, durvalumab, and avelumab, all demonstrated deep and durable responses in NSCLC patients who responded.[3–5] Table 10.1 illustrates promising clinical efficacy in a number of early phase studies with PD-1 blockade in heavily pretreated advanced NSCLC patients with objective response rate (ORR) ranging from 12% to 23%, median overall survival (OS) of 8.4–16 months, 1 year survival rate of 36%–63%, 2 year survival rate of 24%–30%, and 3 year survival rate of 18%–19%.[5–11]

There are now four randomized phase III studies demonstrating overall survival benefit over docetaxel (12.2–13.8 months vs. 8.5–9.6 months) in previously treated NSCLC, and three of the studies included pulmonary adenocarcinoma (Table 10.2).[12–14] The ORR was higher in patients receiving antibodies blocking the PD1 pathway than docetaxel, 14%–19% versus 9%–13%, but there was no difference in the median progression-free survival (PFS) in patients receiving the checkpoint inhibitors or docetaxel. This was mainly due to the fact that disease progression in substantial proportion of patients with heavily pretreated NSCLC would be expected within 6 or 9 weeks when the first response assessment was performed.

CheckMate 057 recruited 582 patients with only nonsquamous NSCLC. The updated data, with over 3-year median follow-up, demonstrated 3-year survival rate of 18% in patients who received nivolumab versus 9% in patients who received docetaxel with a hazard ratio (HR) of 0.73.[15] The other two studies recruited both squamous and nonsquamous NSCLC. With stratification by histology, 74% (628) of patients in the OAK study had nonsquamous NSCLC, and median overall survival in this subgroup receiving atezolizumab and docetaxel was 15.6 months and 11.2 months, respectively, with HR of 0.73.[14] In the KEYNOTE 010 study, all patients receiving either pembrolizumab or docetaxel needed to have PD-L1 of at least 1%,[13] while the other two studies recruited both PD-L1 positive and negative patients. Of 1034 patients in the KEYNOTE 010 study, 68.4% (708) had adenocarcinoma histology and HR for OS was 0.63 favoring pembrolizumab. The adjusted HR for OS by histology comparing nonsquamous with squamous in patients receiving pembrolizumab was 0.60 favoring nonsquamous with $P < .0001$.[16] Patients in KEYNOTE 010 were randomized to receive two doses of pembrolizumab 10 or 2 mg/kg or chemotherapy with docetaxel. There was no significant difference in clinical outcome with the two doses, consistent with the earlier reported data from KEYNOTE 001 showing no exposure dependency on efficacy or safety and supporting the use of 2 mg/kg dose of pembrolizumab.[17] All three randomized phase III studies demonstrated remarkable 2 year overall survival rate of around 30% in previously treated NSCLC patients with PD-1 blockade.[15,16,18] The large real-world experience in 1588 previously treated NSCLC patients receiving up to 2 years of nivolumab 3 mg/kg through the Italian Expanded Access Program was similar to the data from CheckMate 057 with an ORR of 18%, disease control rate (DCR) of 44%, 1 year OS rate of 48%, and median OS of 11.3 months.[19]

After failure of platinum-doublet chemotherapy and maintenance pemetrexed (or platinum-doublet chemotherapy with bevacizumab and maintenance bevacizumab) in patients with advanced pulmonary adenocarcinoma without oncogenic driver mutations, an anti-PD1 or anti-PD-L1 agent is now the established standard of care as second-line systemic treatment.

TREATMENT-NAÏVE ADVANCED NON–SMALL CELL LUNG CANCER
Early Phase Studies in Treatment-Naïve NSCLC

The longest follow-up data with first-line PD-1 blockade was from the KEYNOTE 001 study demonstrating impressive median overall survival of 22.3 months in 101 treatment-naïve advanced NSCLC patients unselected by PD-L1 status treated with pembrolizumab.[8] The subset of patients with nonsquamous NSCLC receiving first-line pembrolizumab had a median overall survival of 28.4 months and 3-year survival rate of 30.6%.[8] A smaller first-line study with nivolumab with shorter median follow-up also demonstrated similar median overall survival of 21.8 months in unselected patients with 1 and 2 year survival rates of 73% and 44%, respectively.[20] Both studies showed higher response rates and survival rates, longer median PFS and OS in patients with high level of PD-L1 expression of >50% (Table 10.3). First-line pembrolizumab provided response rate of 66.7% with median PFS of 12.5 months, median OS of 34.9 months, and 2 year survival rate of 66.7% in patients with high PD-L1 of at least 50% using DAKO 22C3 antibody.[8,21] A cohort of the BIRCH study recruited treatment-naïve advanced NSCLC patients, with at least 5% PD-L1 staining in tumor or immune cells using Ventana SP142 antibody (TC2/3 or IC2/3) to receive anti-PD-L1 immunotherapy atezolizumab. Of the 138 patients, 77% had nonsquamous histology.[22] Around half of the patients (47%) had higher PD-L1 tumor cell expression of at least 50% or immune cell expression of at least 10% (TC3 or IC3).[22] Although the response rate was higher in

TABLE 10.1

Clinical Efficacy in Early Phase Studies of PD-1 Pathway Blockade in Previously Treated Non–Small Cell Lung Cancer

	No. of Pt	mFU	ORR (%)	DOR	mPFS (m)	mOS (m)	1 y OS (%)	18 m OS	2 y OS	3 y OS
Nivolumab[6]	129	39m	17.1	17.0 m	2.3	9.9	42		24%	18%
Pembrolizumab[7,8]	449	34.5 m	22.7	33.3 m	2.9	10.5	47	36.6%	29.9%	19%
Atezolizumab[9,10,10a]	88	49.9 m	23	16.4 m	4.0	16.0	63		37%	28%
Durvalumab[11]	240	29.4 m	11.2	NR	1.5	10.2	47.3	38%		
Avelumab[5]	184	8.8 m	12	NR	2.7	8.4	36			

1 y OS, 1 year overall survival; *18 m OS*, 18 month overall survival; *2 y OS*, 2 year overall survival rate; *3 y OS*, 3 year overall survival rate; *DOR*, duration of response; *mFU*, median follow-up; *No. of pt*, number of patients; *ORR*, objective response rate; *mOS*, median overall survival; *mPFS*, median progression-free survival.

TABLE 10.2

Randomized Phase 3 Studies in Previously Treated Non–Small Cell Lung Cancer

Study	Immunotherapy	Number of Pts Non-sq/Total	PD-L1	ORR (I–O vs. Docetaxel)	Median PFS (I–O vs. Docetaxel) HR	Median PFS (I–O vs. Docetaxel)	Median OS (I–O vs. Docetaxel) HR	Median OS (I–O vs. Docetaxel)	2 y OS (%)
CM057[12,15]	Nivolumab	582/582	Any	19% versus 12%	0.92	2.3 versus 4.2 m	0.73	12.2 versus 9.4 m	29
KN010[13,16]	Pembrolizumab	812/1034	>1%	18% versus 9%	1.09	4.0 versus 4.0 m	0.61	12.7 versus 8.5 m	~31
OAK[14,18]	Atezolizumab	628/850	Any	14% versus 13%	0.95	2.8 versus 4.0 m	0.73	13.8 versus 9.6 m	31

2 y OS, 2 year overall survival; *non-sq*, nonsquamous; *I-O*, immunotherapy; *ORR*, objective response rate; *OS*, overall survival; *PFS*, progression-free survival; *pts*, patients.

TABLE 10.3
Clinical Efficacy of Anti-PD1 or Anti-PDL1 in Early Phase Studies of Treated Naïve Non–Small Cell Lung Cancer

Study		No. of Pts (Non-sq %)	mFU	PD-L1 Level	ORR (%)	DOR	mPFS	mOS	1 y OS	18 m OS	2 y OS	3 y OS
Nivolumab[20,24]	CM012	52 (75%)	22 m	Any	23	NR	3.6 m	21.8 m	73%		44%	
				>5%	31	NR	3.5 m		73%	54%		
				>50%	50	NR	8.3 m	NR	83%			
Pembrolizumab[7,8,21]	KN001	101 (78%)	34.5 m	Any	40.6	16.7 m	6.1 m	22.3 m	70%	58.1%	49%	26.4%
				>50%	66.7		12.5 m	34.9 m	84%	72.7%	66.7%	25.2%
Atezolizumab[22,23]	BIRCH	138 (77%)	34.3 m	>5% TC2/3	26	14.5 m	7.6 m	24.0 m	66.4%		50%	
				>50% T3	35	16.5 m	7.3 m	26.9 m	61.5%		52%	
Durvalumab[25,26]	Study 1108	49 (51%)	17.3 m	>25%	28.6		4.0	21.0 m	72%			
Avelumab[27]	JAVELIN	156 (67%)		Any	22.4		4.1 m					

18 m OS, 18 month overall survival rate; *1 y OS*, 1 year overall survival rate; *2 y OS*, 2 year overall survival rate; *3 y OS*, 3 year overall survival rate; *DOR*, duration of response; *mFU*, median follow-up; *mOS*, median overall survival; *mPFS*, median progression free survival; *No. of pts*, number of patients; *Non-sq*, Nnon-squamous; *ORR*, objective response rate.

patients with higher PD-L1 expression (35% vs. 26%), the survival outcome was similar in patients with TC3 or IC3 and TC2/3 or IC2/3 (mPFS 7.3 months vs. 7.6 months, mOS 26.9 months vs. 24 months, 2 year survival 52% vs. 50% respectively).[23]

On the whole, studies with first-line nivolumab, pembrolizumab, atezolizumab, and durvalumab consistently demonstrated higher response rates in patients with higher PD-L1 expression. One year survival rate with various anti-PD1 or anti-PD-L1 was very promising around 70%–80%, particularly in patients with PD-L1 expressing NSCLC (Table 10.3)[7,8,20–27] The PD-L1 cut points, however, were different in the various early-phase studies, therefore leading to different study designs for first-line randomized phase III studies.

Randomized Phase III Studies in Treatment-Naïve NSCLC

The response rate for standard first-line platinum doublet chemotherapy in advanced NSCLC patients was around 30%.[28] Data from earlier phase studies suggested that the response rate to first-line monotherapy blocking PD-1 pathway was generally lower than 30% in unselected patients. Therefore, it was thought to be important to enrich the population of patients with higher response rate to be treated with anti-PD1 or anti-PD-L1. There are now two reported randomized phase III studies investigating monotherapy anti-PD1 in first-line setting.

In the KEYNOTE 024 study, 305 patients with treatment-naïve stage IV NSCLC expressing PD-L1 in at least 50% of tumor cells (using DAKO IHC 22C3 antibody), but without EGFR mutation or ALK translocation, were randomized to receive a flat dose of pembrolizumab 200 mg or 4–6 cycles of platinum-doublet chemotherapy with the option of maintenance pemetrexed.[29] Upon disease progression, patients who were randomized to the chemotherapy arm could consider crossing over to receive pembrolizumab. Among 1934 patients screened, 1653 had adequate tissue for PD-L1 testing and 30% were found to have PD-L1 expression of ≥50%.[29,30] Pembrolizumab provided significantly improved outcome with higher response rate (45% vs. 28%), longer median PFS (10.3 months vs. 6.0 months), longer median OS (30 months vs. 14.2 months), and higher 2-year survival rate (51.5% vs. 34.5%) despite 62.3% of patients in the chemotherapy arm effectively crossing over to receive pembrolizumab or other PD1 blocking antibodies.[29,31] HR for PFS in the entire population of 305 patients was 0.50, while the HR in the 81.6%

patients with nonsquamous NSCLC was similar at 0.55.[29] Interestingly, the median time to response was the same in both arms, at the time of the first follow-up imaging at 2.2 months,[29] showing that first-line pembrolizumab produced responses as quickly as chemotherapy. In view of the substantial cross-over rate, there was always a question if it is essential for pembrolizumab to be considered in the first-line setting and this has been addressed by evaluating progression after the next line of therapy (PFS2). PFS2 reflecting the time from randomization to disease progression or death after the start of second-line treatment was superior in pembrolizumab arm, with longer median PFS2 (21.5 months vs. 8.5 months, HR 0.46), higher 1 and 2 year PFS2 rates (70.3% vs. 54.8%, 51.5% vs. 34.5%, respectively),[32,33] supporting the value of administering pembrolizumab in first-line setting to patients with PD-L1 of at least 50%. Patient reported outcome was one of the secondary endpoints. In addition to superior clinical efficacy, health-related quality of life was also better with improved symptom and function scores as well as longer time to deterioration of chest symptoms in patients treated with pembrolizumab than those treated with chemotherapy.[34]

CheckMate 026, another randomized phase III study for treatment-naïve advanced NSCLC patients, had similar study design to KEYNOTE 024, but with nivolumab 3 mg/kg and a different predetermined PD-L1 level of 5% (using DAKO 28-8 antibody) for primary endpoint PFS assessment.[35] The 541 patients recruited to CheckMate 026 required to have PD-L1 of ≥1% and also absence of EGFR and ALK aberration. Patients were stratified by histology at randomization with 76% being nonsquamous NSCLC. Upon disease progression, around 60% of patients on the chemotherapy arm effectively crossed over to receive nivolumab as second-line treatment. In contrast to KEYNOTE 024, there was no difference in PFS, OS, or ORR between first-line nivolumab and platinum-doublet chemotherapy.[35,36] With the same cut point of 5% in CheckMate 057 study, nivolumab provided longer PFS and OS in previously treated patients compared with docetaxel.[12] As the standard comparator with platinum-doublet chemotherapy in first-line study is much more active than single-agent docetaxel in the second-line population, a higher level of PD-L1 expression would be required to be more adequately enrich the population. This was supported by the fact that the ORR of 26% in the nivolumab arm in CheckMate 026 was numerically lower than the ORR of 32.5% in the chemotherapy arm.[35,36] In

KEYNOTE 024 study with PD-L1 of $\geq$50%, the ORR of 45% was higher in pembrolizumab arm than ORR of 28% in chemotherapy arm.[29] However, there was no evidence of any trend favoring nivolumab in the 214 patients with PD-L1 of $\geq$50% (88 in nivolumab arm, 126 in chemotherapy arm) in the CheckMate 026 study.[36] There has been much speculation as to the reasons beyond lower PD-L1 cut point for the differences in outcome between the two studies. The imbalance of baseline characteristics might be a contributor. Retrospectively, patients with high mutation burden receiving first-line nivolumab were found to have superior PFS over chemotherapy (9.7 months vs. 5.8 months, HR 0.62), although there was no difference in OS.[35,37]

A press release in July 2017 announced that first-line monotherapy durvalumab did not meet the primary endpoint of PFS in patients with PD-L1 of >25% (using VENTANA SP263 antibody) as compared with platinum-doublet chemotherapy in the MYSTIC study. The analysis of coprimary endpoint of OS is pending.

Combination of Chemotherapy and Checkpoint Inhibition

In contrast to the initial concern that chemotherapy might lead to immunosuppression, in vivo studies demonstrated synergy combining chemotherapy with immunotherapy.[38] The promising clinical benefit of combining chemotherapy with PD-1 checkpoint inhibitor was first suggested by cohort G of the randomized phase II study KEYNOTE 21.[39] One hundred and twenty-three treatment-naïve patients with nonsquamous NSCLC, but without EGFR mutation or ALK translocation, were randomized to receive four cycles of carboplatin and pemetrexed with or without pembrolizumab.[39] Patients in the combination arm continued pembrolizumab for up to 2 years. Patients on chemotherapy alone arm could crossover to receive pembrolizumab at time of disease progression. Combination of chemotherapy with pembrolizumab provided superior ORR (56.7% vs. 31.7%) and median PFS (19 months vs. 8.9 months, HR 0.54).[40] With longer median follow-up of 18.7 months, the updated data showed promising improvement of OS with HR reducing from 0.9 as in the initially published data to 0.59.[40] The median OS in the combination arm was not reached, while the median OS of 20.9 months in chemotherapy alone arm was much longer than expected due to substantial crossover of 75% to receive an anti-PD1 or anti-PD-L1 agent as second-line treatment.[40] Interestingly, the time to response was faster in the combination arm (1.5 months vs. 2.7 months).[39]

The ORR was similar in patients with PD-L1 of <1% or $\geq$1% (57% vs. 54%), but much higher at 80% in patients with PD-L1 $\geq$50%.[41] However, the impact of PD-L1 status has to be interpreted with caution, in view of the small number of patients in each PD-L1 subgroups.

The first reported phase III study to investigate combination of chemotherapy with checkpoint inhibitor in nonsquamous NSCLC was IMPOWER 150. There were three treatment arms randomizing 1202 patients to receive carboplatin + paclitaxel ± bevacizumab with or without atezolizumab.[42] The addition of atezolizumab to carboplatin + paclitaxel + bevacizumab led to superior median PFS (8.3 months vs. 6.8 months, HR 0.617), 6-month PFS (67% vs. 56%), and 12-month PFS (37% vs. 18%) when compared with chemotherapy and bevacizumab alone.[42] The magnitude of benefit was higher in patients with high T effector gene signature with median PFS of 11.3 months, 6-month PFS of 72%, and 12-month PFS of 46%. The ORR was impressive at 64% in the entire population and 69% in patients with high T effector gene signature. The preliminary median OS was also longer in the atezolizumab arm, 19.2 months versus 14.4 months.[42] PFS benefit (HR 0.59) was also observed in the 13% patients in the study who had EGFR mutation or ALK translocation. HR was even better 0.41 in those with actionable EGFR mutations, exon 19 deletion or L858R mutation. Patients with oncogenic driver mutations generally have lower tumor mutation burden and the impressive efficacy in this subgroup of patients may be due to the addition of bevacizumab.[42a]

The longest follow-up data on first-line combination treatment with chemotherapy and PD1 pathway blockade were from CheckMate 012 demonstrating 3-year overall survival rate of 25% in NSCLC patients with both squamous and nonsquamous histology.[43]

The coprimary endpoints PFS and OS were met with HR of 0.52 and 0.49 respectively in another phase III study (KEYNOTE 189) in metastatic non-squamous NSCLC, with the same design as the phase II study KEYNOTE 21G comparing pembrolizumab with placebo in addition to chemotherapy, cisplatin or carboplatin, and pemetrexed. OS benefit was evident irrespective of PD-L1 status with HR 0.59 for PD-L1 <1%, HR 0.55 for PD-L1 1-49% and HR 0.42 for PD-L1 >50%. ORR was higher in the combination chemotherapy and pembrolizumab arm than chemotherapy alone arm (47.6% vs 18.9%) with ORR of 61.4% in patients with PD-L1 >50%. There is no head to head comparison between monotherapy pembrolizumab and combination chemotherapy with pembrolizumab in patients with PD-L1 >50%. As the PFS curves separated earlier with the combination pembrolizumab plus chemotherapy than monotherapy pembrolizumab, combination treatment may be preferable for patients with high disease burden. Apart from slightly increased incidence of renal toxicity (5.2%) with the combination treatment of chemotherapy plus pembrolizumab, the safety profile was similar to that of monotherapy pembrolizumab. It is reassuring that patient reported outcomes showed improved function/QoL and a delay in the development of chest symptoms by adding pembrolizumab to chemotherapy.[43a,43b]

UNRESECTABLE STAGE III NON–SMALL CELL LUNG CANCER
Combination of Radiation and Immunotherapy

Synergistic effects from combining radiation and checkpoint inhibitors improve antitumor immune response locally and occasionally at distant sites. Although this abscopal effect is rather uncommon, it has been increasingly reported where systemic tumor response occurs with distant tumor regression outside the radiation field. Radiation may promote the release of tumor antigen, induce inflammatory cytokines, upregulate tumor cell expression of PD-L1, and suppress Tregs activity, thereby enhancing immune response.[44–46]

Concurrent chemotherapy and thoracic radiation therapy followed by consolidation anti-PD-L1 agent was investigated in the PACIFIC study. Seven hundred and thirteen unresectable stage III NSCLC patients without disease progression after concurrent chemoradiation were randomized 2:1 to receive durvalumab 10 mg/kg or placebo every 2 weeks for up to 12 months. Patients were not selected according to PD-L1 status. Durvalumab provided superior efficacy over placebo with higher 18-month PFS rate of 44.2% versus 27% and improved median PFS of over 11 months from 5.6 to 16.8 months with a remarkable HR of 0.52 and a P value of <.0001.[47] Nonsquamous cell NSCLC patients comprised 54% of the entire population, and HR for PFS in this subset was 0.45, similar to the overall HR. In the literature, the PFS in patients with locally advanced NSCLC receiving definitive concurrent chemoradiation is around 8 months,[48] which is consistent with the standard-of-care arm in the PACIFIC study, as patients in the study were randomized up to 42 days after the completion of their chemoradiation. The poor outcome from concurrent chemoradiation in locally advanced NSCLC is not only because of failure

to eliminate local disease but also development of distant metastases. Patients receiving durvalumab had longer median time to distant metastasis or death, 23.2 months versus 14.6 months, with a lower incidence of new lesions, including new brain metastases compared with patients receiving placebo.[47,49] The patient reported outcomes data demonstrated maintenance of health-related quality of life and function in patients receiving durvalumab.[50] Unlike the KEYNOTE 024 study demonstrating improvement of quality of life in stage IV NSCLC receiving pembrolizumab,[34] the patients in PACIFIC study who had earlier stage disease without progression after definitive local treatment were expected to have little cancer-related symptoms. Therefore, the addition of durvalumab for 12 months without compromising quality of life further supports the clinical value of consolidation durvalumab in unresectable stage III NSCLC.

SAFETY AND MANAGEMENT OF TOXICITY

All early-phase studies of PD-1 or PD-L1 inhibitors did not reach a maximally tolerated dose with very few treatment-related grade 3 to 4 toxicities. The commonest adverse event was grade 1 to 2 fatigue generally occurring in 20% of patients.[3,5,12–14,47] Other common adverse events including grade 1 to 2 decreased appetite, nausea, diarrhea, and pruritis were usually seen in <15% of patients.

The irAEs were also relatively low in frequency with the majority being grade 1 and 2. The commonest was grade 1 to 2 hypothyroidism occurring in around 6%–8% of patients, while up to 4% of patients experienced other immune-mediated toxicities including hyperthyroidism, skin reactions, pneumonitis, colitis, arthritis, and other endocrinopathies, e.g., hypophysitis, hypoadrenalism, type 1 diabetes mellitus. Less frequent irAE included myocarditis, pancreatitis, nephritis, vasculitis, hemolytic anemia, and neurologic toxicities such as encephalitis, Guillian-Barre syndrome, peripheral neuropathy, and myasthenia gravis. The immune-mediated inflammation can literally involve any organ and tissue. Median time to onset of the various irAE and the duration of the toxicities are variable and may become apparent only after treatment is stopped. Some events such as endocrinopathies can be permanent resulting in the need for life-long hormone replacement. Therefore clinicians always need to be on alert to recognize the diverse symptoms and signs of the potential immune-mediated toxicities. Regular blood tests at least once a month to check thyroid-stimulating hormone (TSH), blood cell count, renal and liver functions are recommended. Symptoms of other endocrinopathies, e.g., hypophysitis or hypoadrenalism can be vague and nonspecific. Although the incidence of grade 3 or 4 irAE is low with single agent anti-PD-1 or anti-PD-L1, occasionally the toxicity can be severe and life-threatening. As most toxicities are reversible by steroids, the key to the management of irAEs is early recognition and prompt initiation of steroids. Raising awareness and educating patients, carers, nursing staff, and junior doctors are essential. Moreover, involvement of multidisciplinary specialists (e.g., dermatologist, pulmonologist, gastroenterologist, endocrinologist, neurologist, and immunologist) in the management of various irAE is imperative. At the time of presentation of certain irAEs, e.g., pneumonitis or colitis, infection needs to be excluded and empirical antibiotics may be considered in additional to the use of steroids.

The starting dose of steroid depends on the severity and the organ involved. For most grade 2 irAE, the starting dose of oral prednisone is usually 0.5—1 mg/kg and symptom improvement is to be expected within a few days. Upon improvement, it is vital to taper the dose of steroid slowly over no less than 1 month. If without improvement within 3 days, or in the event of grade 3 toxicity, hospital admission is warranted to commence intravenous methylprednisolone 1—2 mg/kg or higher dose 2—4 mg/kg for pneumonitis. Other immunosuppressive drugs, e.g., infliximab 5 mg/kg would need to be initiated if symptoms of irAE persist or worsen. As infliximab may cause hepatotoxicity, mycophenolate mofetil is used instead in high-grade immune-mediated hepatitis. The checkpoint inhibitor needs to be permanently discontinued after the large majority of grade 3 irAEs, even when symptoms improve to <grade 1. While dampening down the inflammatory toxicity, it is reassuring that the use of steroid did not have any impact on antitumor activity of the immune checkpoint inhibitors.[51] Recently, ESMO guidelines for the practical management of specific irAEs have been published.[52]

Lung cancer patients often have prior exposure to cigarette smoking and may be treated with thoracic radiation. The incidence of immune-mediated pneumonitis tends to be higher in damaged lungs than other cancer types, with approximately 4% any grade and 2% grade 3/4. Among the NSCLC patients in the phase I nivolumab study, two treatment-related deaths were due to pneumonitis occurring early in the trial.[6] Very few grade 5 pneumonitis were reported in later studies due to higher awareness and appropriate steroid management. Unlike other drug-related pneumonitis, the

interstitial radiologic changes can be focal or diffuse, unilateral, or bilateral. All patients in the PACIFIC study had received radical dose thoracic radiation prior to receiving durvalumab or placebo, the incidence of any grade pneumonitis (including radiation pneumonitis) was higher in the durvalumab arm (33.9% vs. 24.8%), but the incidence was similarly low for grade 3/4 pneumonitis in the two arms (3.4% vs. 2.6%).[47]

In the three studies combining immune checkpoint inhibitor with chemotherapy (KEYNOTE 21G, KEYNOTE 189 and IMPOWER 150), apart from higher frequency of hypothyroidism (13%—15%) than the historic incidence for monotherapy, the incidence of other irAEs was similar to monotherapy.[39,42]

BIOMARKERS

Although drugs targeting the PD-1 pathway have revolutionized treatment for NSCLC including pulmonary adenocarcinoma, unfortunately the majority of patients do not respond to anti-PD1 or anti-PD-L1 monotherapy. As responders usually have durable response, it is important to define predictive biomarkers to identify the patients who will likely benefit from PD-1 blockade and also to identify those who will unlikely benefit to avoid toxicity from ineffective treatment and to lessen financial burden. Much work has been done in this area investigating the role of clinicopathologic parameters, PD-L1 immunohistochemistry, tumor mutational load, and immune gene expression signature.

Clinicopathologic Markers
Smoking status

Although the proportion of never smokers is higher in pulmonary adenocarcinoma than squamous cell cancer, the majority of patients with pulmonary adenocarcinoma are still former or current smokers. With higher mutational load due to the carcinogenic effect of tobacco,[53] smoking history may be a clinical predictor for higher response rates to checkpoint inhibitors. In the earlier phase studies with monotherapy anti-PD1 or anti-PD-L1, the ORR in current/former smokers was higher than never smokers 23.4% versus 10.4% in KEYNOTE 001 with pembrolizuamb,[54] 26% versus 10% in phase Ia study with atezolizumab.[9] In randomized phase III CheckMate 057 study, the HR for OS favored nivolumab over docetaxel in current/former smokers with 0.70 versus 1.02 in nonsmokers.[12] In the OAK study, although the ORR was also higher in smokers than nonsmokers 16% versus 6% in the atezolizumab arm, HR for OS was similar comparing atezolizumab with docetaxel in both smokers and nonsmokers 0.74 versus 0.71.[14,55] The magnitude of PFS benefit from pembrolizumab over first-line chemotherapy in KEYNOTE 024 was bigger in former and current smokers than never smokers with HR of 0.47 and 0.68 versus 0.90, respectively.[29] However, in PACIFIC study with stratification by smoking status at randomization, nonsmokers with stage III NSCLC still derived significant benefit from consolidation durvalumab after concurrent chemoradiation with HR of 0.29.[47]

EGFR Status

Around 20% of pulmonary adenocarcinomas harbor sensitizing EGFR mutation. The prevalence is higher in the Asian population. In the earlier studies, patients with EGFR mutation positive disease were found to have less benefit from PD-1 blockade than wild-type, with ORR 17% versus 23% with atezolizumab,[56] 7.8% versus 21.6% with pembrolizumab in KEYNOTE 001 study,[54] 6.7% versus 19.6% with durvalumab in study 1108.[25] In contrast to EGFR wild type, the overall survival in previously treated patients with EGFR-mutant NSCLC treated with anti-PD1 or anti-PD-L1 agents was not any better than docetaxel in the randomized phase III studies. The HR for OS in patients with EGFR mutant versus EGFR wild type was 1.18 versus 0.66 with nivolumab in CheckMate 057[12], 1.79 versus 0.83 with pembrolizumab in KEYNOTE 010[13] and 1.24 versus 0.69 with atezolizumab in OAK study.[14] The adjusted HR for OS comparing EGFR wild type versus mutant was 0.66 with P value of .0132.[16] In the first-line JAVELIN study with avelumab, no response was evident in the 5% of patients with EGFR-mutant disease.[5] Therefore, patients with EGFR mutation or ALK translocation were excluded in first-line phase III studies, KEYNOTE 024, CheckMate 026, and MYSTIC. However, the first-line cohort in BIRCH suggested that patients with EGFR-mutant NSCLC after having failed prior EGFR tyrosine kinase inhibitors had similar median overall survival as wild type, 28.5 months versus 20.1 months.[23] Interestingly, in stage III NSCLC, consolidation durvalumab was of benefit in both EGFR mutation positive and negative disease with HR of 0.76 and 0.47, respectively. However, this has to be interpreted with caution due to small sample size with only 9% of patients being EGFR mutation positive and the confidence interval for EGFR-mutant subgroup crossed 1.0.[47]

PD-L1 Expression

PD-L1 expression was first reported to be associated with higher response rates to atezolizumab in 53 NSCLC patients with ORR of 31% in PD-L1 ≥1%, 46% in PD-L1 ≥5%, and 83% in PD-L1 ≥10%.[9] In the first cohort of 38 patients in KEYNOTE 001, higher response rate to pembrolizumab was also noted with ORR of 67% versus 4% above and below a potential cut point of PD-L1, respectively.[57] Further research was conducted to validate this potential cut point in the large phase 1b KEYNOTE 001 study with altogether 550 patients among six expansion cohorts. PD-L1 status using DAKO IHC 22C3 antibody was initially assessed in a training set of 182 patients and then in an independent validation set of 313 patients. The cut point of 50% was selected from the training set based on scientifically derived receiver operating characteristics (ROC) curve with true positive and false negative rates.[3,58] The most effective and practical scoring system of PD-L1 level was determined to be the percentage of tumor cells with membranous staining at any intensity. The ORR in patients with PD-L1 ≥50% in the validation set was higher at 45.2% versus 16.5% and 10.7% in patients with PD-L1 1%–49% and <1%, respectively.[3,58] The ORR increased with increasing quartiles of PD-L1 levels. Longer PFS (6.3 months vs. 3.3 months) and OS (NR vs. 8.8 months) were also evident in patients with PD-L1 ≥50% as compared with lower levels.[3] With longer follow-up of 34.5 months, the median OS for treatment-naïve and previously treated patients with PD-L1 ≥50% were incredible at 34.9 and 15.4 months, respectively.[8]

High level of PD-L1 expression on tumor cells by immunohistochemistry has since been shown to be associated with improved clinical efficacy, ORR, PFS, and OS when compared with low level or negative PD-L1 in many previously treated NSCLC studies (Table 10.4). With long-term follow-up, nivolumab and pembrolizumab provided impressive 3 year survival rate of 39% and 30%, respectively, to previously treated NSCLC patients with high level of PD-L1 expression of ≥50%.[8,15]

However, the PD-L1 status for different anti-PD1 (nivolumab, pembrolizumab) or anti-PD-L1 (durvalumab, atezolizumab, and avelumab) drugs was determined by five different companion PD-L1 antibodies (DAKO 28-8, DAKO 22C3, VENTANA SP263, VENTANA SP142, and VENTANA SP73–10) on two different platforms with various cut points (Table 10.4). Therefore it is crucial to standardize PD-L1 assays, and the earlier 4 PD-L1 antibodies were evaluated in 39 tumor samples by three pathologists in the first phase of the Blueprint PD-L1 IHC Assay Comparison Project.[59] A larger panel of 25 international pathologists in phase II of the Blueprint

TABLE 10.4
Efficacy of Anti-PD1 or Anti-PDL1 in Previously Treated Patients With High PD-L1 Advanced Non−Small Cell Lung Cancer

	Study (Phase)	Pt's Number: Total (Non-sq %)	PD-L1 Antibody	Scoring Method	High PD-L1 Cut-point	Prevalence (%)	ORR (%)	mPFS	MOS (HR—high versus low PD-L1)	1 y OS (%)	2 y OS
Nivolumab	CM057[12] (Ph 3)	231 (100%)	DAKO IHC 22-8	TC	≥10%	37	37	5.0 m	19.9 m (HR 0.40)	~66	
Pembrolizumab	KN001[3,7,8] (Ph 1)	396 (82%)	DAKO IHC 22C3	TC	≥50%	34.8	38.3	4.3 m	15.4 m	~54	38.6%
Pembrolizumab	KN010[13,16] (Ph 3)	690 (70%)	DAKO IHC 22C3	TC	≥50%	28	30	5.0 m	14.9 m (HR 0.62)	~54	
Atezolizumab	PCD4989g[81] (Ph 1)	89 (74%)	Ventana SP142	TC/IC	≥50%/≥10% (TC3/IC3)	24.7	50	7.0 m	20 m	72	42%
Atezolizumab	POPLAR[61] (Ph 2)	144 (66%)	Ventana SP142	TC/IC	≥50%/≥10% (TC3/IC3)	16	38	7.8 m	15.5 m	~64	
Atezolizumab	OAK[14,18] (Ph 3)	425 (74%)	Ventana SP172	TC/IC	≥50%/≥10% (TC3/IC3)	17	31		20.5 m	69	43%
Durvalumab	Study 1108[11,82] (Ph 1)	240 (47.1%)	Ventana SP263	TC	≥25%	51.5	20	2.2 m	15.4 m	56	
Durvalumab	ATLANTIC[83] (Ph 2)	265 (79.2%)	Ventana SP263	TC	≥25%	33.4	16.4	3.3 m	10.9 m	48	
Avelumab	JAVELIN[5] (Ph 1)	142 (65%)	DAKO IHC73-10	TC	≥1%	85.9	14	2.8 m	8.9 m	39	
Avelumab	JAVELIN[5] (Ph 1)	142 (65%)	DAKO IHC73-10	TC	≥25%	37.3	17	2.8 m	8.4 m	28	

1 y OS, 1 year overall survival rate; 2 y OS, 2 year overall survival rate; IC, immune cell; mOS, median overall survival; mPFS, median progression-free survival; Non-sq, nonsquamous; Pt's, Patient's; TC, tumor cell.

Project scored all five PD-L1 antibodies staining 81 tumor samples and largely affirmed the phase I results.[60] The performance of three antibodies, IHC 28-8, IHC 22C3, and SP263 was similar, while SP73−10 stained more tumor cells and SP142 had consistently lower percentage of tumor cell staining in the corresponding tumor samples.[59,60] The latter is also the antibody with additional scoring criteria to include percentage of tumor area with immune cells infiltration which may compensate the lower staining in tumor cells. However, the scoring of immune cells with all five antibodies was found to be more difficult than tumor cell staining[59,60] and therefore lower interobserver concordance. With similar performance in tumor cell staining, the cut points would be comparable among the 3 PD-L1 antibodies 28-8, 22C3, and SP263. However, the cut point chosen for each of the three drugs was not necessarily the same, e.g., 1%, 5%, and 10% for nivolumab; 1% and 50% for pembrolizumab; 25% for durvalumab.

In CheckMate 057, the magnitude of survival benefit of nivolumab over docetaxel was bigger with higher PD-L1 cut point (HR of 0.59, 0.43, 0.40 for cut points of 1%, 5%, 10%, respectively).[12] In contrast, patients with <1%, <5%, or <10% of PD-L1 had no survival improvement over docetaxel, although not worse.[12] Similarly, in KEYNOTE 010, the magnitude of survival benefit of pembrolizumab over docetaxel was higher in patients with higher PD-L1 of ≥50% (HR 0.53) than lower level of 1%−49% (HR 0.76).[13] In the phase I study with durvalumab as second-line treatment, the median survival was also longer in patients with PD-L1 ≥25% (15.4 months) than PD-L1 <25% (7.6 months).[11]

In the randomized phase II study POPLAR, atezolizumab was superior to docetaxel if PD-L1 was positive with TC (tumor cell staining) or IC (immune cell staining) ≥1% (HR 0.59). The benefit was greater if TC or IC was ≥5% (HR 0.54), and more so with higher cut point of PD-L1 TC ≥50% or IC ≥10% (HR 0.49). However, there was no difference in overall survival in patients with PD-L1 negative disease (TC and IC <1%) receiving atezolizumab or docetaxel (HR 1.04).[61] Interestingly, patients with PD-L1 negative disease using the same antibody SP142 and same scoring criteria in the randomized phase III study OAK, atezolizumab provided superior survival benefit over docetaxel irrespective of PD-L1 status with HR of 0.75 for patients with PD-L1 negative disease (TC and IC <1%) and HR of 0.74 for those with PD-L1 positive disease (TC or IC ≥1%).[14] The benefit remained the largest for the highest level of PD-L1 (TC ≥50% or IC ≥10%) with HR of 0.41.[14] Retrospective comparison of the two antibodies SP142 and 22C3 was performed in a subset of 400 out of 850 patients from the OAK study, and it is comforting to see that similar survival benefit was achieved in the patients with PD-L1 negative disease assessed by DAKO IHC 22C3 antibody.[62]

Other practical challenging questions in implementing PD-L1 testing include the feasibility to use the antibodies on other technical staining platforms, inter- and intraobserver reproducibility, and the type of tissue sample. In a French Harmonization Study, the three antibodies 28-8, 22C3, and SP263 demonstrated similar analytic performance on five DAKO or VENTANA platforms with SP263 having the highest concordance across the various platforms, while lowest concordance was evident for immune cell staining.[63] In another study, there was high interobserver (>80%) and intraobserver (∼90%) concordance evaluating 120 samples with 1% and 50% cut points using DAKO IHC 22C3 antibody among 10 pathologists.[64]

As PD-L1 expression may be dynamic changing over time, some of the earlier studies requested mandatory fresh biopsy for PD-L1 assessment. In KEYNOTE 010, around half of the patients submitted archival tissue and half submitted fresh biopsies. It was reassuring that the survival benefit of pembrolizumab over docetaxel was similar, irrespective of archival or fresh tissue.[13] The phase II Blueprint Comparison Project included 22 cytology samples and the reliability was not as strong as tissue samples requiring further validation.[60] An atlas of PD-L1 IHC testing in lung cancer has been produced by IASLC to guide clinicians and pathologists.

Unlike oncogenic mutation−driven biomarkers, NSCLC patients with PD-L1 negative disease can still respond to any of the anti-PD1 or anti-PD-L1 checkpoint inhibitors, although with lower response rate. Irrespective of PD-L1 status, the responders usually have durable duration of response with prolonged survival. Although PD-L1 expression is not an ideal biomarker and cannot capture all the responders, it is still the most studied, clinically validated, and practical biomarker to date to enrich the population for treatment response and would be essential to select patients for first-line anti-PD-1 monotherapy. PD-L1 status is useful to guide appropriate timing of treatment with monotherapy but is not essential to select patients for second-line treatment after failure to platinum-based chemotherapy. The role of PD-L1 status will be defined further in many ongoing phase III first-line combination studies with chemotherapy and anti-PD-1 or anti-PD-L1.

Tumor Mutation Burden

Across human cancer types, pulmonary adenocarcinoma is ranked third in the prevalence of somatic mutations following melanoma and pulmonary squamous cell cancer[53] likely due to exposure to mutagens such as cigarette smoking, although the number of mutations varies significantly between individual tumors. Higher mutational prevalence leads to larger number of neoantigen formation with increased tumor immunogenicity and thereby potentially higher sensitivity to checkpoint inhibition. In a retrospective study, tumors from 34 patients treated with pembrolizumab were assessed with whole exome sequencing and longer PFS was evident with HR of 0.19 in patients with high versus low nonsynonymous mutation burden.[65]

In CheckMate 026 study, 312 of 541 treatment-naïve patients had matched DNA from tumor and blood for retrospective exploratory tumor mutation burden (TMB) analysis. In patients with high TMB, nivolumab provided superior PFS over chemotherapy with HR of 0.62, but it was the reverse in patients with the lower two tertiles of TMB.[35,37] Interestingly, there was absolutely no correlation between TMB and PD-L1 expression.[37] Similar ORR to chemotherapy were seen in patients with high TMB and low PD-L1 1%–49% or low TMB with high PD-L1 of at least 50% treated with nivolumab (32% and 34%, respectively). Patients with both low PD-L1 and TMB had the lowest ORR of only 16%, while patients with both high PD-L1 and TMB had much higher ORR of 75% and longer PFS than the other three groups.[37] However, we need to be mindful that there were only 16 patients in this group, making up only 10% of the analyzed patients.

Retrospective assessment of TMB in tumor tissue by the FoundationOne-targeted sequencing panel was also found to be associated with improved survival outcome of atezolizumab in treatment-naïve and previously treated NSCLC patients from POPLAR and BIRCH studies.[66] In contrast, TMB had no impact on the efficacy of docetaxel,[66] indicating that it was not a prognostic biomarker.

More recently, TMB was shown to be measurable in blood, making the test less invasive. Cut point of 16 for blood-based TMB in predicting PFS benefit from atezolizumab over docetaxel was selected in the test set from the POPLAR study and validated in the OAK study (HR 0.65).[67] Of 229 evaluable patients, 13% having high bTMB >16 and high PD-L1 expression (TC >50% or IC >10%) derived the greatest benefit from atezolizumab with HR of 0.38 for PFS and HR of 0.23 for OS.[67]

In non-squamous NSCLC patients with PD-L1 <1% but with high tumor mutation burden (≥10mut/Mb) in Checkmate 227 study, first-line combination immunotherapy nivolumab and ipilimumab without chemotherapy improved PFS over chemotherapy with HR of 0.55. In contrast, those with low tumor mutation burden (<10mut/Mb) and negative PD-L1 (<1%), there was no difference in PFS comparing combination nivolumab and ipilimumab to chemotherapy. High tumor mutation burden may guide treatment with combination immunotherapy sparing chemotherapy particularly in those with PD-L1 <1%.[67a]

T-Effector Gene Signature Expression

Another biomarker was also investigated in several atezolizumab studies. Higher expression of T-effector and interferon-γ gene signature (comprising CD8A, GZMA, GZMB, IFNγ, EOMES, CXCL9, CXCL10, TBX21 genes), reflecting preexisting immune competency, was associated with improved OS (HR 0.43) in patients treated with atezolizumab from the POPLAR study.[61] Similarly in patients from the randomized OAK study, T-effector (Teff) signature (comprising three genes PD-L1, CXCL9, and IFNγ) >median was associated with superior PFS (HR 0.73) and OS (HR 0.59).[68] With bigger magnitude of benefit and similar prevalence of Teff signature > median (50% of patients), Teff appears to be a more sensitive biomarker than PD-L1 expression in predicting benefit from atezolizumab.[68] The clinical value of Teff signature was further evaluated prospectively in the IMPOWER 150 study. Adding atezolizumab to chemotherapy and bevacizumab in patients with higher Teff signature expression was associated with bigger magnitude of PFS benefit (HR 0.51) than those with lower Teff signature (HR 0.76).[42]

Other potential biomarkers including DNA repair mismatch defect, immune competency in tumor microenvironment, other ligands to immune checkpoint inhibitors, etc. are being explored in ongoing research, with the hope to select the right patients more effectively for immunotherapy.

TREATMENT DURATION

Although pseudoprogression is rare in NSCLC, it has been well recognized that patients may still derive clinical benefit from immunotherapy when there is minor radiologic disease progression by RECIST measurements. If patients remain clinically well, treatment beyond progression can be considered. Patients with worsening symptoms, particularly with deteriorating function may have hyperprogression, a phenomenon where rapid disease progression occurs after commencement of immunotherapy.

In the randomized phase II POPLAR study, 45.9% patients were treated with atezolizumab beyond progression and median OS in these patients was 11.3 months from the time of disease progression.[69] In the OAK study, 7% of patients were found to have subsequent reduction in the size of the target lesions consistent with the concept of pseudoprogression, while 49% of patients had stable target lesions. Median OS was extended in the patients who continued atezolizumab beyond radiologic progression, 12.7 months versus 8.8 months.[70]

The optimal treatment duration with an anti-PD1 or anti-PD-L1 drug has not been determined. Many clinical studies have incorporated in the study design a finite maximal treatment duration of 12 months or 24 months and would allow the option of retreatment upon subsequent disease progression.

In the CheckMate 153 study, 220 patients after having received 12 months of nivolumab were randomized to continue or to stop treatment. The 1-year PFS rate was higher (65% vs. 40%) and median PFS was longer (not reached vs. 10.3 months) with HR of 0.42 in the continuous arm,[71] indicating that 1 year treatment in the nonprogressors was not adequate. This applied to both nonsquamous and squamous histology with HR 0.46 and 0.41, and irrespective to PD-L1 status.[71] There was a trend for improved OS in the continuous arm with HR 0.63, and follow-up for OS analysis is ongoing. However, it must be cautioned that treatment duration was not the primary endpoint of this trial. Larger trials adequately powered to detect noninferiority are required to establish the feasibility of stopping treatment in patients who achieve an excellent response.

ONGOING STUDIES/FUTURE DIRECTIONS

Positive phase III trials have been reported for 4 PD-1/PD-L1 checkpoint inhibitors (nivolumab, pembrolizumab, atezolizumab, durvalumab) in stage IV and stage III NSCLCs. These have resulted in regulatory approval in the United States, Europe, and other countries. Currently there are more than 30 phase III trials recruiting or pending activation, further evaluating immune checkpoint inhibitors in NSCLC (www.clintrials.gov, accessed on December 18, 2017). A summary of the key trials is presented in

Table 10.5a–c. Trials restricted to squamous cell histology are not included. The table presents the experimental arm or arms, the standard-of-care comparator, and the primary endpoints. All trials have multiple secondary endpoints which may include subgroup analysis based on predefined PD-L1 expression levels using different immunohistochemistry stains and cut-offs.

The first group of trials (Table 10.5a) compares a single agent PD-1/PD-L1 inhibitor either alone or with chemotherapy to standard-of-care chemotherapy. Chemotherapy is a platinum doublet for first-line treatment trials and (as comparator) docetaxel for second-/third-line treatment trials. The majority of these studies follows the design of previously successful randomized trials and evaluates other PD-1/PD-L1 antibodies, some developed in emerging markets and with trials restricted to those markets (BGB-A317 and SHR1210 in China, BCD-100 in Russia/Belarus). Given the close similarity of these PD-1 and PD-L1 antibodies to existing approved ones it is likely that these trials will ultimately report similar results and hopefully extend the availability of checkpoint inhibitors to patients in countries where access is currently limited.

One noteworthy trial is comparing atezolizumab with standard-of-care platinum-doublet chemotherapy in a patient group selected on the basis of high TMB in circulating DNA measured from a baseline blood sample (NCT03178552). This selection is based on retrospective analysis of blood samples from patients on randomized trials of atezolizumab versus second-/third-line chemotherapy. Using a proprietary TMB assay, patients with TMB ≥16 showed the lowest HRs for both PFS and OS for atezolizumab compared with docetaxel and was superior to PD-L1 immunohistochemistry using SP142 and 22C3. If the distribution of blood-based TMB in previously untreated patients reflects that seen in patients who have received chemotherapy, then approximately 30% of patients will fall into this high TMB group.

The second group of trials (Table 10.5b) is evaluating checkpoint inhibitors in earlier stage NSCLC, predominantly following curative surgery and adjuvant chemotherapy. These four trials (NCT02486718 planned 1127 patients, NCT02504372 planned 1380 patients, NCT02595944 planned 714 patients, NCT02273375 planned 1100 patients), all evaluating 1 year of single agent PD-1 or PD-L1 inhibitor, will eventually provide a dataset of >4000 patients hopefully allowing precise estimate of treatment efficacy

TABLE 10.5
Ongoing Phase III Trials

Study Drug(s)	Comparator	Disease Stage	Primary Endpoint(s)	Status
STAGE IV—CHECKPOINT INHIBITOR ± CHEMOTHERAPY				
Avelumab	Chemotherapy	IV, first line	PFS, OS	NCT02576574, recruiting
REGN2810	Chemotherapy	IV, first line	PFS	NCT03088540, recruiting
Atezolizumab + chemotherapy	Chemotherapy	IV, nonsquamous, first line	PFS, OS	NCT02657434, recruiting
Atezolizumab	Chemotherapy	IV, nonsquamous, first line	OS	NCT02409342, recruiting
Pembrolizumab + chemotherapy	Chemotherapy	IV, nonsquamous first line,	OS, PFS	NCT02578680, recruiting
Durvalumab	Chemotherapy	IV, first line, PD-L1 $\geq$25%	PFS, OS	NCT03003962, recruiting
Atezolizumab	Chemotherapy	IV, first line, TMB high based on ctDNA	PFS	NCT03178552, recruiting
BGB-A317	Chemotherapy	IV, second/third line	OS	NCT03358875, recruiting
BCD-100	Chemotherapy	IV, second line	OS	NCT03288870, pending activation
SHR-1210 + chemotherapy	Chemotherapy	IV, first line	PFS	NCT03134872, recruiting
Pembrolizumab	Chemotherapy	IV, second/third line, PD-L1 $\geq$1%	OS, PFS	NCT02864394, recruiting
STAGE I–III NSCLC				
Atezolizumab	Observation	IB-IIIA, adjuvant postsurgery and adjuvant chemotherapy	Disease-free survival	NCT02486718, recruiting
Pembrolizumab	Observation	IB-IIIA, adjuvant postsurgery ± adjuvant chemotherapy	Disease-free survival	NCT02504372, recruiting
Nivolumab	Observation	IB-IIIA, adjuvant postsurgery and adjuvant chemotherapy	Disease-free survival, OS	NCT02595944, recruiting
Durvalumab	Observation	IB-IIIA, adjuvant postsurgery ± adjuvant chemotherapy	Disease-free survival	NCT02273375, recruiting
Nivolumab + ipilimumab	Chemotherapy	IB-IIIA, neoadjuvant presurgery	Event free survival, pathologic CR	NCT02998528, recruiting
Nivolumab	Observation	IIIA/IIIB after concurrent chemotherapy/radiation	OS, PFS	NCT02768558, not recruiting

STAGE IV—IMMUNE CHECKPOINT COMBINATIONS

Intervention	Comparator	Setting	Endpoint	Trial
Nivolumab + ipilimumab; nivolumab + chemotherapy; nivolumab	Chemotherapy	IV, first line	OS, PFS	NCT02477826, recruited
Nivolumab + ipilimumab + chemotherapy	Chemotherapy	IV, first line	OS	NCT03215706, recruiting
Nivolumab + ipilimumab	Chemotherapy	IV, first line, PS 2 or age >70	OS	NCT03351361, pending activation
Nivolumab + epacadostat + chemotherapy; nivolumab + chemotherapy	Chemotherapy	IV, first line, PD-L1 0%–49%	OS, PFS	NCT03348904, pending activation
Pembrolizumab + epacadostat	Pembrolizumab	IV, first line, PD-L1 ≥50%	PFS, OS	NCT03322540, pending activation
Pembrolizumab + epacadostat + chemotherapy; pembrolizumab + epacadostat	Pembrolizumab + chemotherapy	IV, first line	OS, PFS	NCT03322566, pending activation
Pembrolizumab + ipilimumab	Pembrolizumab	IV, first line, PD-L1 ≥50%	PFS, OS	NCT03302234, recruiting
REGN2810 + ipilimumab + chemotherapy; REGN2810 + chemotherapy	Chemotherapy	IV, first line	PFS	NCT03409614, Pending activation
Durvalumab + tremelimumab	Chemotherapy	IV, first line	OS	NCT02542293, recruiting
Durvalumab + tremelimumab + chemotherapy; durvalumab + chemotherapy	Chemotherapy	IV, first line	PFS	NCT03164616, recruiting
Nivolumab + ipilimumab; nivolumab + chemotherapy	Chemotherapy	IV, EGFR mut, T790 m −ve after 1st line TKI	PFS	NCT02864251, recruiting

OS, overall survival; PFS, progression-free survival.

across multiple subgroups. The availability of tissue from a prior resection rather than the small biopsies usually collected in stage IV NSCLC trials should also lead to discovery and validation of new predictive tissue immune and other biomarkers in the adjuvant treatment setting, and potentially for later-stage NSCLC patients.

A small phase II study of neoadjuvant nivolumab has reported impressive activity including pathologic complete responses,[72] and currently neoadjuvant treatment with checkpoint inhibitors is being tested in one large randomized study (NCT02998528, CHECKMATE 816) with a planned accrual of 642 patients who will receive prior to surgery either standard-of-care chemotherapy, chemotherapy with nivolumab, or the combination of nivolumab and the CTLA-4 checkpoint inhibitor ipilimumab. Data from the coprimary endpoint of pathologic CR rate is planned in 2020.

There is one trial (NCT02768558, RTOG 35-05) which attempts to evaluate 12-months treatment with nivolumab after concurrent chemotherapy and thoracic irradiation for stage III NSCLC. However, the positive results from durvalumab may limit enrollment and the trial is currently not recruiting.

Single-agent checkpoint inhibition benefits only a minority of patients with NSCLC. Conceptually, resistance to immune checkpoint inhibitors may reflect the absence of the ability to generate a T cell response or the de novo upregulation of additional negative checkpoints than the PD-1/PD-L1 checkpoint which would confer an intrinsic resistance. Acquired resistance could also develop because of upregulation of additional negative checkpoints and also following acquisition of new molecular abnormalities inhibiting T cell responses.[73,74]

Table 10.5c presents phase III trials testing the addition of another immune checkpoint inhibitor to a PD-1 or PD-L1 agent. These trials have combined these drugs with either a CTLA-4 inhibitor (ipilimumab or tremelimumab) or epacadostat, an inhibitor of the immunosuppressive enzyme indoleamine 2, 3-dioxygenase 1 (IDO-1).

Although the CTLA-4 inhibitor ipilimumab provided negligible antitumor activity in advanced NSCLC,[1] the combination of CTLA-4 and PD-1/PD-L1 blockade is logical, as CTLA-4 inhibition mainly takes place during priming phase in the lymph nodes, while PD-1/PD-L1 blockade occurs in the effector phase within the tumor microenvironment.[75] In metastatic melanoma, the combination of ipilimumab and

nivolumab has produced longer PFS and overall survival than single-agent nivolumab but with a higher rate of grade 3 and 4 immune-related toxicities.[76] This combination was investigated in first-line NSCLC, but the dose and schedule approved in melanoma proved unacceptably toxic in NSCLC patients.[77] Subsequent modifications principally reducing the dose and frequency of administration of ipilimumab result in a combination that has entered phase III studies. Interestingly, although the anti-PD-1/CTLA4 combination may be expected to be particularly promising in negative or low PD-L1 expressing NSCLC, initial results have reported high response rates particularly with high PD-L1 expression.[78] A recent press release announced that combination of nivolumab 3 mg/kg every 2 weeks with low dose ipilimumab 1 mg/kg every 6 weeks as first-line treatment improved PFS over chemotherapy in advanced NSCLC patients with high TMB irrespective of PD-L1 expression. A different combination of the anti-PD-L1 durvalumab and anti-CTLA4 tremelimumab has been investigated in previously treated NSCLC in a phase Ib study[79] and is also in phase III. These studies should define the role of combined PD-1 or PD-L1 plus CTLA-4 inhibition in first-line NSCLC. One study is testing nivolumab plus ipilimumab in EGFR-mutant NSCLC with non-T790M resistance after first-line tyrosine kinase inhibitor. This is the only large study evaluating combined immunotherapy in a molecularly selected adenocarcinoma subgroup, which as discussed above may have less benefit from single-agent PD-1 blockade. The combination of PD-1 inhibition with IDO-1 inhibition has progressed rapidly from early phase to phase III trials. Initial reports of pembrolizumab and epacadostat have shown promising activity in chemotherapy-treated patients who had not received a PD-1 or PD-L1 inhibitor with a response rate of 40% and a DCR of 60% including durable responses.[80] Unlike the anti-PD-1/CTLA4 combination, pembolizumab/epacadostat appears well tolerated with immune-related events not appreciably greater than expected with PD-1 inhibition alone.

There are currently over 100 earlier phase trials evaluating PD-1/PD-L1 inhibitors in combination with other agents in advanced NSCLC. The "partners" in these trials include chemotherapy regimens, radiation especially stereotactic irradiation, vaccines, cytokines such as IL-15 and IL-10, small molecular DNA repair pathway inhibitors, antiangiogenic therapies, histone deacetylase inhibitors, and oncolytic viruses.

Combination trials in specific molecular subtypes include partnering with EGFR inhibitors, ALK/ROS inhibitors, TRK inhibitors, and RAS inhibitors. There are also multiple small trials in early-stage NSCLC combining checkpoint inhibitors with curative treatments including surgery; stereotactic radiation; and combinations of chemotherapy, radiation, and surgery. Postcurative treatment trials usually have endpoints of safety, whereas neoadjuvant trials evaluate feasibility, and surrogate endpoints such as pathologic response as well as sequential tissue analysis for markers of checkpoint efficacy. One planned trial will evaluate nivolumab as a potential preventive agent in patients at high risk of developing lung cancer (NCT03347838).

Additionally, there are even more trials evaluating combinations of inhibitory checkpoint antagonists (anti-PD-1 plus anti-LAG-3, anti-PD-1 plus anti-TIM-3, anti-PD-1 plus TIGIT, etc.), combinations of inhibitory checkpoint antagonists and agonist antibodies to stimulatory checkpoints (anti-PD-L1 plus OX-40, anti-PD-1 plus GITR, etc.), and combinations of checkpoint inhibition and other immunotherapy where NSCLC is a planned "expansion" cohort or one of a few restricted eligible tumor types. Consequently, we can expect the rapid appearance of new data and promising preliminary results which will strain the resources available to conduct phase III studies. It is therefore essential to continue to refine and develop baseline predictive biomarkers for benefit from single-agent PD-1/PD-L1 inhibition, so patients who will not benefit can bypass these drugs and proceed to potentially more active combinations in clinical trials. Such biomarkers are likely to include more comprehensive profiling techniques of biopsy tissue, circulating tumor material (cells, exosomes, DNA), and the patient's immune system and microbiome. Truly personalized immunotherapy will result and fully realize the potential of harnessing the immune system to cure lung cancer.

Practical Approaches to the Use of Immunotherapy in Pulmonary Adenocarcinoma

1. Exclude patients with previous history of pneumonitis, pulmonary fibrosis, and autoimmune disease requiring steroid treatment within last 2 years.
2. Advanced pulmonary adenocarcinoma (Fig. 10.1)
   a. PD-L1 IHC is currently the most practical biomarker and is to be assessed at the time of diagnosis of stage IV NSCLC together with molecular analysis at minimum EGFR, ALK, and ROS-1 to determine timing of immunotherapy.
   b. If without actionable driver mutations and PD-L1 is ≥50%, then the current standard treatment is monotherapy pembrolizumab and possibly consider combination platinum-pemetrexed chemotherapy with pembrolizumab.
   c. If without actionable driver mutations and PD-L1 is <50%, not for monotherapy pembrolizumab, and the current standard treatment is combination platinum-pemetrexed chemotherapy with pembrolizumab.
   d. If without driver mutations and no prior anti-PD1 or anti-PD-L1, but prior platinum-doublet chemotherapy ± maintenance pemetrexed and ± bevacizumab, the current standard second-line treatment is nivolumab or atezolizumab for all comers or pembrolizumab for PD-L1 ≥1%.
   e. If EGFR mutant, immunotherapy should not be considered until after failing EGFR tyrosine kinase inhibitors including osimertinib for T790M positive disease and standard platinum-doublet chemotherapy ± maintenance pemetrexed. Combination of carboplatin/paclitaxel/atezolizumab/bevacizumab may be considered after all available EGFR TKIs.
   f. If ALK or ROS-1 translocation positive, immunotherapy should not be considered until after failing ALK tyrosine kinase inhibitors and standard platinum-doublet chemotherapy with maintenance pemetrexed. Combination of carboplatin/paclitaxel/atezolizumab/bevacizumab may be considered after all available ALK TKIs.
   g. If positive for other oncogenic drivers with actionable targets, treat with approved targeted therapies until resistance, then treat with platinum-doublet chemotherapy prior to considering immunotherapy.
   h. If without driver mutations and prior first-line treatment with anti-PD1 or anti-PD-L1, current standard second-line treatment is platinum-doublet chemotherapy with maintenance pemetrexed (or platinum-doublet chemotherapy with bevacizumab) and then docetaxel (or pemetrexed, if no prior pemetrexed).
3. Stage III unresectable NSCLC including pulmonary adenocarcinoma. If no disease progression after definitive concurrent chemoradiation, the new standard treatment is consolidation durvalumab for 12 months, irrespective of driver mutations and PD-L1 status.
4. Resectable early-stage NSCLC including pulmonary adenocarcinoma. There is no currently established role for immunotherapy, awaiting results from ongoing trials.

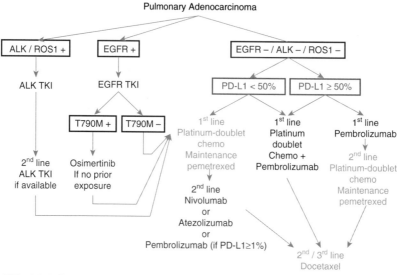

FIG. 10.1 Practical management approach for stage IV pulmonary adenocarcinoma.

REFERENCES

1. Lynch TJ, Bondarenko I, Luft A, et al. Ipilimumab in combination with paclitaxel and carboplatin as first-line treatment in stage IIIB/iv non–small-cell lung cancer: results from a randomized, double-blind, multicenter phase ii study. *J Clin Oncol.* 2012;30(17):2046–2054.
2. Brahmer JR, Tykodi SS, Chow LQM, et al. Safety and activity of anti–PD-L1 antibody in patients with advanced cancer. *New Engl J Med.* 2012;366(26):2455–2465.
3. Garon EB, Rizvi NA, Hui R, et al. Pembrolizumab for the treatment of non-small-cell lung cancer. *N Engl J Med.* 2015;372(21):2018–2028.
4. Herbst RS, Soria JC, Kowanetz M, et al. Predictive correlates of response to the anti-PD-L1 antibody MPDL3280A in cancer patients. *Nature.* 2014;515(7528):563–567.
5. Gulley JL, Rajan A, Spigel DR, et al. Avelumab for patients with previously treated metastatic or recurrent non-small-cell lung cancer (JAVELIN Solid Tumor): dose-expansion cohort of a multicentre, open-label, phase 1b trial. *The Lancet Oncol.* 2017;18(5):599–610.
6. Gettinger SN, Horn L, Gandhi L, et al. Overall survival and long-term safety of nivolumab (Anti-Programmed death 1 antibody, BMS-936558, ONO-4538) in patients with previously treated advanced non-small-cell lung cancer. *J Clin Oncol.* 2015;33(18):2004–2012.
7. Hui R, Gandhi L, Costa EC, et al. Long-term OS for patients with advanced NSCLC enrolled in the KEYNOTE-001 study of pembrolizumab (pembro). *J Clin Oncol.* 2016; 34(suppl 15):9026.
8. Leighl NB, Hellmann MD, Hui R, et al. KEYNOTE-001: 3-year overall survival for patients with advanced NSCLC treated with pembrolizumab. *J Clin Oncol.* 2017; 35(suppl 15):9011.
9. Soria JC, Cruz C, Bahleda R, et al. Clinical activity, safety and biomarkers of PD-L1 blockade in non-small cell lung cancer (NSCLC): additional Analyses from a clinical study of the engineered antibody MPDL3280A (Anti-PDL1). In: *Paper Presented at: European Cancer Congress.* 2013.
10. Horn L, Spigel DR, Gettinger SN, et al. Clinical activity, safety and predictive biomarkers of the engineered antibody MPDL3280A (anti-PDL1) in non-small cell lung cancer (NSCLC): update from a phase Ia study. *J Clin Oncol.* 2015;33(suppl 15):8029.
10a. Horn L, et al. Safety and Clinical Activity of Atezolizumab Monotherapy in Metastatic Non-Small Cell Lung Cancer: From a Phase I Study. *Submitted for Publication.* 2018.
11. Balmanoukian AS, Antonia SJ, Hwu W-J, et al. Updated safety and clinical activity of durvalumab monotherapy in previously treated patients with stage IIIB/IV NSCLC. *J Clin Oncol.* 2017;35(suppl 15):9085.
12. Borghaei H, Paz-Ares L, Horn L, et al. Nivolumab versus docetaxel in advanced nonsquamous non-small-cell lung cancer. *N Engl J Med.* 2015;373(17):1627–1639.
13. Herbst RS, Baas P, Kim D-W, et al. Pembrolizumab versus docetaxel for previously treated, PD-L1-positive, advanced non-small-cell lung cancer (KEYNOTE-010): a randomised controlled trial. *Lancet.* 2016;387(10027): 1540–1550.
14. Rittmeyer A, Barlesi F, Waterkamp D, et al. Atezolizumab versus docetaxel in patients with previously treated non-small-cell lung cancer (OAK): a phase 3, open-label, multicentre randomised controlled trial. *Lancet.* 2017; 389(10066):255–265.
15. Felip Font E, Gettinger SN, Burgio MA, et al. 1301PDThree-year follow-up from CheckMate 017/057: nivolumab

versus docetaxel in patients with previously treated advanced non-small cell lung cancer (NSCLC). *Ann Oncol.* 2017;28(suppl 5): mdx380.004-mdx380.004.

16. Herbst RS, Baas P, Kim D-W, et al. Factors associated with better overall survival (OS) in patients with previously treated, PD-L1−expressing, advanced NSCLC: Multivariate analysis of KEYNOTE-010. *J Clin Oncol.* 2017; 35(suppl 15):9090.

17. Chatterjee M, Turner DC, Felip E, et al. Systematic evaluation of pembrolizumab dosing in patients with advanced non-small-cell lung cancer. *Ann Oncol.* 2016;27(7): 1291−1298.

18. Satouchi M, Fehrenbacher L, Dols MC, et al. OA 17.07 long-term survival in atezolizumab-treated patients with 2L+ NSCLC from Ph iii randomized OAK study. *J Thorac Oncol.* 2017;12(11):S1794.

19. Grossi F, Crinò L, Delmonte A, et al. MA 10.06 real-world results in non-squamous non-small cell lung cancer patients: Italian nivolumab Expanded access Program. *J Thorac Oncol.* 2017;12(11):S1841.

20. Gettinger S, Rizvi NA, Chow LQ, et al. Nivolumab monotherapy for first-line treatment of advanced non-small-cell lung cancer. *J Clin Oncol.* 2016;34(25):2980−2987.

21. Hui R, Garon EB, Goldman JW, et al. Pembrolizumab as first-line therapy for patients with PD-L1-positive advanced non-small cell lung cancer: a phase 1 trial. *Ann Oncol.* 2017;28(4):874−881.

22. Garassino M, Rizvi N, Besse B, et al. OA03.02 atezolizumab as 1L therapy for advanced NSCLC in PD-L1−selected patients: updated ORR, PFS and OS Data from the BIRCH study. *J Thorac Oncol.* 2017;12(1): S251−S252.

23. Carcereny E, Felip E, Reck M, et al. OA 17.02 updated efficacy results from the BIRCH study: first-line atezolizumab therapy in PD-L1−selected patients with advanced NSCLC. *J Thorac Oncol.* 2017;12(11):S1791−S1792.

24. Gettinger S, Rizvi N, Chow L, et al. OA03.01 first-line nivolumab monotherapy and Nivolumab plus ipilimumab in patients with advanced NSCLC: long-term outcomes from CheckMate 012. *J Thorac Oncol.* 2017;12(1): S250−S251.

25. Antonia SJ, Brahmer JR, Khleif S, et al. Phase 1/2 study of the safety and clinical activity of durvalumab in patients with non-small cell lung cancer (NSCLC). *Ann Oncol.* 2016;27(suppl 6):1216PD.

26. Antonia SJ, Brahmer JR, Balmanoukian AS, et al. Safety and clinical activity of first-line durvalumab in advanced NSCLC: updated results from a Phase 1/2 study. *J Clin Oncol.* 2017;35(suppl 15):e20504.

27. Jerusalem G, Chen F, Spigel D, et al. OA03.03 JAVELIN solid tumor: safety and Clinical Activity of avelumab (Anti-PD-L1) as first-line treatment in Patients with advanced NSCLC. *J Thorac Oncol.* 2017;12(1):S252.

28. Scagliotti GV, Parikh P, von Pawel J, et al. Phase III study comparing cisplatin plus gemcitabine with cisplatin plus pemetrexed in chemotherapy-naive patients with advanced-stage non-small-cell lung cancer. *J Clin Oncol.* 2008;26(21):3543−3551.

29. Reck M, Rodriguez-Abreu D, Robinson AG, et al. Pembrolizumab versus chemotherapy for PD-L1-positive non-small-cell lung cancer. *N Engl J Med.* 2016;375(19): 1823−1833.

30. Reck M, Rodríguez-Abreu D, Robinson A, et al. 437O KEYNOTE-024: pembrolizumab (pembro) vs platinum-based chemotherapy (chemo) as first-line therapy for advanced NSCLC with a PD-L1 tumor proportion score (TPS) ≥50%. *Ann Oncol.* 2016;27(suppl 9): mdw594.001-mdw594.001.

31. Brahmer J, Rodríguez-Abreu D, Robinson A, et al. OA 17.06 updated analysis of KEYNOTE-024: pembrolizumab vs platinum-based chemotherapy for advanced NSCLC with PD-L1 TPS ≥50%. *J Thorac Oncol.* 2017; 12(11):S1793−S1794.

32. Brahmer JR, Rodriguez-Abreu D, Robinson AG, et al. Progression after the next line of therapy (PFS2) and updated OS among patients (pts) with advanced NSCLC and PD-L1 tumor proportion score (TPS) ≥50% enrolled in KEY-NOTE-024. *J Clin Oncol.* 2017;35(suppl 15):9000.

33. Brahmer J, Rodríguez-Abreu D, Robinson A, et al. Progression after the next line of therapy (PFS2) and updated OS among patients with advanced NSCLC and PD-L1 TPS >50% enrolled in KEYNOTE-024. In: *Paper Presented at: The Clinical Oncology Society of Australia Annual Scientific Meeting; 13th November 2017.* 2017.

34. Brahmer JR, Rodríguez-Abreu D, Robinson AG, et al. Health-related quality-of-life results for pembrolizumab versus chemotherapy in advanced, PD-L1-positive NSCLC (KEYNOTE-024): a multicentre, international, randomised, open-label phase 3 trial. *The Lancet Oncol.* 2017; 18(12):1600−1609.

35. Carbone DP, Reck M, Paz-Ares L, et al. First-line nivolumab in stage iv or recurrent non-small-cell lung cancer. *N Engl J Med.* 2017;376(25):2415−2426.

36. Socinski M, Creelan B, Horn L, et al. NSCLC, metastatic-CheckMate 026: a phase 3 trial of nivolumab vs investigator's choice (IC) of platinum-based doublet chemotherapy (PT-DC) as first-line therapy for stage iv/recurrent programmed death ligand 1 (PD-L1)−positive NSCLC. *Ann Oncol.* 2016;27(suppl 6):LBA7_PR-LBA7_PR.

37. Peters S, Creelan B, Hellmann MD, et al. Abstract CT082: impact of tumor mutation burden on the efficacy of first-line nivolumab in stage iv or recurrent non-small cell lung cancer: an exploratory analysis of CheckMate 026. *Cancer Res.* 2017;77(Supplement 13):CT082-CT082.

38. Nowak AK, Robinson BWS, Lake RA. Synergy between chemotherapy and immunotherapy in the treatment of established Murine solid tumors. *Cancer Res.* 2003;63: 4490−4496.

39. Langer CJ, Gadgeel SM, Borghaei H, et al. Carboplatin and pemetrexed with or without pembrolizumab for advanced, non-squamous non-small-cell lung cancer: a randomised, phase 2 cohort of the open-label KEYNOTE-021 study. *The Lancet Oncol.* 2016;17(11): 1497−1508.

40. Borghaei H, Langer CJ, Gadgeel S, et al. LBA49Updated results from KEYNOTE-021 cohort G: a randomized, phase 2

study of pemetrexed and carboplatin (PC) with or without pembrolizumab (pembro) as first-line therapy for advanced nonsquamous NSCLC. *Ann Oncol.* 2017; 28(suppl 5):mdx440.052-mdx440.052.

41. Langer C, Gaddgeel SM, Borghaei H, et al. Randomized, phase 2 study of carboplatin and pemetrexed with or without pembrolizumab as first-line therapy for advanced NSCLC: KEYNOTE-021 cohort G. *Ann Oncol.* 2016; 27(suppl 6):LBA46_PR-LBA46_PR.

42. Reck M, Socinski M, Cappuzzo F, et al. Primary PFS and safety Analyses of a randomised phase iii study of carboplatin + paclitaxel +/- bevacizumab, with or without atezolizumab in 1L non-squamous metastatic NSCLC (IMpower150). In: *Paper Presented at: ESMO Immuno-oncology Congress; December 7, 2017.* 2017.

42a. Kowanetz M, Socinski MA, Zou W, et al. IMpower 150: Efficacy of Atezolizumab Plus Bevacizumab and Chemotherapy in 1L Metastatic Nonsquamous NSCLC Across Key Subgroups. *AACR Annual Meeting Proceedings.* 2018. Abstract CT076.

43. Juergens R, Hellmann M, Brahmer J, et al. OA 17.03 first-line nivolumab plus platinum-based doublet chemotherapy for advanced NSCLC: CheckMate 012 3-year update. *J Thorac Oncol.* 2017;12(11):S1792-S1793.

43a. Gandhi L, Rodriguez-Abreu D, Gadgeel S, et al. Pembrolizumab plus chemotherapy in metastatic non-small cell lung cancer. *N Engl J Med.* 2018;378(22):2078-2092.

43b. Grassino MC, Rodriguez-Abreu D, Gadgeel S, et al. Health-related quality of life in the KEYNOTE-189 study of pembrolizumab or placebo plus pemetrexed and platinum for metastatic NSCLC. *ASCO.* 2018. Abstract 9021.

44. Kalbasi A, June CH, Haas N, Vapiwala N. Radiation and immunotherapy: a synergistic combination. *J Clin Invest.* 2013;123(7):2756-2763.

45. Tang C, Wang X, Soh H, et al. Combining radiation and immunotherapy: a new systemic therapy for solid tumors? *Cancer Immunol Res.* 2014;2(9):831-838.

46. Daly ME, Monjazeb AM, Kelly K. Clinical trials Integrating immunotherapy and radiation for non-small-cell lung cancer. *J Thorac Oncol.* 2015;10(12):1685-1693.

47. Antonia SJ, Villegas A, Daniel D, et al. Durvalumab after Chemoradiotherapy in stage iii non-small-cell lung cancer. *N Engl J Med.* 2017;377(20):1919-1929.

48. Ahn JS, Ahn YC, Kim JH, et al. Multinational randomized phase iii trial with or without consolidation chemotherapy using docetaxel and cisplatin after concurrent chemoradiation in Inoperable stage iii non-small-cell lung cancer: KCSG-LU05-04. *J Clin Oncol.* 2015;33(24):2660-2666.

49. Paz-Ares L, Villegas A, Daniel D, et al. LBA1_PRPACIFIC: a double-blind, placebo-controlled phase III study of durvalumab after chemoradiation therapy (CRT) in patients with stage III, locally advanced, unresectable NSCLC. *Ann Oncol.* 2017;28(suppl 5):mdx440.049-mdx440.049.

50. Hui R, Özgüroğlu M, Daniel D, et al. PL 02.02 patient-reported outcomes with durvalumab after chemoradiation in locally advanced, unresectable NSCLC: data from PACIFIC. *J Thorac Oncol.* 2017;12(11):S1604.

51. Leighl N, Gandhi L, Hellmann M, et al. Pembrolizumab for NSCLC: immune-mediated adverse events and Corticosteroid Use. In: *Paper Presented at: World Conference on Lung Cancer.* 2015.

52. Haanen J, Carbonnel F, Robert C, et al. Management of toxicities from immunotherapy: ESMO Clinical Practice Guidelines for diagnosis, treatment and follow-up. *Ann Oncol.* 2017;28(suppl 4):iv119-iv142.

53. Alexandrov LB, Nik-Zainal S, Wedge DC, et al. Signatures of mutational processes in human cancer. *Nature.* 2013; 500(7463):415-421.

54. Hellmann M, Garon EB, Gandhi L, et al. Efficacy of pembrolizumab in key subgroups of patients with advanced NSCLC. In: *Paper Presented at: World Conference on Lung Cancer.* 2015.

55. Gadgeel S, Ciardiello F, Rittmeyer A, et al. PL04a.02: OAK, a randomized Ph iii Study of Atezolizumab vs docetaxel in Patients with advanced NSCLC: results from subgroup Analyses. *J Thorac Oncol.* 2017;12(1):S9-S10.

56. Horn L, Herbst RS, Spigel DR, et al. An analysis of the relationship of clinical activity to baseline EGFR status, PD-L1 expression and prior treatment history in patients with non-small cell lung cancer (NSCLC) following PD-L1 blockade with MPDL3280A (Anti-PDL1). In: *Paper Presented at: World Conference on Lung Cancer.* 2013.

57. Garon EB, Balmanoukian A, Hamid O, et al. Preliminary clinical safety and activity of MK-3475 monotherapy for the treatment of previously treated patients with non-small cell lung cancer (NSCLC). In: *Paper Presented at: World Conference on Lung Cancer.* 2013.

58. Garon EB, Rizvi N, Hui R, et al. Abstract CT104: efficacy of pembrolizumab (MK-3475) and relationship with PD-L1 expression in patients with non-small cell lung cancer: Findings from KEYNOTE-001). *Cancer Res.* 2015; 75(Supplement 15):CT104-CT104.

59. Hirsch FR, McElhinny A, Stanforth D, et al. PD-L1 immunohistochemistry assays for lung cancer: results from phase 1 of the Blueprint PD-L1 IHC assay comparison Project. *J Thorac Oncol.* 2017;12(2):208-222.

60. Tsao M, Kerr K, Yatabe Y, Hirsch FR. PL 03.03 Blueprint 2: PD-L1 immunohistochemistry Comparability study in real-life, clinical samples. *J Thorac Oncol.* 2017;12(11): S1606.

61. Fehrenbacher L, Spira A, Ballinger M, et al. Atezolizumab versus docetaxel for patients with previously treated non-small-cell lung cancer (POPLAR): a multicentre, open-label, phase 2 randomised controlled trial. *Lancet.* 2016; 387(10030):1837-1846.

62. Gadgeel S, Kowanetz M, Zou W, et al. 1296OClinical efficacy of atezolizumab (Atezo) in PD-L1 subgroups defined by SP142 and 22C3 IHC assays in 2L+ NSCLC: results from the randomized OAK study. *Ann Oncol.* 2017; 28(suppl 5):mdx380.001-mdx380.001.

63. Adam J, Rouquette I, Damotte D, et al. PL04a.04: multi-centric French Harmonization Study for PD-L1 IHC Testing in NSCLC. *J Thorac Oncol.* 2017;12(1):S11-S12.

64. Cooper WA, Russell PA, Cherian M, et al. Intra- and inter-observer reproducibility assessment of PD-L1 biomarker

in non-small cell lung cancer. *Clin Cancer Res.* 2017; 23(16):4569−4577.

65. Rizvi NA, Hellmann MD, Snyder A, et al. Mutational landscape determines sensitivity to PD-1 blockade in non−small cell lung cancer. *Science.* 2015;348(6230): 124−128.

66. Kowanetz M, Zou W, Shames D, et al. OA20.01 tumor mutation burden (TMB) is associated with improved efficacy of atezolizumab in 1L and 2L+ NSCLC patients. *J Thorac Oncol.* 2017;12(1):S321−S322.

67. Gandara DR, Kowanetz M, Mok TSK, et al. 1295OBlood-based biomarkers for cancer immunotherapy: tumor mutational burden in blood (bTMB) is associated with improved atezolizumab (atezo) efficacy in 2L+ NSCLC (POPLAR and OAK). *Ann Oncol.* 2017;28(suppl 15): mdx380-mdx380.

67a. Hellmann M, Ciuleanu T, Pluzanski A, et al. Nivolumab + Ipilimumab vs Platinum-Doublet Chemotherapy as First-line Treatment for Advanced Non-Small Cell Lung Cancer: Initial Results From CheckMate. *AACR Annual Meeting Proceedings.* 2018;227. Abstract CT077.

68. Kowanetz M, Zou W, McCleland M, et al. MA 05.09 pre-existing Immunity measured by Teff gene expression in tumor tissue is associated with Atezolizumad efficacy in NSCLC. *J Thorac Oncol.* 2017;12(11):S1817−S1818.

69. Mazieres J, Fehrenbacher L, Rittmeyer A, et al. Non-classical response measured by immune-modified RECIST and post-progression treatment effects of atezolizumab in 2L/3L NSCLC: results from the randomized phase II study POPLAR. *J Clin Oncol.* 2016;34(suppl 15):9032.

70. Gandara DR, Pawel JV, Sullivan RN, et al. Impact of atezolizumab (atezo) treatment beyond disease progression (TBP) in advanced NSCLC: results from the randomized phase III OAK study. *J Clin Oncol.* 2017;35(suppl 15):9001.

71. Spigel DR, McLeod M, Hussein MA, et al. 1297ORandomized results of fixed-duration (1-yr) vs continuous nivolumab in patients (pts) with advanced non-small cell lung cancer (NSCLC). *Ann Oncol.* 2017;28(suppl 5): mdx380.002-mdx380.002.

72. Chaft JE, Forde PM, Smith KN, et al. Neoadjuvant nivolumab in early-stage, resectable non-small cell lung cancers. *J Clin Oncol.* 2017;35(suppl 15):8508.

73. Sharma P, Hu-Lieskovan S, Wargo JA, Ribas A. Primary, Adaptive, and Acquired resistance to cancer immunotherapy. *Cell.* 2017;168(4):707−723.

74. Gettinger S, Choi J, Hastings K, et al. Impaired HLA Class I antigen Processing and presentation as a Mechanism of Acquired resistance to immune checkpoint inhibitors in lung cancer. *Cancer Discov.* 2017;7(12):1420−1435.

75. Ribas A. Tumor immunotherapy Directed at PD-1. *New Engl J Med.* 2012;366(26):2517−2519.

76. Wolchok JD, Chiarion-Sileni V, Gonzalez R, et al. Overall survival with combined nivolumab and ipilimumab in advanced melanoma. *New Engl J Med.* 2017;377(14): 1345−1356.

77. Hellmann MD, Gettinger SN, Goldman JW, et al. Check-Mate 012: safety and efficacy of first-line (1L) nivolumab (nivo; N) and ipilimumab (ipi; I) in advanced (adv) NSCLC. *J Clin Oncol.* 2016;34(suppl 15):3001.

78. Hellmann MD, Rizvi NA, Goldman JW, et al. Nivolumab plus ipilimumab as first-line treatment for advanced non-small-cell lung cancer (CheckMate 012): results of an open-label, phase 1, multicohort study. *The Lancet Oncol.* 2017;18(1):31−41.

79. Antonia S, Goldberg SB, Balmanoukian A, et al. Safety and antitumour activity of durvalumab plus tremelimumab in non-small cell lung cancer: a multicentre, phase 1b study. *The Lancet Oncol.* 2016;17(3):299−308.

80. Gangadhar TC, Schneider BJ, Bauer TM, et al. Efficacy and safety of epacadostat plus pembrolizumab treatment of NSCLC: preliminary phase 1/2 results of ECHO-202/KEY-NOTE-037. In: *Paper Presented at: American Society of Medical Oncology Annual Meeting.* 2017.

81. Gordon MS, Herbst RS, Horn L, et al. Long-term safety and clinical activity of atezolizumab monotherapy in metastatic NSCLC: Final results from a phase Ia study. In: *Paper Presented at: IASLC Chicago Multidisciplinary Symposium in Thoracic Oncology.* 2016.

82. Rizvi NA, Brahmer JR, Ou S-HI, et al. Safety and clinical activity of MEDI4736, an anti-programmed cell death-ligand 1 (PD-L1) antibody, in patients with non-small cell lung cancer (NSCLC). *J Clin Oncol.* 2015; 33(suppl 15):8032.

83. Garassino M, Vansteenkiste J, Kim J-H, et al. PL04a.03: durvalumab in ≥3rd-Line Locally Advanced or metastatic, EGFR/ALK wild-type NSCLC: results from the phase 2 ATLANTIC study. *J Thorac Oncol.* 2017;12(1):S10−S11.

Index

A

Acinar/papillary predominant adenocarcinoma, 16
Activated killer T-cells and dendritic cells (AKT-DC), 48
Adenocarcinoma in situ (AIS), 13
Adenocarcinoma(s), 13, 14t
  histology, 87
  subtype classification
    acinar/papillary predominant adenocarcinoma, 16
    invasive mucinous adenocarcinoma, 16
    lepidic predominant adenocarcinoma, 16
    micropapillary and solid predominant adenocarcinoma, 16
Adenosine monophosphate kinase (AMPK), 18
Adenosine triphosphate (ATP), 19
Adenosquamous carcinoma, 14t
Adjuvant chemotherapy, 67, 70
  in NSCLC, 35–38
Adjuvant Lung Cancer Enrichment Marker Identification and Sequencing Trial (ALCHEMIST), 46, 123
Adjuvant Lung Project Italy (ALPI), 36
Adjuvant Navelbine International Trialist Association trial (ANITA), 36–37, 65, 66t
Adjuvant radiation therapy, 41–42
Adjuvant therapy, 122–123
  in non–small-cell lung cancer, 35
ADJUVANT trial, 45
Ado-trastuzumab emtansine (T-DM1), 145–146
Adoptive immunotherapy (AI), 48
Advanced ALK positive NSCLC, early-stage and locally, 140
Advanced-stage ALK patient, approach to, 134
AF-001JP trial, 136
Afatinib, 145–146
AI. See Adoptive immunotherapy (AI)
AIS. See Adenocarcinoma in situ (AIS)
AJCC. See American Joint Committee on Cancer (AJCC)
AKT-DC. See Activated killer T-cells and dendritic cells (AKT-DC)

ALCHEMIST. See Adjuvant Lung Cancer Enrichment Marker Identification and Sequencing Trial (ALCHEMIST)
Alectinib, 136, 139–140
ALEX trial, 136–137
ALK. See Alkaline lymphoma kinase (ALK); Anaplastic lymphoma kinase (ALK)
Alkaline lymphoma kinase (ALK), 87, 116
ALPI. See Adjuvant Lung Project Italy (ALPI)
American Joint Committee on Cancer (AJCC), 16
  eighth edition, 16–17
American Society of Clinical Oncology (ASCO), 94
American Thoracic Society (ATS), 13
AMG 337, 145
AMPK. See Adenosine monophosphate kinase (AMPK)
Amplification-refractory mutation system (ARMS), 20
Anaplastic lymphoma kinase (ALK), 18, 20–21, 61t, 72, 133, 143
  gene rearranged NSCLC
    AF-001JP trial, 136
    alectinib, 136
    ALEX trial, 136–137
    approach to advanced-stage ALK patient, 134
    ceritinib, 137
    clinical features of ALK positive NSCLC, 133
    CNS metastases, 139–140
    crizotinib, 134
    early-stage and locally advanced ALK positive NSCLC, 140
    future directions, 140
    JALEX trial, 136–137
    next-generation ALK inhibitors in crizotinib-treated patients, 134
    next-generation ALK TKIs as frontline therapy, 134
    non-ALK-directed therapy, 139
    other drugs, 137–138
    patients management with oligometastatic disease, 140
    resistance to next-generation ALK inhibitors, 138
    sequence of ALK inhibitors, 138

Anaplastic lymphoma kinase (ALK) (Continued)
    testing for ALK, 133–134
    and ROS1 testing, 21–23
      break apart FISH assay, 21–22
      fusion protein detection of ALK and ROS1 by IHC, 22
      NGS, 22–23
      RT-PCR, 22
ANITA. See Adjuvant Navelbine International Trialist Association trial (ANITA)
Anti-PD1 agent, 159–161
Anti-PDL-1 agents, 151–152, 159–161
Antiangiogenic agents, 87
Antiimmune checkpoint inhibitor molecules, 25
Area under curve (AUC), 105–106
ARMS. See Amplification-refractory mutation system (ARMS)
ASCEND-4 trial, 137
ASCO. See American Society of Clinical Oncology (ASCO)
Atezolizumab, 94–95, 109, 111–112, 121–122, 151–152, 154t, 155, 163
ATLANTIC trial, 122
ATP. See Adenosine triphosphate (ATP)
ATS. See American Thoracic Society (ATS)
AUC. See Area under curve (AUC)
AVAiL trial, 90, 96
Avelumab, 151–152, 154t, 155

B

B-raf proto oncogene, serine/threonine kinase (BRAF), 23, 61t, 144
Basaloid squamous cell carcinomas, 60
BED. See Biologic effective dose (BED)
Bevacizumab, 71–72, 89–91, 121
Biologic effective dose (BED), 67–68
Biomarkers, 158–162. See also Clinicopathologic markers
  clinicopathologic markers, 158–159
  PD-L1 expression, 159–161
  T-effector gene signature expression, 162
  tumor mutation burden, 162
BLOOM trial, 119–120

Note: Page numbers followed by "f" indicate figures, "t" indicate tables and "b" indicate boxes.

BRAF. See B-raf proto oncogene, serine/threonine kinase (BRAF)
Bronchioid. *See* Terminal respiratory unit (TRU)
Bypass pathway activation, 19

C
Cabozantinib, 145
CALGB. *See* Cancer and Leukemia Group B (CALGB)
Cancer, genomic profile of, 103
Cancer and Leukemia Group B (CALGB), 8, 68
CALGB9633 trial, 38, 40–41
Cannabinoids, 62
CAP. *See* Cyclophosphamide (CAP)
Capmatinib, 145
Carbon ions, 75
Carboplatin, 88, 89t
Cardiopulmonary exercise testing, 3
Cardiovascular risk assessment, 3
Cell-free DNA (cfDNA), 118–119
CellSearch System, 24
Central nervous system (CNS), 65–66, 116, 123–124, 134–135
metastases, 124, 139–140
Ceritinib, 44, 137, 143–144
Cetuximab, 71, 107
cfDNA. *See* Cell-free DNA (cfDNA)
CheckMate-026 trial, 49–50, 93, 155–156
CheckMate-057 trial, 121–122, 161
Checkpoint inhibition, combination of chemotherapy and, 156–157
Chemotherapy, 63, 87–89, 163
choice, 39–41
combination of checkpoint inhibition and, 156–157
duration, 89
Chemotherapy for Early Stages Trial (CHEST), 42
Chromosomal translocations, 87
CI. *See* Confidence interval (CI)
Circulating tumor cells (CTCs), 24
Circulating tumor DNA (ctDNA), 24, 35
Cisplatin, 87–88, 89t
Clinical target volume (CTV), 74
Clinicopathologic markers. *See also* Biomarkers
EGFR status, 159
smoking status, 158–159
CNS. *See* Central nervous system (CNS)
Cobas EGFR Mutation Test, 20
Combination chemotherapy, 105–107
Computed tomography (CT), 1, 58
Concurrent chemoradiotherapy, 68–69
Concurrent chemotherapy, 157
Confidence interval (CI), 35
Consolidation chemotherapy, 70

Cost-effectiveness model, 92–93
CP-358, 115
CP-774, 115
Crizotinib, 23, 44, 140, 145
next-generation ALK inhibitors in crizotinib-treated patients, 134, 138f–139f
CT. *See* Computed tomography (CT)
CTCs. *See* Circulating tumor cells (CTCs)
ctDNA. *See* Circulating tumor DNA (ctDNA)
CTLA-4 inhibitor. *See* Cytotoxic T-lymphocyte antigen-4 inhibitor (CTLA-4 inhibitor)
CTONG 1104 (ADJUVANT trial), 45, 123
CTV. *See* Clinical target volume (CTV)
Cyclophosphamide (CAP), 35
Cytokines, 166–167
Cytotoxic chemotherapy, 120–121. *See also* Immunotherapy
docetaxel, 103–104
other cytotoxic agents, 104–105
pemetrexed, 104
Cytotoxic T-lymphocyte antigen-4 inhibitor (CTLA-4 inhibitor), 93, 151, 166

D
Dacomitinib, 145
Dako 22C3 IHC assay, 106–107
DAKO IHC 22C3 antibody, 159
DC-CIK. *See* DCs and cytokine-induced killer cells (DC-CIK)
DCR. *See* Disease control rate (DCR)
3DCRT. *See* Three-dimensional conformal radiotherapy (3DCRT)
DCs and cytokine-induced killer cells (DC-CIK), 48
DFS. *See* Disease-free survival (DFS)
Diarrhea, 126
Diffusion capacity for carbon monoxide (DLCO), 3
Digital PCR, 24
Disease control rate (DCR), 152
Disease-free survival (DFS), 16, 36, 122–123
DLCO. *See* Diffusion capacity for carbon monoxide (DLCO)
Docetaxel, 88, 103–104
Downstream pathway activation, 19
3DPT. *See* 3-D proton therapy (3DPT)
Driver oncogenes, 23–24
BRAF, 23
HER2, 23–24
KRAS gene, 23
MET, 23
NTRK1, 23
RET, 23
Dronabinol, 62
Drug-related pneumonitis, 158
Durvalumab, 94–95, 122, 139, 151–152, 154t, 155, 157, 163

E
Early-stage lung cancer, 4, 4t
Eastern Cooperative Oncology Group (ECOG), 35–36, 65–66, 88
EBUS. *See* Endobronchial ultrasound (EBUS)
EBUS-TBNA. *See* Endobronchial ultrasound–guided transbronchial needle aspiration (EBUS-TBNA)
Echinoderm microtubule-associated protein-like 4 (EML4), 133
Echinoderm microtubule–associated protein–like 4 anaplastic lymphoma kinase (EML4-ALK), 44
ECOG. *See* Eastern Cooperative Oncology Group (ECOG)
ECOG 4599 trial, 90
EGF. *See* Epidermal growth factor (EGF)
EGFR. *See* Epidermal growth factor receptor (EGFR)
Electromagnetic navigational bronchoscopy (ENB), 2
EML4-ALK. *See* Echinoderm microtubule–associated protein–like 4 anaplastic lymphoma kinase (EML4-ALK)
EML4. *See* Echinoderm microtubule-associated protein-like 4 (EML4)
EMT. *See* Epithelial to mesenchymal transition (EMT)
ENB. *See* Electromagnetic navigational bronchoscopy (ENB)
Endobronchial biopsy, 1–2
Endobronchial ultrasound (EBUS), 2
Endobronchial ultrasound–guided transbronchial needle aspiration (EBUS-TBNA), 60
Endocrinopathies, 157–158
Endoscopic ultrasound–guided fine needle aspiration (EUS-FNA), 60
Ensartinib, 138
Entrectenib, 23
Epidermal growth factor (EGF), 18, 115
Epidermal growth factor receptor (EGFR), 18–20, 44, 61t, 70, 87, 106–107, 115, 143
activation
of bypass pathways, 19
of downstream pathways, 19
adjuvant therapy, 122–123
CNS metastases, 124
cytotoxic chemotherapy, 120–121
development of third-generation EGFR TKIs, 118–120
diagnosis, 116
EGFR TKI gefitinib, 116
EGFR–mutant NSCLC, 115
epidemiology, 115–116
exon 20 insertion mutations, 125
histologic transformation, 19
immune therapy, 121–122

Epidermal growth factor receptor
(EGFR) (*Continued*)
  mutation testing
    nontargeted assays, 20
    targeted assays, 20
  resistance to first-and second-
    generation TKIs, 118–120
  secondary resistance mutations, 19
  small-cell lung cancer transformation,
    124–125
  treatment, 116–118
    first-and second-generation EGFR
      TKIs, 116–118
    beyond progression and
      oligoprogressive disease,
      123–124
    of selected TKI toxicities,
      125–126
Epithelial to mesenchymal transition
  (EMT), 19, 118
ERBB1 gene. *See* Epidermal growth
  factor receptor (EGFR)
ErbB1 receptor, 115
ERBB2 gene, 23–24
ERK pathways. *See* Extracellular
  signal–related kinase pathways
  (ERK pathways)
Erlotinib, 71, 92, 115–117
ERS. *See* European Respiratory Society
  (ERS)
Etoposide, 87
European Big Lung Trial, 36
European Respiratory Society (ERS),
  13
EUS-FNA. *See* Endoscopic
  ultrasound–guided fine needle
  aspiration (EUS-FNA)
Exon 20 insertion mutations, 125
Extended cervical mediastinoscopy,
  59
Extracellular signal–related kinase
  pathways (ERK pathways), 109

F
FDA. *See* US Food and Drug
  Administration (FDA)
FEV1. *See* Forced expiratory volume in
  1 (FEV1)
Fiberoptic bronchoscopy with
  bronchoalveolar lavage, 60
Fibroblast growth factor receptor 1–3
  (FGFR1–3), 108
Fine needle aspiration (FNA), 2
First-generation EGFR TKIs, 116–118
  resistance to, 118–120
First-line therapy, 103
  for wild-type patients, 87
    bevacizumab, 89–91
    chemotherapy, 87–89
    decision tree for patients with
      newly diagnosed lung
      adenocarcinoma, 99f
    duration of chemotherapy, 89
    elderly patients, 95–96

First-line therapy (*Continued*)
  first-line regimens for lung
    adenocarcinoma, 98t
  immunotherapy, 93–95
  impaired performance status,
    96–98
  maintenance therapy, 91–93
Fluorescence in situ hybridization
  (FISH), 18, 21–22, 45, 133
FNA. *See* Fine needle aspiration (FNA)
Folate antimetabolite pemetrexed,
  104
Forced expiratory volume in 1 (FEV1),
  3
Fusion protein detection of *ALK* and
  ROS1 by IHC, 22

G
Gastrointestinal symptoms
  (GI symptoms), 135
Gefitinib, 71, 116–117
Gemcitabine, 88, 89t, 104
Gene-rearranged tumors, 16
Genomic profile of cancer, 103
GI symptoms. *See* Gastrointestinal
  symptoms (GI symptoms)
Glesatinib, 145
GOIRC 02–2006 study,
  105–106
Gross tumor volume, 74

H
Hazard ratio (HR), 64, 117, 152
Hematoxylin and eosin (H & E),
  25–26
HER1 gene. *See* Epidermal growth
  factor receptor (EGFR)
HER2 gene. *See* Human epidermal
  growth factor receptor 2 gene
  (HER2 gene)
Histologic transformation, 19
Horner syndrome, 59
HR. *See* Hazard ratio (HR)
hsp90 inhibitor, 125
Human epidermal growth factor
  receptor 2 gene (HER2 gene),
  23–24, 61t, 117, 145–146
Hypofractionation, 67–68

I
IALT. *See* International Adjuvant Lung
  Cancer Trial (IALT)
IASLC. *See* International Association
  for Study of Lung Cancer (IASLC)
ICs. *See* Immune cells (ICs)
IDO-1. *See* Indoleamine 2,3-
  dioxygenase 1 (IDO-1)
Ifosfamide, 87
IHC. *See* Immunohistochemistry
  (IHC)
IMA. *See* Invasive mucinous
  adenocarcinoma (IMA)
Imaging, 59
Immune cells (ICs), 48

Immune checkpoint inhibitors, 26t
  biomarkers, 158–162
  ongoing studies/future directions,
    163–167, 164t–165t
    practical management approach,
      168f
  previously treated advanced NSCLC,
    151–152
    clinical efficacy in early phase
      studies of PD-1 pathway
      blockade, 153t
    randomized phase 3 studies in,
      153t
  pulmonary adenocarcinoma
    treatment with, 151
  safety and management of toxicity,
    157–158
  treatment duration, 162–163
  treatment-naïve advanced NSCLC,
    152–157
  unresectable stage III NSCLC, 157
Immune therapy, 121–122
Immune-related adverse events
  (ir-AEs), 110, 151
Immunohistochemistry (IHC), 45, 60,
  133
  assay, 106–107
  fusion protein detection of *ALK* and
    ROS1 by, 22
Immunotherapy, 47–48, 72–73, 87,
  93–95, 94t, 109–112. *See also*
  Cytotoxic chemotherapy
  atezolizumab, 111–112
  combination of radiation and, 157
  combining radiotherapy and, 73
  nivolumab, 110
  PD-L1, 72–73
  pembrolizumab, 110–111
  phase III adjuvant immunotherapy
    trials, 49t
  practical approaches in pulmonary
    adenocarcinoma, 167b
Indoleamine 2,3-dioxygenase 1
  (IDO-1), 166
Induction chemotherapy, 63
Intensity-modulated radiotherapy
  planning, 74
International Adjuvant Lung Cancer
  Trial (IALT), 36, 66
International Association for Study of
  Lung Cancer (IASLC), 13, 16,
  133
Invasive mucinous adenocarcinoma
  (IMA), 13–16, 14t
IPASS trial, 117
Ipilimumab, 166
ir-AEs. *See* Immune-related adverse
  events (ir-AEs)
Irinotecan, 105

J
JALEX trial, 136–137
Japan Lung Cancer Research Group
  (JLCRG), 38

K

Karnofsky PS (KPS), 68
KCSG-LU05−04 trial, 70
KEYNOTE-010 trial, 110−111,
   121−122, 152
Kirsten rat sarcoma 2 viral oncogene
   homolog gene (*KRAS* gene), 23,
   109

L

LACE. *See* Lung Adjuvant Cisplatin
   Evaluation (LACE)
LACE metaanalysis, 39
Lactic dehydrogenase (LDH), 151
LAK-IL-2. *See* Lymphokin−activated
   killer cells and interleukin-2
   (LAK-IL-2)
LANSCLC. *See* Locally advanced
   non−small-cell lung cancer
   (LANSCLC)
Lapatinib, 145−146
Large-cell lung carcinoma, 14t, 60
Larotrectinib, 146
LAT. *See* Local(ly) ablative therapy
   (LAT)
LDH. *See* Lactic dehydrogenase (LDH)
Lepidic predominant
   adenocarcinoma, 16
Liquid biopsies, 24−25, 116,
   118−119
   assessing tumor burden, 25
   characterizing resistance
      mechanisms, 25
   clinical applications, 24
   CTCs, 24
   ctDNA, 24
   monitoring response to therapy, 25
   targeting multiple molecular
      alterations, 24
   targeting specific molecular
      alterations, 24
Local recurrence (LR), 41−42
Local(ly) ablative therapy (LAT),
   123−124, 140
Locally advanced lung cancer, 4
Locally advanced non−small-cell lung
   cancer (LANSCLC), 57−58
   adenocarcinoma, 60
   immunotherapy, 72−73
   large-cell lung carcinoma, 60
   lymph node stations in lung cancer,
      58f
   management, 62
   modalities
      carbon ions, 75
      photons, 74
      protons, 74−75
   molecular analysis, 60, 61t
   paraneoplastic syndromes, 59
   radiotherapy, 73
   resectable, 63−64
   screening, 58
   squamous cell carcinoma, 60
   staging

Locally advanced non−small-cell lung
   cancer (LANSCLC) (*Continued*)
      pleural invasion, 60
      primary tumor, 62t
      regional lymph node, 62t
      superior sulcus tumors, 64−67
   symptoms, 59
   targeted therapies, 70−72
   unresectable, 67−70
   volumes
      CTV, 74
      gross tumor volume, 74
      PTV, 74
   workup, 59−60
      EBUS-TBNA, 60
      fiberoptic bronchoscopy with
         bronchoalveolar lavage, 60
      imaging, 59
      mediastinoscopy, 59
      sputum cytology, 59
Lorlatinib, 138
LR. *See* Local recurrence (LR)
LUME-Lung 1 trial, 108
Luminespib, 125
Lung adenocarcinoma
   combination chemotherapy,
      105−107
   cytotoxic chemotherapy, 103−105
   immunotherapy, 109−112
   oncogenic driver mutations and
      molecular testing in, 18
   pathological staging, 16−17
   targeted agents, 107−109
Lung Adjuvant Cisplatin Evaluation
   (LACE), 37, 66−67
Lung cancer, 13, 87, 143
   in nonsmokers, 57
   surgical approach to, 6−8
      open lobectomy, 6
      robotic lobectomy, 7−8
      uniportal and subxiphoid
         lobectomy, 8
      VATS lobectomy, 6−7
   surgical management, 4−6
      early-stage lung cancer, 4
      locally advanced lung cancer, 4
      N2 disease, 4−5
      oligometastatic disease, 5−6
      superior sulcus tumors, 5
      T3N1 tumors, 4
      T4 tumors, 5
LUX-Lung 3 trial, 117−118
LUX-Lung 6 trial, 117−118
Lymph node resection extent, 8−9
Lymphokin−activated killer cells and
   interleukin-2 (LAK-IL-2), 48

M

MAGE-A3. *See* Melanoma-associated
   antigen-A3 (MAGE-A3)
Magnetic resonance imaging (MRI),
   59
Maintenance therapy, 91−93
Major pathologic response (MPR), 49

MAPK. *See* Mitogen-activated protein
   kinase (MAPK)
Massive parallel sequencing
   technology, 18
Mediastinoscopy, 2, 59
MEK. *See* Mitogen-activated protein
   kinase kinase (MEK)
Melanoma, 151
Melanoma-associated antigen-A3
   (MAGE-A3), 47−48
Merestinib, 145
Mesenchymal−epithelial transition
   (MET), 23, 61t, 144−145
   gene copy number, 144
MET. *See* Mesenchymal−epithelial
   transition (MET)
MIA. *See* Minimally invasive
   adenocarcinoma (MIA)
Micropapillary and solid
   predominant adenocarcinoma,
   16
MILES trial, 96
Minimally invasive adenocarcinoma
   (MIA), 13
Minimally invasive surgery, 7
Mitogen-activated protein kinase
   (MAPK), 144
Mitogen-activated protein kinase
   kinase (MEK), 109, 144
   second-line checkpoint inhibitors in
      NSCLC, 109t
Mitomycin C, 87
Mitomycin C, vindesine, and cisplatin
   (MVP), 36
Molecular analysis of NSCLC, 60, 61t
Molecular testing
   in lung adenocarcinoma, 18
   methods, 18
Molecularly targeted therapy,
   44−47
   Phase III adjuvant EGFR TKI trials in
      EGFR-mutated NSCLC, 47t
   phase III adjuvant EKGF TKI trials,
      46t
Monoclonal antibodies, 109
Monotherapy, 103−105
MPR. *See* Major pathologic response
   (MPR)
MRI. *See* Magnetic resonance imaging
   (MRI)
Multidisciplinary approach, 1
Multiple randomized clinical trials, 88
Multitargeted TKIs, 145
MVP. *See* Mitomycin C; vindesine, and
   cisplatin (MVP)

N

N2 disease, 4−5
NanoString system, 22
NATCH trial. *See* Neoadjuvant vs.
   Adjuvant Taxol/Carbo Hope trial
   (NATCH trial)
National Cancer Institute of Canada
   (NCIC), 36−37

National Cancer Institute of Canada
Clinical Trials Group (NCIC CTG),
107
Navigational bronchoscopy, 1
NCIC. *See* National Cancer Institute of
Canada (NCIC)
NCIC CTG. *See* National Cancer
Institute of Canada Clinical Trials
Group (NCIC CTG)
Neoadjuvant chemotherapy, 42—43
Neoadjuvant immunotherapy, 49—50
phase II neoadjuvant
immunotherapy trials, 50t
Neoadjuvant *vs.* Adjuvant Taxol/
Carbo Hope trial (NATCH trial), 42
Neratinib, 145—146
Neuroendocrine tumors, 13
Neurotrophin 3, 146
Neurotrophin tyrosine kinase receptor
(NTRK), 146
*NTRK*1, 23
NTRK—mutated NSCLC, 146
Next-generation ALK inhibitors
in crizotinib-treated patients, 134,
138f—139f
next-generation ALK TKIs as frontline
therapy, 134
resistance to, 138
Next-generation sequencing (NGS),
22—23, 116, 134
Nintedanib, 108
Nivolumab, 25, 109—110, 121—122,
154t, 155, 163
Nodal Stations, 57—58
Non-ALK-directed therapy, 139
Non-shedding tumor, 119
Noninvasive tumors, 13
Nonmucinous adenocarcinoma, 14t
Nonrandomized series, 5
Non—small-cell lung cancer (NSCLC),
4, 13, 35, 87, 103, 115, 133, 143,
151. *See also* Locally advanced
non—small-cell lung cancer
(LA-NSCLC)
adjuvant chemotherapy, 35—38
adjuvant radiation therapy,
41—42
choice of chemotherapy, 39—41
immunotherapy, 47—48
molecularly targeted therapy,
44—47
neoadjuvant chemotherapy, 42—43
neoadjuvant immunotherapy,
49—50
NTRK—mutated NSCLC, 146
stage I disease, 38—39
phase III adjuvant trials, 40t
treatment-naïve advanced NSCLC,
152—157
Nontargeted assays, 20
NSCLC. *See* Non—small-cell lung
cancer (NSCLC)
NTRK. *See* Neurotrophin tyrosine
kinase receptor (NTRK)

O
Objective response rate (ORR), 87—88,
143—144, 151—152
Oligometastatic disease, 5—6
patients management with, 140
Oligoprogressive disease, 123—124
Oncogenic driver mutations in lung
adenocarcinoma, 18
Open lobectomy, 6
ORR. *See* Objective response rate
(ORR)
OS. *See* Overall survival (OS)
Osimertinib, 119—120, 122, 126
Overall survival (OS), 35, 62, 117,
144, 151—152
Oxaliplatin, 106

P
Paclitaxel, 88, 105
Pancoast tumors. *See also* Superior
sulcus tumors
Pancost tumors. *See* Superior sulcus
tumors
Paraneoplastic syndromes, 59
Pathologic mediastinal assessment,
2—3
Pathological staging of lung
adenocarcinoma—AJCC eighth
edition, 16—17
PCR. *See* Polymerase chain reaction
(PCR)
PD-1. *See* Programmed death-1
(PD-1)
PD-L1. *See* Programmed death ligand
1 (PD-L1)
PDGFR. *See* Platelet-derived growth
factor receptor (PDGFR)
Pembrolizumab, 25, 93, 109—111,
121—122, 151—155, 154t, 163
Pemetrexed, 91, 104
Performance status (PS), 59
PET. *See* Positron emission
tomography (PET)
PFS. *See* Progression-free survival
(PFS)
Phase I KEYNOTE-001 trial, 110
Photons therapy, 74
PI subtype. *See* Proximal
inflammatory subtype (PI subtype)
Planned target volume (PTV), 74
Platelet-derived growth factor receptor
(PDGFR), 108
Platinum
agent, 96
doublet chemotherapy, 106, 109
platinum-based chemotherapy, 44
Pleural invasion, 60
Pneumocyte markers, 13—16
Polymerase chain reaction (PCR),
116
PCR-based detection methods, 24
POPLAR trial, 161
PORT. *See* Postoperative radiation
therapy (PORT)

Positron emission tomography (PET),
1, 59
Posterolateral thoracotomy, 6
Postoperative chemoradiation, 65—66
Postoperative radiation therapy
(PORT), 41, 63, 65
PP subtype. *See* Proximal proliferative
subtype (PP subtype)
PROCLAIM trial, 69
Program death ligand 1. *See*
Programmed death ligand 1
(PD-L1)
Programmed death ligand 1 (PD-L1),
25—26, 48, 72—73, 93, 106—107,
121
expression, 159—161
efficacy of anti-PD1 or anti-PDL1,
160t
immune checkpoint inhibitors, 26t
inhibitors, 25, 109
testing, 25—26
Programmed death-1 (PD-1), 48, 72,
93, 106—107, 109, 151
Progression-free survival (PFS), 36, 64,
117, 134, 143, 152
Proto-oncogene tyrosine-protein
kinase ROS (ROS-1), 61t
Protons therapy, 74—75
Proximal inflammatory subtype
(PI subtype), 18
Proximal proliferative subtype
(PP subtype), 18
PS. *See* Performance status (PS)
PTV. *See* Planned target volume (PTV)
Pulmonary adenocarcinoma, 1, 13,
103—104, 106—107, 109
ALK and *ROS*1 testing, 21—23
biomarkers, 158—162
clinical relevance of adenocarcinoma
subtype classification, 16
driver oncogenes, 23—24
EGFR, 18—20
histological classification, 13—16
major classification of pulmonary
NSCCs, 14t
liquid biopsies, 24—25
molecular classification, 17
NSCLC
previously treated advanced,
151—152
treatment-naïve advanced NSCLC,
152—157
unresectable stage III NSCLC,
157
oncogenic driver mutations and
molecular testing, 18
ongoing studies/future directions,
163—167, 164t—165t
pathological staging of lung
adenocarcinoma—AJCC eighth
edition, 16—17
PD-L1, 25—26
safety and management of toxicity,
157—158

Pulmonary adenocarcinoma (*Continued*)
 subtypes, 15f
 transcriptomic classifications, 17—18
 treatment duration, 162—163
 treatment with immune checkpoint inhibitors, 151
Pulmonary function
 assessment, 3—4
 testing, 3
Pyrosequencing method, 20

Q

Qiagen. *See* Therascreen EGFR RCQ PCR kit
Quantitative radionucluclide scan, 3

R

RADIANT trial, 122—123
Radiation, 65
 combination of immunotherapy and, 157
Radiation Therapy Oncology Group (RTOG), 65—66
Radiotherapy, 73
 combining immunotherapy and, 73
Ramucirumab, 108
Randomized phase III INTEREST trial, 107
Randomized phase III REVEL trial, 108
Randomized phase III studies in treatment-naïve NSCLC, 155—156
RAS. *See* Rat sarcoma viral oncogene homolog (RAS)
Rat sarcoma viral oncogene homolog (RAS), 61t
Rearranged during transfection (RET), 108
Receiver operating characteristics (ROC), 159
Receptor tyrosine kinase (RTK), 20
 fusion tumors, 23
Recurrence-free survival (RFS), 36—37
Resectable LA-NSCLC, 63—64. *See also* Unresectable LA-NSCLC
 induction chemotherapy, 63
 trimodality, 63—64
Resectional biopsy, 1
Resistance
 to first-and second-generation TKIs, 118—120
 mechanism characterization, 25
 to next-generation ALK inhibitors, 138
RET. *See* Rearranged during transfection (RET)
RET gene, 23, 61t, 145
Reverse transcription-polymerase chain reaction (RT-PCR), 22, 134
RFS. *See* Recurrence-free survival (RFS)
Robotic lobectomy, 7—8, 7f
Robotic surgery, 7

ROC. *See* Receiver operating characteristics (ROC)
ROS-1. *See* Proto-oncogene tyrosine-protein kinase ROS (ROS-1)
ROS1 gene, 18, 21, 143—144
 ALK and, 21—23
RT-PCR. *See* Reverse transcription-polymerase chain reaction (RT-PCR)
RTK. *See* Receptor tyrosine kinase (RTK)
RTOG. *See* Radiation Therapy Oncology Group (RTOG)

S

S49076 inhibitor, 145
Salivary gland type carcinoma, 13
Sanger sequencing, 18
SAR125844, 145
Sarcomatoid carcinoma, 13, 14t
Savolitinib, 145
SBRT. *See* Stereotactic body radiation therapy (SBRT)
SCC. *See* Squamous cell lung cancer (SCC)
SCIS. *See* Squamous in situ carcinoma (SCIS)
SCLC. *See* Small cell lung carcinoma (SCLC)
Second-generation EGFR TKIs, 116—118
 resistance to, 118—120
Second-line checkpoint inhibitors in NSCLC, 109t
Second-line therapy, 103
Secondary resistance mutations, 19
Sentinel lymph node biopsy (SNLB), 9
"Sequencing strategy", 120
Sequential chemoradiation, 68
Sequential chemoradiotherapy, 68—69
Sitravatinib, 145
Small cell lung carcinoma (SCLC), 19
Small-cell lung cancer transformation, 124—125
Smoking, 57
 cessation, 3, 62
SNLB. *See* Sentinel lymph node biopsy (SNLB)
Southwest Oncology Group (SWOG), 42, 63—64
Spread through air spaces (STAS), 16
Sputum cytology, 59
Squamoid. *See* Proximal inflammatory subtype (PI subtype)
Squamous cell carcinoma, 14t, 60
Squamous cell lung cancer (SCC), 116
Squamous in situ carcinoma (SCIS), 16—17
SRS. *See* Stereotactic radiosurgery (SRS)
STAS. *See* Spread through air spaces (STAS)

Stereotactic body radiation therapy (SBRT), 73
Stereotactic radiosurgery (SRS), 124
STK11 suppressor, 18
Sublobar resection, 8, 8t
Subxiphoid lobectomy, 8
Superior sulcus tumors, 5, 5f, 64—67
 adjuvant chemotherapy, 66—67
 postoperative chemoradiation, 65—66
 postoperative radiation therapy, 65
 radiation alone, 65
Superior vena cava (SVC), 5
Surgical lung biopsy, 2
Surgical management of pulmonary adenocarcinoma
 assessing surgical candidacy, 3—4
  assessment of cardiovascular risk, 3
  assessment of pulmonary function, 3—4
  smoking cessation, 3
 extent of lymph node resection, 8—9
 extent of resection, 8
 of lung cancer, 4—6
 staging, 1—3
  endobronchial and transbronchial biopsy, 1—2
  imaging, 1
  pathologic mediastinal assessment, 2—3
  surgical lung biopsy, 2
  tissue diagnosis for suspected lung cancer, 1
 surgical approach to lung cancer, 6—8
SVC. *See* Superior vena cava (SVC)
SWOG. *See* Southwest Oncology Group (SWOG)
Systemic therapy, 87

T

T-effector (Teff), 162
 gene signature expression, 162
T3N1 tumors, 4
T4 tumors, 5
T790M gatekeeper resistance mutation, 119
TAILOR trial, 107
Targetable drugs, 23
Targeted agents
 EGFR, 107
 MEK, 109
 VEGF, 107—109
Targeted assays, 20
Targeted therapy, 70—72, 103
 ALK, 72
 bevacizumab and thalidomide, 71—72
 cetuximab, 71
 EGFR, 70
 erlotinib, 71
 gefitinib, 71
 in non—small-cell lung cancer
  BRAF, 144
  HER2, 145—146

Targeted therapy (*Continued*)
  NTRK–mutated NSCLC, 146
  RET, 145
  ROS1, 143–144
Targeting multiple molecular
  alterations, 24
Targeting specific molecular
  alterations, 24
TCGA. *See* The Cancer Genome Atlas
  (TCGA)
TCs. *See* Tumor cells (TCs)
Teff. *See* T-effector (Teff)
Tepotinib, 145
Terminal respiratory unit (TRU), 18
TGF. *See* Transforming growth factor
  (TGF)
Thalidomide, 71–72
The Cancer Genome Atlas (TCGA), 17
Therascreen EGFR RCQ PCR kit, 20
Third-generation
  chemotherapy, 88
  EGFR TKIs development,
    118–120
Thoracic radiation therapy, 157
Thoracic radiotherapy, 70
Thoracic revised cardiac risk index, 3
Thoracoscopic equipment, 4
3-D proton therapy (3DPT), 75
3-D radiotherapy planning, 74
Three-dimensional conformal
  radiotherapy (3DCRT), 67
Thyroid transcription factor 1 (TTF-1),
  13–16, 60
Thyroid-stimulating hormone (TSH),
  157–158
TIL-rIL-2. *See* Tumor-infiltrating
  lymphocytes and recombinant IL-2
  (TIL-rIL-2)
Tissue diagnosis for suspected lung
  cancer, 1
Tivantinib, 145
TKI. *See* Tyrosine kinase inhibitor
  (TKI)
TMB analysis. *See* Tumor mutation
  burden analysis (TMB analysis)
Tooth-lid factor, 115
Topoisomerase-I inhibitor topotecan,
  105

Toxicity, safety and management of,
  157–158
TRACERx study, 25
Transbronchial biopsy, 1–2
Transcriptomic classifications, 17–18
  PI, 18
  PP subtype, 18
  TRU, 18
Transesophageal EUS-FNA, 60
Transforming growth factor (TGF),
  115
  TGF-α, 115
Trastuzumab, 145–146
Treatment beyond progression,
  123–124
Treatment-naïve advanced NSCLC
  combination of chemotherapy and
    checkpoint inhibition, 156–157
  early phase studies in, 152–155
    clinical efficacy of anti-PD1 or anti-
      PDL1 in, 154t
  randomized phase III studies in,
    155–156
Trimodality, 63–64
Tropomyosin-related kinase (TRK),
  146
TRU. *See* Terminal respiratory unit
  (TRU)
TSH. *See* Thyroid-stimulating
  hormone (TSH)
TTF-1. *See* Thyroid transcription factor
  1 (TTF-1)
Tumor cells (TCs), 48
Tumor mutation burden analysis
  (TMB analysis), 49–50, 139, 162
Tumor-associated antigens, 25
Tumor-infiltrating lymphocytes and
  recombinant IL-2 (TIL-rIL-2), 48
2-D radiotherapy planning, 74
Tyrosine kinase inhibitor (TKI), 115,
  133, 143
  treatment of selected TKI toxicities,
    125–126

U

UFT. *See* Uracil and tegafur (UFT)
Union for International Cancer
  Control (UICC), 16

Uniportal lobectomy, 8
Unresectable LA-NSCLC, 67–70.
  See also Resectable LA-NSCLC
  consolidation chemotherapy, 70
  radiation alone, 67–68
  sequential and concurrent
    chemoradiotherapy, 68–69
  sequential chemoradiation,
    68
Unresectable stage III NSCLC, 157
  combination of radiation and
    immunotherapy, 157
Uracil and tegafur (UFT), 38
US Food and Drug Administration
  (FDA), 21–22, 71

V

VAF. *See* Variant allele frequencies
  (VAF)
Val600Gly, 20
Vandetanib, 108
Variant allele frequencies (VAF), 25
Vascular endothelial growth factor
  (VEGF), 71, 89–90, 107–109
Vascular permeability factor, 71
VATS lobectomy. *See* Video-assisted
  thoracoscopic surgery lobectomy
  (VATS lobectomy)
VEGF. *See* Vascular endothelial growth
  factor (VEGF)
Ventana SP142 antibody,
  152–155
Ventana SP142 IHC assay, 111
VENTANA SP263 antibody, 156,
  159–161
Video-assisted thoracoscopic surgery
  lobectomy (VATS lobectomy), 2,
  6–7, 6f–7f
Vinblastine, 87
Vinorelbine, 88, 95, 105

W

Wild-type patients, 87
WJTOG 9904 trial, 95
World Health Organization (WHO),
  13

Printed in the United States
By Bookmasters